Catalyst

To John and Mary
With appreciation of your friendship and kindness throughout my career.
With best wishes

CATALYST

The Medical Memoirs of a World Anaesthetist

Kester

Kester Brown

AM, MB.ChB, MD (Melbourne), FANZCA, FRCA, FCA(SA).
Director of Anaesthesia, Royal Childrens Hospital, Melbourne 1974-2000
President World Federation of Societies of Anaesthesiologists 2000-2004

Published by Brolga Publishing Pty Ltd
ABN 46 063 962 443
PO Box 12544 A'Beckett Street Melbourne 8006
Victoria Australia
E-mail: bepublished@brolgapublishing.com.au

National Library of Australia
Cataloguing-in-Publication entry

Brown, Kester,
Catalyst : the medical memoirs of a world anaesthetist

ISBN 1 920785 38 8

1. Brown, Kester, 1935- . 2. Anesthesia - History.
3. Anesthesiology - History. 4. Anesthesiology.
5. Anesthesiologists. I. Title.

617.962

Printed in China

Cover design by Trish Hart
Typeset by Diana Evans

Dedication

These memoirs are dedicated to:

My wife, Janet,
with gratitude for her patience and support through
an adventurous and demanding life.

My Parents,
who taught, encouraged and inspired me,

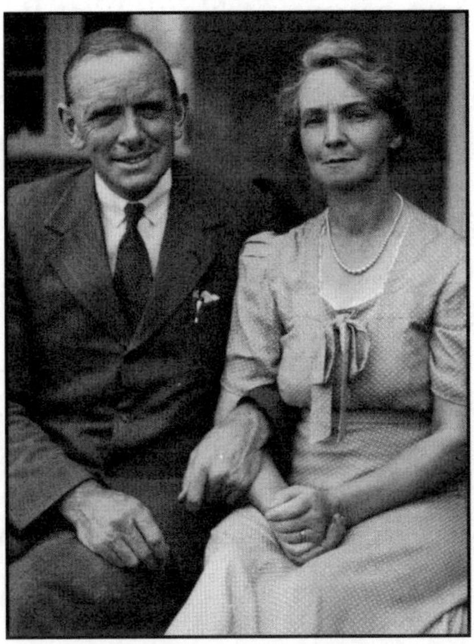

My colleagues.
who supported me so that I could achieve all I did

and
All those people from whom I learned
so that I could teach and help others.

Illustrations

The illustrations are numbered and referenced in the text by the number in brackets.

Colour illustrations are numbered C— and referred in the text (figure C—).

Cover Legend

1. With children patients at North West River, Labrador in 1959.
2. Tumutumu Hospital, Kenya — Mens' ward designed and built by the author's father, with the original corrugated iron ward behind.
3. Indians in canoe at Davis Inlet in Labrador.
4. Cessna 185 at Arctic Sound on the Arctic coast.
5. President's medal of the WFSA.
6. Gilbert Brown ASA Award designed by A Mazarros.
7. Teaching how to hold a mask on the face.
8. Riding an elephant in Bangkok.
9. The author giving an anaesthetic.
10. The "Koala" chairing a session at an ASA meeting.

Acknowledgements

Telling my tales to people on aeroplanes led to the suggestion that I should write my autobiography. The first was Sonia Davies with whom I chatted on my way back from Wellington. She was Minister of Health in New Zealand at the time. She told me that she had written her autobiography, *Bread and Roses*. It is a very interesting story about a woman who was ahead of her time in many ways. For some years I pondered the possibility but it was not until I had stopped full time work that it became possible. When I told a friend that I thought I should write two books he told me that was a bit presumptuous! Later when I sent him some chapters for his comments he said that I should write two or three books! John Roberts, former Editor in Chief of Anaesthesia and Intensive Care, has kindly written the Foreword. My co-author on our paediatric anaesthesia textbook, *Anaesthesia for Children*, Graham Fisk, and his wife Flora, both gave me some helpful comments. Ian McKenzie, co-editor on *Acute Pain Management in Children* made some useful suggestions. Wendy Sutherland reviewed the original text and suggested that maybe it should be split in two. Many other friends including Anne Bryan, Janice Peeler, Haydn Perndt, Ian Lack, Jane McConnell, Peter Howe, my brother Monty and some of my children read, made comments and discussed parts of my memoirs, many of which will appear in another book.

One day one of our anaesthetic registrars, following some discussion on a topic of anaesthetic interest, said I should write a book about these. I suddenly realized the solution to my problem was to write one on the various aspects of my medical career as an anaesthetist with all its wide ramifications. It would be full of useful and interesting information for anaesthetists, trainees and many others. It is my memoirs rather than autobiography because it contains much information about others with whom I came in contact as well as telling my story.

A special thanks goes to those who contributed to the text

— John Inkster on Philip Ayre; a poem by Justin Kelly, some comments from a citation by Michael Hodgson and an appreciation from Anneke Meursing, which I have included in the final chapter. My nephew, Ken Brown, drew the cartoon.

Diana Evans reviewed the manuscript and made some useful suggestions which helped me to highlight various topics and make the text more coherent. She and Wendy Aird have been responsible for the layout and the illustrations. Peta Philp, Alvin Aquino and Robert Reitmaier in the RCH Educational Resources Centre, took hours to scan and organize the photographs with me. Most of the photographs are my own or were taken for me. Some groups come from the RCH Anaesthetic Department collection. No. 59 is reprinted from one of my papers with permission from Anaesthesia and Intensive Care. Trish Hart has helped with the cover design.

Mark Zocchi from Brolga Publishing has co-ordinated and directed the production. I am very grateful to them all.

Kester Brown

Contents

Foreword

This remarkable chronicle details a life characterised by a deep and abiding care and concern for others — patients, friends, colleagues, trainees and the broad community of anaesthesia worldwide.

T.C.K.Brown, known universally as Kester, is a unique individual who is liked, loved, respected and even revered by those who know him as well as by a vast number of people whose only contact with him has been as an audience member at a multitude of his lectures or as readers of his many scientific papers and textbooks. For the non-cognoscenti, reading this book will reveal what others already know — that Kester packed more productive activity into his lifetime to date than any three or four of us average mortals. How he has done it I know not but the contents of this work indicate the why of such a full life. It all gives one more than a tinge of regret in having led a much more prosaic and much less productive existence but it is hoped that the absorption of even only a portion of his underlying raison d'être will benefit many in the earlier stages of their medical careers before they succumb to the comfortable ennui of middle and later professional life.

This book is only part of the story, concentrating on his professional life. An inveterate traveller to exotic and challenging locations the peripatetic Kester has taken full advantage of opportunities to indulge his love of the outdoors, of photography, painting and establishing rapport with the locals. The account of that harvest of journeys will be a treat to savour in the future. Hopefully at that time he will let us have the secret of travelling light — his trusty bag and parka which have accompanied him to diverse places such as Petra, Antarctica, Machu Pichu in Peru, Labrador and the top of Kilimanjaro.

But now join Kester for a roller-coaster ride of experience from Kenya to Scotland and Yellowknife in the Canadian North West Territories to a long and prestigious tenure at the Royal

Childrens Hospital in Melbourne. You will learn how to organize a department, conceive and conduct scientific/clinical research and its implementation and how to organize and direct a meeting. Teaching takes a high profile as does involvement in the complexities of national, international and world societies of Anaesthetists. He has received accolades and high awards in abundance and then capped things off by being elected President of the World Federation of Societies of Anaesthesiologists.

Now read on!

John Roberts,
Editor Emeritus,
Anaesthesia and Intensive Care

Preface

Life is like a tree which grows and branches, as activities and interests develop. The main branch tells the story of my professional life as a doctor and anaesthetist. It recounts important developments and events. It tells about many of the anaesthetists (=anaesthesiologists) with whom I have worked and people that I have met, sometimes in strange or amusing situations. This part will contribute something to the history of anaesthesia in the second half of the twentieth century.

Another branch reviews much of the interesting clinical work with which I have been involved and research that was done in association with it. Some of these ideas and findings were original, some useful to pass on to others.

Teaching became an interest and then a passion. It is the third branch. Over the years I have been involved with training about five hundred anaesthetists from all over the world and taught many more. I have passed on many "pearls" to them — interesting or useful ideas — to help them to understand and hence perform their work better. I have also tried to broaden their horizons and inspire them to contribute, for this makes life more interesting.

Finally, anaesthetists and doctors are often asked to administer and organize. I was involved in administration at the Royal Childrens Hospital, Melbourne for many years. I participated in national College and Society affairs and eventually, for 20 years, in the World Federation of Societies of Anaesthesiologists, of which I eventually became President. These activities gave me many insights and the opportunity to meet many people.

Because of these multiple facets in my life this book is necessarily divided into segments — I have had too varied a life which branched into so many different areas that some of them will have to form another book.

My life, which I have enjoyed, encompassed growing up in

Africa, being a student in Scotland, working as a General Practitioner / anaesthetist in a remote community in the far north of Canada and ending up as Director of the Anaesthetic Department in one of the world's major childrens hospitals.

Opportunities arose to train and work in good centres at an exciting time when some major developments were occurring — the beginnings of paediatric intensive care, infant cardiac surgery and the increased survival of premature infants. Many advances were made during my career and I was fortunate to be involved in research on several of these.

I am passing on my experience and ideas to you, my reader.

Kester Brown AM.
Melbourne, June 2004

EARLY YEARS

Chapter 1
The Beginnings

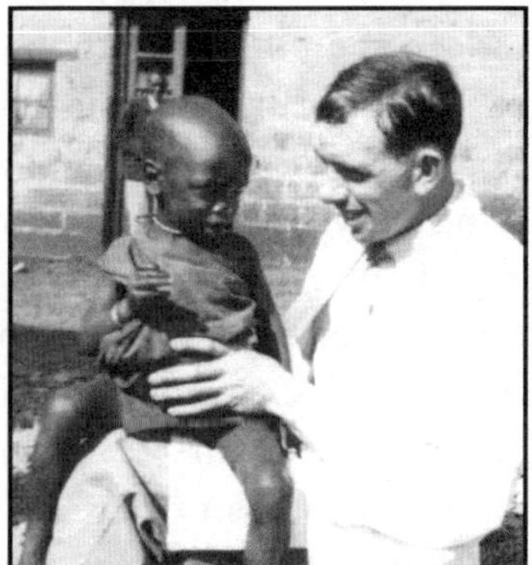

1. Dr Monteith Brown, my father, with a young patient (1930s).

My father, Monteith Brown, was a doctor, one of those old fashioned kind who could turn his hand to almost anything. After completing his degree in Glasgow he returned to his home town of Stirling in central Scotland to do his pre-registration year before leaving for Kenya in 1925 to become a mission doctor. He met my mother, who came from Strathpeffer in the Scottish Highlands, on the ship and they were married two years later. My older brother, Monty, and sister, Catherine, were born six and a half and five years before me so much of my childhood was spent on my own because they had to go away to school where they boarded. My mother taught me until I was nine years old when I was sent to school in Nairobi, which was 140 kilometres away. After that I was at home only during school holidays.

Monteith Brown, began at Kikuyu Hospital, about 30 km from Nairobi, but spent most of his working life at Tumutumu.

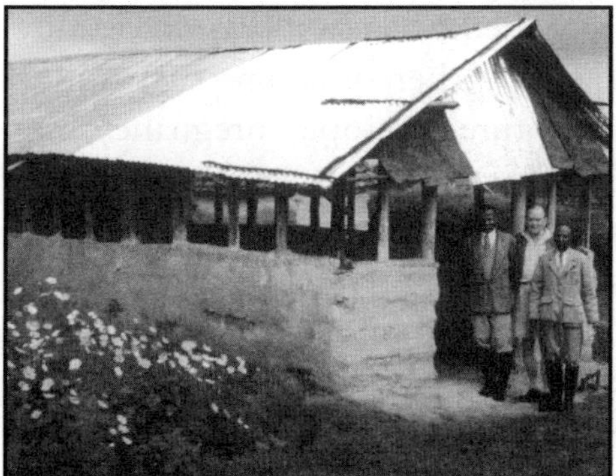

2. My father and dressers Johnstone and Samueli at Ngorano out-dispensary.

It was a beautiful place situated 50 km south of Mt. Kenya which rises over 5,000m in the centre of Kenya. It was in our house which looked out on this magnificent view that I was born in December 1935.

He ran a 120 bed hospital there with an adjacent 20 bed leper colony for 30 years, mostly as the only doctor. He had one or two Scottish nurses at any one time and they trained their own staff — medical dressers or assistants and nurses. He had to oversee six dispensaries and midwifery centres around the district, run by these medical assistants and midwives. There was a paucity of medical care in the country. Much of it was provided by missions.

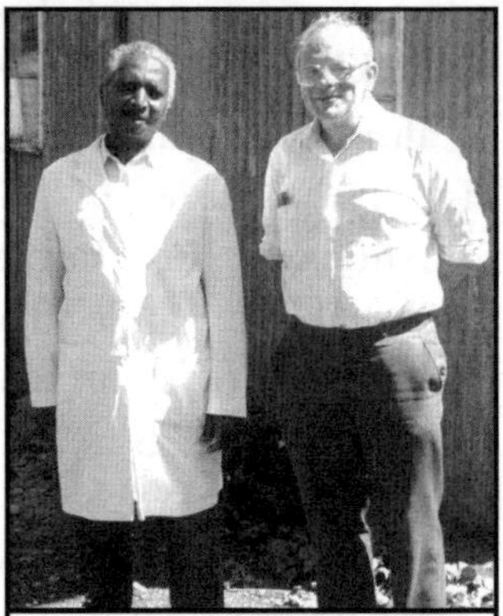

3. With Epafara, who first showed me an anaesthetic being administered.

One of these medical assistants, Epafara, also acted as an anaesthetist, using ethyl chloride for induction followed by breathing air which was drawn over ether and trilene in vaporizing bottles. Seeing this simple technique was my first exposure to anesthesia. The patient was an infant with intussusception where the gut telescopes into itself causing a bowel obstruction and the potential for ischaemia (lack of blood supply) to the gut if not treated. I was fourteen. Having had this introduction I have always been able to appreciate that simple anaesthetics such as ether can be given by non physicians who are trained to do it. When there is nobody else available there is no choice. Later I saw other operations. One I remember clearly was a 16 year old girl who had 33 spear wounds inflicted on her during the Maumau uprising during the Emergency in the 1950s. It was the first time that I saw saline given intravenously. It was rarely used because it was not readily available made up as it is today. In other situations such intra-abdominal bleeding from a ruptured ectopic pregnancy my father collected the blood, filtered it through gauze and ran it back into the patient's veins. This was 40–50 years before cell savers came into common use.

About that time Dapsone and Solapsone, which were drugs that could cure leprosy, became available. My mother used to visit the lepers weekly to supervise drug administration and check haemoglobin levels in case bone marrow depression resulted in anaemia. This was done with a finger prick (if they had fingers) with the drop placed on blotting paper and compared to a colour scale. Since Biblical times leprosy had been a terrible disease which had made sufferers outcasts. Its various forms left the victim with hideous skin lesions or neurological damage causing numbness, gradual loss of digits following trauma because they could not feel, or even blindness. In our group we had one who had lost his sight, one who had terrible lesions on her face and ears which made her look hideous and another young fellow who had lost his fingers. He was clever and became their teacher holding the chalk between the stumps of his two hands so he could write on the blackboard. I think my mother helped him to get started.

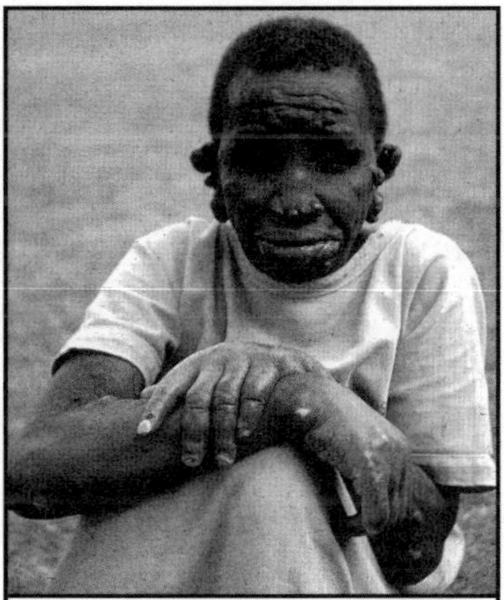

4. One of the patients with lepromatous leprosy.

During his first leave back to Scotland in 1929, when my brother was born, my father did six months training in ophthalmology. He learnt how to do cataract operations which enabled him to give sight back to many people who were becoming blind. I saw him do one of these operations in a patient who had come 600 kilometres from the coast to seek his help. Thirty five years after his death in 1968 my brother met an ophthalmologist who told him people still talked about Dr. Brown's skill at doing cataracts all those years before.

It was hardly surprising, after all this exposure, that I should think of nothing but medicine for my future career. I hit an obstacle when I finished the school certificate as my teachers did not think I was good enough to continue science. I told the headmaster that I had to as I intended to become a doctor. He allowed me to continue. I managed to get through my Higher School Certificate and gain university entrance, although if it had been like it is today, in a very competitive world, I would probably not have made it. I am sure many potentially good doctors have missed out in recent times to people with high marks but not necessarily the qualities to make good doctors.

And so in August 1954 I set out by ship from my home in

Kenya to Scotland to attend St. Andrews University. I had selected it because it was small and my brother had been there. There were 1200 students in St. Andrews and 1200 in Dundee where we went for the clinical half of our course. Although the University is nearly 600 years old St. Andrews is probably better known as the home of golf. I was also offered a place at St. Thomas' Hospital in London which I turned down. Our school was always offered a place there for any budding doctor. There were no others in my year who were interested.

The change from the beautiful climate of the Kenya Highlands to the miserable cold winters of Scotland was not easy to accept, although I seemed to feel the cold less than many of the locals, at least for the first couple of years. It was as if I had enough stored heat to keep me going for a while.

I look back on my university years with pleasure — good social life, plenty of activities to experience, meeting some nice girls and playing hockey for the University. I was captain for two years and also captained Scottish Universities. I was President of the University Sports Union in my fifth year.

It was not all plain sailing. I decided early on that the distractions could be devastating so I would plan to do 20 hours study a week outside classes which occupied much of the day. It was a good discipline to develop. I also learnt how to take a short sleep before dinner so that I would have a clear head to study in the evening.

I found physiology difficult to understand until one day in third year we were taken to the Perth Infirmary where we saw patients. Suddenly it became obvious what the thyroid gland did when we saw patients side by side with too much and too little thyroid hormone with one of the students in the middle who was normal. Teaching physiology in isolation is hopeless for medical students. Years later I instituted a course in our department to relate basic science to paediatric anaesthesia for third year medical students to fill this deficiency. One of these, who was on the point of giving up because he could not see the relevance of his medical basic science course, changed his mind after attending ours. Fortunately, we had no degree examinations in second year. I did poorly and, with some others who failed, had to write an essay on the physiology of human survival, a subject which continued to interest me for the remainder of my life.

My anatomy dissecting partner was Alastair Breckenridge. He was difficult to work with because he took over the dissection most of the time. We all thought he would become a professor and he did — of Pharmacology at Liverpool University where I met him again many years later. Our Professor, Walmsley, was a beady eyed man who seemed to look right through us. After failing yet another term exam having performed badly in the oral where I developed thought block, he called me into his office. He told me he thought I was working too hard and should buy a fishing rod and go to the Highlands and do some fishing. How could he come to that correct conclusion? In my third year I had a brief spell when I thought I would throw it all in and go home to Kenya but my parents came on leave and I managed to persist and finish.

At the end of third year I thought it would be useful to gain some experience working in a hospital. I worked as an orderly at a tuberculosis sanatorium near Edinburgh which proved to be invaluable experience. It made me appreciate the role of nurses which I feel many doctors fail to appreciate fully.

Effective treatment for TB had just been developed so that by the second holidays when I went back in fourth year the hospital was changing to geriatrics. I learnt how to give injections, how to wash and feed patients and also how to talk with them, an essential part of doctoring. I worked with some Edinburgh medical students. One was Arthur Tulloch from the Orkney islands. I met him three times by chance in Canada where he became an anaesthetist. Many years later I was told by Angela Enright who was Chair of the WFSA Education Committee that he was one of the best teachers she had.

One of the orderlies who did night duty was Polish. They called him Charlie. He used to get one of the patients to write the night report for him. One night for fun he wrote "Patients slept well and so did Charlie". Poor Charlie was sacked.

In the summer of my fourth year I went back to Kenya and worked with my father which was interesting experience. I was allowed to do the necessary baby deliveries for my university accreditation while I was there. They were often complicated and so I gained invaluable experience. This was useful when I later went into General Practice where I delivered about 50 babies a year.

We had done pathology during fourth year and I had attended post mortem examinations which I found interesting as they showed the disease from which the patient died. There were several occasions during the summer where I was able to help my father by doing some for him at his hospital. One was a boy who had had a very large meal, went next door and ate more and then went out and was playing some vigorous game when he dropped dead. The autopsy showed only that his stomach and intestinal veins were grossly engorged which probably resulted in not enough blood going to the heart to supply the body's needs. One often hears people advising against swimming immediately after eating. It is good advice.

Despite my struggle, I always managed to pass the degree examinations — which were the ones that had to be passed to continue— sometimes with what seemed like an element of luck. Or maybe I was supposed to become a doctor.

I think the most valuable part of my training was the opportunity to do locums during my final two years for the resident doctors in the hospitals when they went on holidays. On these occasions I had the chance to admit, examine and look after the patients under supervision. I learn much better by actually doing practical things than listening to someone lecturing or teaching by the bedside. I wasn't a brilliant student but I did have an enquiring mind. My first little research project was studying the fluid balance in a lady, Mrs Lyon who had cancer. She was on intravenous therapy for ten days. This was so uncommon at the time that the hospital biochemist came round to check the fluid and electrolyte balance each day and order them for the following day. I also noted the patient's temperature and showed how much the fluid requirement increased with raised body temperature.

During the same locum I witnessed a birth of a 26 week fetus. Nobody even contemplated that it could survive in those days. It was sad because Mrs Cross had tried unsuccessfully several times to have a live baby.

I gained wonderful experience doing locums in obstetrics and gynaecology, paediatrics, orthopaedics, medicine and ENT.

The doctor in Strathpeffer, the village in the north of Scotland where my grandmother lived, used to do a list of anaesthetics once a week in Inverness. Sometimes, when I was on holiday there, Dr. Dick used to take me with him.This was another seed sown. Forty years later during an ENT list in Melbourne I found out that the grandfather of the ENT registrar was the surgeon with whom Dr Dick worked in Inverness.

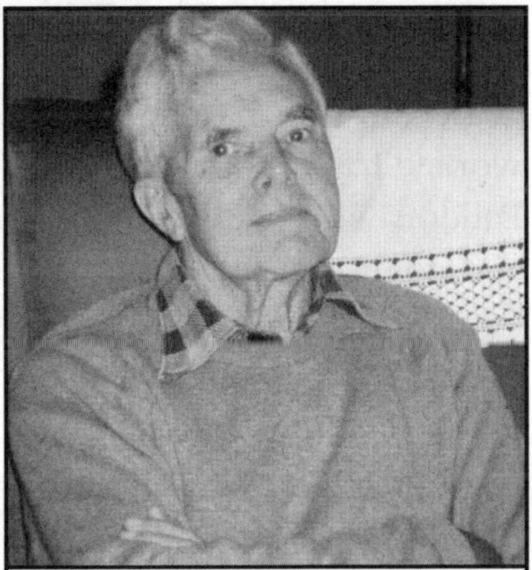

5. Dr David Dick of Strathpeffer.

In our fifth year we had to do twelve anaesthetics. I did these one morning during a tonsillectomy list. We used ethyl chloride and ether and the tonsils were removed very rapidly with a guillotine.

The final and maybe greatest stimulus to my becoming interested in anaesthetics was sharing delightful lodgings with James Forrester during fifth year. His father was senior anesthetist in Glasgow and James often spoke about anaesthesia. I even read Macintosh's book on the subject which would have been unusual for a student.

Our landlord was a Congregational minister, Mr. Donaldson, who taught us a lot about interpersonal relationships and how to communicate with people. Because Catholics were sometimes suspicious of this protestant minister his opening comment might be to ask them why the Pope wore red socks. That broke the ice. He was a wonderful man with a good sense of humour. He had had medical students living with them for the fourteen years he was in Dundee. He told us about one who left his wardrobe full of whisky bottles. He still wondered whether he drank them or put them there as a practical joke! In my final year I had to move because the Donaldsons left Dundee. I shared with Bob Coulthard, staying with an elderly General Practitioner, Dr Chalmers, in Broughty Ferry on the outskirts of

Dundee. His second wife was a younger boisterous Belgian lady with four children. Bob went on to become a criminal psychiatrist in Canada. Living with these interesting landlords was a valuable part of my education.

In my final summer as a student I went to Labrador on the eastern seaboard of Canada to work as a volunteer with the Grenfell Mission which supplied the medical services on the coast. It was a barren, rugged land with scattered settlements. I worked for a month at North West River Hospital with Dr Tony Paddon who had been born and bred there. Then I travelled up and down the northern half of Labrador on the Maraval, a 24m boat equipped with a dispensary and x-ray machine. I x-rayed everyone in northern Labrador as part of the TB screening program. During the year before I spent a morning in the Radiology department in Dundee. I was treated royally. They told me that I was only the seventh student ever to visit them! In Nain we had to reduce and plaster a broken leg. I assisted with a short anesthetic using divinyl ether — the only time I ever saw it used. When I returned to North West River I had a further two weeks at the hospital before going back to Dundee for my final year.

I was very happy to pass my finals as I was due to leave for Canada the next week. I had a rather trying time in the last exam when they changed my final oral time from 2 to 6pm. It was a nerve-wracking wait and I felt like a zombie when the time came. I think it was fortunate that I had done a locum in the Professor's ward.

I decided to go to Canada to intern. I wanted to see some other countries in case I decided eventually not to go back to Kenya. The world was changing at the time and I didn't think I would get any particularly good jobs in Scotland. I had enjoyed Labrador but it was not typical Canada. I had two friends who had gone to Canada, so after some deliberation I applied to and was accepted at Victoria Hospital in London Ontario. They were willing to forward my fare to Canada which was one of the determining factors. My pay was $145 per month.

It was a large hospital affiliated to the University of Western Ontario. It proved to be a good choice. I gained some wonderful experience during my rotating internship, covering all the main fields including two weeks of anaesthetics. I was taught by some very inspiring doctors. The outstanding anaesthetists that I remember were Wolfgang Spoerel, who was the chief and co-authored with Bain the paper describing the Bain circuit; Ron Aitken who anaesthetised for Charlie Drake, a neurosurgeon who was a world leader in basilar artery aneurysm surgery; and Don Catton, the chief resident who went on to become a professor. I remember Al Bruder, another resident, asking me the causes of low blood pressure during anaesthesia. I struggled to answer.

I worked with several other outstanding surgeons — John Coles, the cardiac surgeon, who let me sew up the groin incisions; Bob McFarlane, the plastic surgeon whom I assisted quite often as others did not want to work with him and from whom I learnt some useful things: Tom McLarty, a general surgeon who insisted that I learnt to tie surgical knots well before I worked with him. Among the physicians was a brilliant endocrinologist, Earl Plunkett, who stimulated my interest in this field. He had discovered many undiagnosed hypothyroid patients in the Mental Hospital who recovered with treatment with thyroid hormone.

I never considered the possibility of being anything but a country General Practitioner. I did not think I had the academic ability to pass post graduate examinations.

My next decision was what to do after that. Labrador? Maybe somewhere else in the north? I considered Frobisher Bay but it was a government job and would likely have a lot of red tape. I looked up all the hospitals in Yukon, North West Territories and Alaska. Yellowknife looked interesting — 40 beds, 1200 admissions per year and 150 deliveries — a reasonable amount of work. I read Pierre Berton's *Mysterious North* and was attracted to this out of the way place. So I wrote a letter to "The Doctor, Yellowknife, NWT" and asked if they wanted an assistant. I didn't even know how many doctors they had there. I received a reply that they would be pleased to have me as one of the three doctors was retiring in June. So that was that. Then I met an Australian physiotherapist called Janet Penfold. I asked her to come to the Hospital Ball. Then I had a problem. There was to be a residents Christmas party the following night. Would I risk asking someone I had not been out with for two functions or ask someone else? I took the risk and a few weeks later I asked her if she would like to come to Yellowknife with me. She agreed and we were married in Melbourne, Australia after I completed my internship, before we went north. She is still with me more than forty years later.

In May I had to sit my Licentiate of the Medical Council of Canada examinations to allow me to practice in Canada. Fortunately, I passed them.

I had many interesting patients, some of them very sick. I learnt from one old man, who had one of the early arterial grafts and was very ill afterwards, that the struggle to survive had been worth it to have another three months at home before he died. I also learnt from him that some people behave badly and in uncharacteristic fashion when they are very ill. We should not judge such patients by that behaviour but rather feel more compassionate towards them.

My year in London, Ontario had been a valuable and enjoyable experience. I gained good medical experience, found a wonderful wife and saw the fantastic fall (autumn) colours. I never regretted going there instead of staying in Scotland.

Chapter 2

General Practice in Yellowknife

Yellowknife was a town of 3,500 people when we went there in 1961. It was mainly a gold mining town, but was the centre for flying north into the central Arctic and for the government in the North West Territories. Later it became the capital . There were many interesting people there. One wondered why some of the characters had settled there. There were probably many intriguing stories behind them.

Yellowknife had a Siberian type climate so that in winter we had temperatures of 40°C below zero and sometimes colder. The lakes were frozen for over seven months a year. (Figure C1) House calls on a cold winter night were not easy and I had to leave my car running otherwise it might not start when I finished the visit. When the temperature dropped below -35°C the car tyres froze solid. The flattened side made them thump when one started driving. Normally in winter the cars were plugged into an electricity outlet so that the battery and oil could be kept warm. We arrived in August when the black flies and mosquitoes were still rampant. It is amazing that such creatures can survive in such a harsh climate. The hottest two or three days were about 30°C and people could swim in Frame Lake for about two weeks if they could tolerate the odd leech

Stanton Yellowknife Hospital had 40 beds and was pleasantly situated on the edge of Frame Lake. The other two doctors were George Case, whose father had been a doctor in northern Ontario, and Lloyd Powell, a Jamaican trained at McGill University in Montreal. They were contrasting personalities, one rather rough and the other fairly smooth in their approach to their patients. There was room for me in the middle.

When I arrived I told them that I was interested in anaesthetics — with two weeks training! You are welcome to do them was the reply from the other two. And so I became the anaesthetist to possibly the largest area practice in the world — a major part of the North West Territories. We used ethyl chloride and ether,

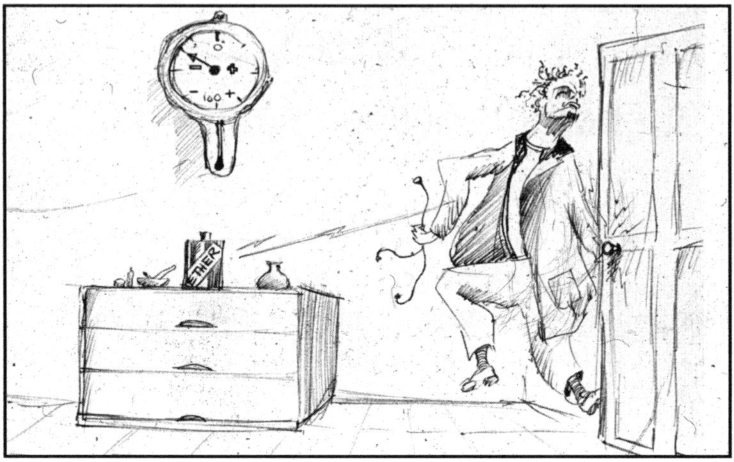

some thiopentone but were not allowed to use cyclopropane, which was widely used then, because it was explosive, particularly in the cold dry climate. In winter we could receive significant static shocks just by touching a door handle or a metal bench.

Cyclopropane has been associated with explosions, the worst of which killed at least six people in Chile in the early 1960s.

My closest to a disaster occurred one day when I was off duty. I went to collect my mail at 10.30am. We had one day off per week unless there was an operation, in which case we went in to the hospital to help. On arrival I was asked where I had been. An operation had been booked on an old Indian to amputate a frost bitten toe. Nobody had told me. When I said we could go ahead they told me we couldn't because the man had died at 10.15am. Had I given his anaesthetic at 10.00 and he had died I would probably been run out of town for killing a patient and would never have considered gaining further training in anaesthesia!

Everyone has a natural time to die. It is unfortunate for the anaesthetist if it happens to be during an anaesthetic because he or she will be blamed. In this case it would not have been my fault.

I saw some amazing medical conditions in my practice. Two old men with hypothermia, one of whom was found drunk in a snow bank, the other, a Norwegian, was found in his hut with pneumonia unable to keep the heater on.

There was a 12 year old girl who presented with horny skin on the back of her Achilles tendons. I had no idea what it could be until the mother asked if it could be anything internal. Then my time with the brilliant endocrinologist, Earl Plunkett, in London came to the fore. She had signs of hypothyroidism. She proved to have the juvenile form. The presentation was very unusual — I have never found anyone who has seen it.

Then out of the north came a 19 year old Inuit (called Eskimos in those days) with a pneumococcal empyema (infected fluid in the chest which compressed the lungs). I was ignorant about giving fluids to replace fluids which were withdrawn — in this case I took 11 pints (5 litres) of purulent fluid from his chest at one time. There was so much that I used a trick I had learnt when interning — I used eight blood bottles which had a negative pressure inside and therefore sucked the fluid out when attached to an intrapleural needle. After I had finished I found a surgical book printed in 1945 (17 years before) describing what I had just seen.

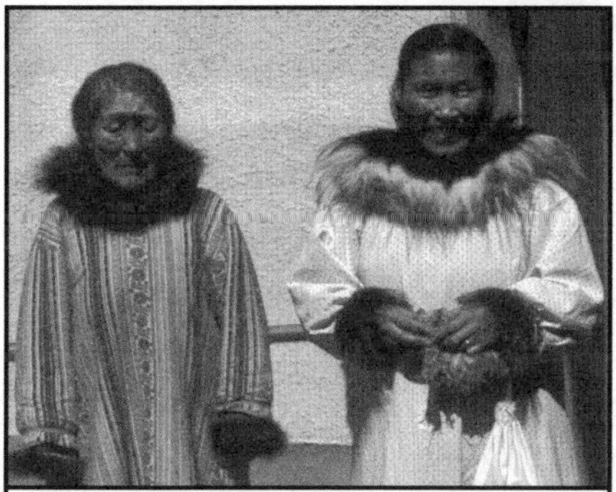

6. Two Eskimo (Inuit) patients from Coppermine in typical dress. The old lady has tattoos on her face.

Another Eskimo child arrived one night with very strange behaviour, writhing on the floor. Had I been practicing when tuberculous meningitis was common I might have recognized that she had the near terminal signs of this condition. She died shortly afterwards.

Imagine having an Indian baby who was given a penicillin injection in the buttock being brought back because she could no longer crawl. I thought the worst — damage to the sciatic nerve. I had no idea what to do so I suggested that if she was not better in two weeks the mother should bring her back. And back she came. Maybe an x Ray would give us a clue. It was sent to Edmonton for a radiologist's opinion. She had scurvy — vitamin C deficiency — because there had been no berries for eight months. Haemorrhages under the periosteum which covers the surface of bones causing pain is a feature of scurvy.

I had done some tonsillectomies in London and so did my own in Yellowknife with Lloyd Powell giving the anaesthetics. I remember having a 25 year old man virtually pain free the day after which seemed unusual.Years later I wondered whether gentle dissection was the key.

My obstetric practice grew steadily after I successfully delivered a nurse who had worked in the doctor's office before I arrived. My experience at Tumutumu (25 deliveries) was helpful in giving me confidence to do this work!

I did some dental work having had some training from Dr Paddon when I was in Labrador. The patients sometimes waited until the dentist left town and then came to see us. One day a girl came in and asked for a full mouth clearance which she needed, and another wanted a temporary filling — Inez Running, who ran our office produced some temporary filling which I heated and packed in the hole. It lasted three weeks!

I saw a refresher course in anaesthesia for G.P.s advertised to be held in Vancouver in March so applied to go. I thought it might be useful. It took us four days to drive out. It was an adventurous trip, much of it still on snow covered roads. It turned out to be a very enlightening experience — not much of a refresher for me — it was mostly new information that I gleaned. The mornings were spent in the operating room and the afternoon at lectures. It was here that I first met Eric Webb, a not very tall, very solid and rather bombastic man who was a wonderful teacher. He taught me how to intubate properly by *putting the tube in from the corner of the mouth so that one could see it going into the larynx*. This was a most important lesson which should be stressed to anyone being taught how to intubate.

Stuart Vandewater, professor from Queens University in Kingston, Ontario was the guest lecturer but after all these years the only thing I remember is a lecture by Bill Brummitt, who subsequently settled in Toronto. He talked about respiratory physiology including alveolar CO2. I recall wondering what on earth he was talking about. My understanding of basic science developed later.

One day during the course the Professor of Medicine, Dr. Kerr, happened to sit next to me at lunch. He had been Sims Travelling Professor to Kenya and was familiar with the part of the country where I grew up. As he left I said to him that some day I might contact him about a training job. I was always an opportunist! Later I did just that and later worked in his department.

The course was a great success and although I was still short on practical experience I continued giving anaesthetics with enthusiasm.

Some months later the other two offered me a partnership but I declined. I had to make more decisions. I was getting into a rut with a comfortable life which included flights around the north. I realised that I really needed some more training and experience. I had been mesmerised by magnificent weather and the beauty of Vancouver during our visit. Only later I found out that it wasn't always like that — in fact it was dull and wet much of the winter. I wrote to Dr. Graves in the Anaesthetic Department at Vancouver General Hospital to see if I could go there for six months. I thought if I followed that with six months medicine that I would be better equipped to continue in general practice. I was accepted so after nearly 17 months we left Yellowknife having had some interesting and wonderful experiences which included the birth of our twins, Catherine and Maryann, in July 1962.

I had flown to several interesting destinations including some trips beyond the Arctic circle where I experienced continuous darkness on Boxing Day in Coppermine. Only a very faint twilight appeared at midday. One night I had to fly out to the radio beacon at Contoyto Lake to pick up an Inuit woman who was reported to have fairly severe abdominal pain. Landing was difficult and bumpy on a strip between flares where the snow was fluted with ridges 20-30 cm high. Fortunately I was flying with a very skilful pilot called Ken Stockall. Another time we flew to the central Arctic and had to pick up some patients, one from an Inuit camp at Arctic Sound.

The North had a special appeal to me enhanced by phenomena like the Northern Lights (aurora borealis) which light up the sky in great coloured waves. Experiencing the cold, freezing of water to two metres of ice, snow in wonderful patterns, and the long nights in winter and days in summer, when it hardly became dark, all fascinated me. It is hard to get up in the morning when the sun doesn't rise until 10.30 am!

Despite all the allures I felt I needed more training and so we moved on to Vancouver.

Chapter 3
Training in Vancouver

We had Christmas in Melbourne, Australia. I arrived for work in Vancouver on January 3rd 1963. (Figure C2) Janet and the twins followed five weeks later as she had to have an operation and the grandparents enjoyed the chance to look after the girls. I was fortunate to have friends with whom I stayed until I found an apartment only three blocks from the hospital. It was an old block with four apartments which has long since gone to make way for a bigger building.

The Vancouver General Hospital was big — 2000 beds covering five city blocks. The operating theatres were scattered in several buildings so we sometimes had to cover large distances during our work. It was a challenging place to train as the equipment was not standardised — on the contrary the anaesthetic machines were intentionally varied so that we would become familiar with all different types. This taught one flexibility but it could be hazardous when the equipment in the anaesthetic room had different connections to the one in the operating room!

My plan was to spend six months there gaining experience in anaesthesia but after three months my boss, Horace (Horky) Graves, approached me to ask if I wished to continue on their training programme. I must have made some favourable impression. I had never before thought that some day I might be a specialist in anything. Maybe anaesthesia was a field that I could encompass. I considered the matter and then told him that I had a number of conditions. First I wanted to return to Kenya so that my family could meet my wife and twin daughters. Second, I wanted to do some medical training in case I decided to return to General Practice and, thirdly, I expected eventually to go to Australia. He was very accommodating. We arranged that after my six months was up at Vancouver General Hospital I would go to the small Childrens Hospital for two months, before going off to Yellowknife for a locum for a month to earn money to pay for our trip to Kenya.

The Childrens Hospital, which was then on East 59th Street, was an enjoyable place to work. It was small — only 80 beds on three wards with one operating theatre. One of the theatre nurses had worked with me when I was in Yellowknife. The staff anaesthetists from the Vancouver General rotated down for a week at a time which meant that I worked with the same person for a whole week.

I began my first research project to find out whether children vomited postoperatively and, if so, how often. We then tried to determine whether there were any predisposing anaesthetic, surgical or patient factors which increased the incidence. This was one of the early studies on this problem in children. Many did vomit as we were using drugs such as ether and cyclopropane which both tended to increase the incidence. Thirty years later this was to become a topic of concern to anaesthetists and the pharmaceutical companies which had developed some relatively effective drugs to prevent vomiting. The predisposing factors are largely the same, the opioid analgesics (pain relievers) such as morphine, still being one of the commonest causes.

I arranged for a medical resident position at the Vancouver General Hospital for the following January. This proved to be invaluable experience with three months in a general medical ward, two months in the clinical investigation unit which was largely endocrinology (diseases caused by hormonal imbalance) and a month in outpatients. There was some good teaching, especially by the dynamic Dr. Bogosh who was a gastroenterologist. He frequently quoted scientific papers which turned out to have been written by himself! There were several others such as Al Cox, a cardiologist, with whom I worked later. When I started I was still uncertain whether I would go back to General Practice or continue with anaesthesia.

I had many patients who were interesting from a medical point of view. One sad situation involved an eighteen year old girl who was a drug addict — it was my first exposure to this problem which was uncommon in those days. She was going to get a "fix" but was picked up by the police. She had some rat poison in her bag to take if this happened to her. She took it — strychnine. This causes most unpleasant muscle spasms with arching of the back in extreme cases — she exhibited this. We gave her huge doses of sedatives to relieve this, although later, when I had more experience, I realized that the spasms could have been more effectively treated with muscle relaxant drugs which are commonly used in anaesthesia to cause paralysis. The patient then has to have her breathing assisted. When she recovered we found out that she had been given drugs when she was twelve and had been an addict since. A sad story. I don't know what happened to her — probably she had a short, sad life.

I was called to see another old lady in Emergency — while recording her electrocardiogram the regular wave form suddenly faded out to a straight line indicating that her heart had stopped. I had witnessed her dying. I did not try to resuscitate her. Cardiac arrest calls had not come into vogue then. When I look back I think how lucky she was that when her time came to die she did so peacefully and with dignity.

After this medical job Dr Graves suggested that I should go to the Veterans Hospital. I told him that I didn't want to go there. So he asked me to go to the Childrens Hospital again for another two months and then return to Vancouver General Hospital. I was delighted. I had another wonderful time at the Childrens Hospital and continued my studies from the previous year on post operative vomiting. Then I had followed 400 patients which was a sizable series at that time. There were no studies specifically on children and although I did not write up the results they provided me with background which I built on years later.

I had read an article about a particular problem related to anaesthesia for burnt patients. It had been reported that patients with extensive burns were liable to have a cardiac arrest following a muscle relaxant called succinylcholine. Several mechanisms were suggested in this paper by Gordon Bush, an anaesthetist from Liverpool, England, who later became a good friend. One theory was that there was a great release of potassium from cells into the blood when this drug was injected into the patients. Nobody had ever studied what this drug did to serum potassium in normal patients, although one study had been done in dogs the previous year, so I made some preliminary studies at the Childrens Hospital. Very little change occurred. This was the beginning of my research on the effect of muscle relaxants in burns, a study which went on for twenty years. Shortly afterwards I received my first research grant for $50 from the British Columbia Medical Research Foundation to study this in normal patients. It paid for the laboratory technician to do the potassium measurements. Small beginnings! I did measurements in three circumstances to see if other factors affected the result. I gave suxamethonium after 1) intravenous induction with thiopentone, 2) an inhalation induction with halothane, and 3) a thiopentone induction followed by 20 minutes of halothane. The results were the same — an insignificant rise of serum potassium of 0.1–0.2 mmol / l. Because the changes were insignificant I did not publish them. I realized two years later when someone from Switzerland published similar results that I should have published mine. Sometimes a negative finding is worth reporting. As far as I know my studies were the first in humans.

The group of anaesthetists at the Vancouver General Hospital was the first in Canada to be contracted to provide the total service for a large hospital. It had been set up by Digby Leigh about 1948. He had been one of the triumvirate in Montreal who had been responsible for running short training courses in anaesthesia for doctors in the armed forces going to World War II. The other two were Wesley Bourne , the doyen of Montreal anaesthesia and Harold Griffiths who became one of the founders and first President of the World Federation of Societies of Anaesthesiologists in 1955. Digby Leigh took several young colleagues with him to Vancouver — John Poole, Horace Graves, Herb Randall, Harold Kester and Eric Webb, all of whom contributed a great deal to my training. Leigh was a forceful character who, in 1952, demanded a separate Department of Anaesthesia and a full chair with the title of Professor. The administration would not bow to this progressive demand so he left and went to Los Angeles where he established a name for himself as one of the early specialist paediatric anaesthetists and author of one of the first books on paediatric anaesthesia, with Kay Belton.

At the Vancouver General Hospital I learnt many things from the large group of anaesthetists — practical anesthesia, how to organize the rosters and the flow of work in the operating rooms, the heady medical politics of a large hospital and much more which was invaluable in later life when I reached positions of responsibility myself.

Looking back over nearly forty years it is interesting how one can remember various things that different people taught me. Eric Webb I have mentioned. He was a shortish, very broad man who needed outsized shirts. He believed that time saved was worth the cost of the couple of speeding fines he paid each year. He was one of the best practical teachers I had and also imbued me with an interest in the history of anaesthesia. John Poole was a kindly, older gentleman with a twinkle in his eye who was a master organizer of the staff. Herb Randall was a good natured man who had done some training with Ralph Waters, one of America's famous early teachers in our specialty. Herb passed on some of his pearls such as replacing cyclopropane with nitrous oxide at the end of an anaesthetic to reduce the likelihood of laryngeal spasm. Cyclopropane declined from its position as the most popular anaesthetic in the hospital to be replaced by halothane during my first six months in Vancouver. Horky Graves was always very good to me, for reasons which I never understood, and agreed to all my rather demanding requests about my training,. He had a tendency to inhibit anyone on the staff who showed signs of investigative flair by giving them undesirable rosters. I found this difficult to understand. Maybe these reactions were to perceived threat. There was none in my case because I had indicated that I would eventually go to Australia.

Jone Chang was a very able and bright younger anaesthetist. It was when working with him one day that I learnt about treating massive blood loss during surgery, an experience which was to prove very useful many times during my career. This was a very rare case of a 34 year old lady who had had a coarctation of her aorta. This is a congenital condition where the aorta, the main blood vessel leaving the heart has a narrowing which causes high blood pressure in the upper body and a low pressure beyond the narrowing due to the constriction. These defects are usually repaired in infancy nowadays but in this lady it wasn't recognised until she was in her thirties. It was following the repair that a weakness in one of the arteries to her gut ruptured due to the increased pressure and she nearly bled to death. Rapid and effective resuscitation and surgery saved her.

Len Jenkins had the only academic attachment with the University and was involved with research in the Pharmacology Department. People training for their fellowship in Anaesthesia could spend up to a year of their four years of training doing research. They also had to do one year of internal medicine which was very valuable in helping them to assess their patients medically before anaesthesia. It was a requirement because Canadian anaesthetists gained their fellowship from the College of Physicians. Len helped me with some of my research including a trial of an anti-vomiting drug. It was a code numbered phenothiazine which proved to be comparable with promethazine (Phenergan) which has anti-emetic properties that reduced the incidence of post-operative vomiting to one third compared to controls in my study.

Len Jenkins was also responsible for our theoretical training. We had one afternoon for tutorials and lectures and another where we each had to present one paper a year. The first year I had to speak on THAM (a buffer that corrects both metabolic and respiratory acidosis), low molecular weight dextran and mannitol. The next year I spoke on syndromes associated with high and low atmospheric pressures which I found interesting as it included topics such as mountain sickness and problems related to building tunnels. I was later able to introduce similar teaching ideas in Australia when I finally settled there. Len later became Professor of Anaesthesia. After he retired he devoted much of his time to painting and writing poetry both of which he did well.

Both Len Jenkins and Jone Chang were involved in developing a test for myasthenia gravis, a condition where there is an abnormality in transmission by acetyl choline of nerve impulses across to the muscle at specialised points known as the neuromuscular junction. This abnormality leads to muscle weakness. Anaesthetists use two types of muscle relaxant drugs to produce paralysis during anaesthesia. These facilitate the insertion of tubes into the trachea without damaging the vocal cords, allows them to control the patient's breathing and relax the muscles so that the surgeons can gain easy access into the body, particularly the abdomen. One type, depolarising relaxants (eg. succinyl choline and decamethonium) act directly on the receptor at the neuromuscular junction to depolarize or stimulate it and then prevents acetyl choline from acting for a few minutes during which the patient remains paralysed. The other type (non-depolarizer) acts by preventing the acetyl choline from reaching the receptor so that muscle contraction cannot occur, and hence results in paralysis until the drug leaves sufficient receptors for normal neuromuscular transmission to return and thence the paralysis ceases. Anticholine-esterase drugs can be given to speed this up. Patients with myasthenia gravis become paralysed with much smaller doses of the latter (non-depolarizing relaxants) and require much larger doses of the depolarizing ones. Decamethonium was used in the test which was being developed. Very small doses were given and the conscious subject had to squeeze a pressure gauge. When weakness began to develop the drug was stopped and the dose recorded. Myasthenic patients required larger doses. I was one of the test subjects! Unfortunately I responded abnormally and needed a bigger dose than expected. This was done awake and afterwards I felt as if someone had hit me on the chest with a sledge hammer — this was muscle aching which can follow the use of depolarizing relaxants. They thought I might be myasthenic but decided to test me again. The next time I tested normal. This was a very interesting observation as I have not come across any research showing such a variable response to a muscle relaxant drug in the same person, particularly when no other drug had been given. It shows that marked individual variation in response can occur. Usually we give an average dose, varying it if there are known factors which modify it. These factors were the subject of some of my later research.

There were many others who contributed to my education. Teachers often don't know what they have contributed to the development of people they are teaching and it can be very gratifying for them to hear occasionally that they have helped in some way. Many years later when I was visiting Vancouver I phoned some of them for a chat and to express my gratitude.

A period of research came about in a very unusual way. The plan for me to return to the Vancouver General Hospital (VGH) after the second spell at the Childrens Hospital changed after meeting Al Cox, a cardiologist, at afternoon coffee one day. When I asked if he had been doing anything interesting lately he told me that he had been to Seattle to buy a treadmill to do exercise studies, first on firemen volunteers and later on patients. It sounded interesting, especially when I found out that he was looking for a research assistant. After some negotiation, Dr. Graves again acceded to my next request and so I became a research assistant in the Department of Medicine where Al Cox was Assistant Professor. This proved to be some of the most valuable experience that I gained.

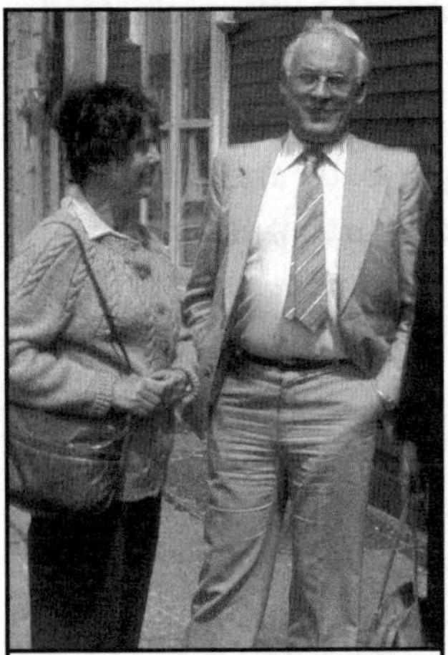
7. Al Cox with his wife, Peg in 1985.

There were two main research projects with which I was involved. One was running firemen on the treadmill, increasing the speed and incline every three minutes. The firemen volunteered because it was very important to maintain fitness in their erratic work. We ran them until they felt they could go no longer — at this point their heart rate had reached its maximum. The men ranged in age from twenties to fifties. We demonstrated that maximum heart rate declined with age from nearly 200 beats per minute in young 20 year-olds to 150–160 per minute by sixty. This limitation is one factor why older people have less reserve for exercise. We were almost ready to publish our results when a Danish group published similar findings for the first time. So I learnt about missing being first to describe something!

We also studied blood sugar during these exercise studies. It was fascinating because it demonstrated how wonderfully the body controls its environment and modifies it to the circumstances. The various hormones that control blood sugar readjusted so that the glucose released from the liver exactly matched the increased amount the body needed during exercise, and thus the blood glucose remained steady. However, when one stopped exercising suddenly the blood level rose as utilization decreased. It gradually readjusted back to normal as the mechanisms releasing glucose from the liver were switched off. An interesting aside to this is that one of the theories of satiety (not feeling hungry) was that when blood sugar reached a certain level hunger ceased. It is common not to experience hunger immediately after strenuous exercise.

The other project involved making glass microelectrodes with a 0.5 micron tip, filling the minute tube with a conductive solution and then impaling it into atrial cells from a rabbit heart. These were kept beating in an electrolyte bath and we studied the effects of some drugs that affect the heart contraction. The electrodes were made by heating a fine glass tube and pulling it as it melted. One could vary the heat applied and the tension with which it was pulled. When these were right the tube broke leaving a fine tip of the diameter required. We then had to fill them, using a vacuum chamber, with strong potassium chloride solution to conduct the action potential from the cell to the electrical recording apparatus. For three months I spent hours pulling these electrodes — about 300 in all — but I could not obtain normal sized action potentials. It was exceedingly frustrating. In those days we had to weigh the chemicals and make the solution for the tissue bath. When I eventually had to make a new solution I found that my predecessor had not taken into consideration that calcium was divalent and therefore had half the concentration needed in the solution. This was a disaster as calcium in adequate concentration is essential for normal contraction and hence normal action potentials. Suddenly my action potentials were the size that they should have been. It was a joyous occasion! It was also a *lesson in patience* which is essential if one is going to withstand the frustration that can occur in research. It taught me infinite patience so that in later years when research projects went on for years or difficulties arose I could tolerate the delays.

During my time with Al Cox he took six weeks off to go to Chicago to do a course in medical education. He brought back some very revolutionary ideas. In the following weeks we had many discussions about education which I believe had an influence on my life as this became one of my great interests.

Before leaving for his course he said that while he was away I could do a project of my own using the microelectrode experimental model. I planned to study the effects of the muscle relaxant, succinyl choline, which I had studied in relation to its effect on serum potassium. Structurally this drug was like two molecules of the transmitter, acetyl choline, which conducts impulses from the vagus nerve endings to the heart, causing it to slow. I wondered if the slowing effect of the drug was directly on the heart muscle or due to its similarity in structure to acetyl choline. Then I read about the first report that the local anaesthetic, lignocaine, has an effect on the heart which inhibited irregularities in heart rhythm. This created a dilemma — which would I study? I eventually chose the succinylcholine one which showed no direct action occurred so the slowing is due to the structural similarity to the natural transmitter, acetyl choline. I often wonder what would have happened if I had made the other choice because I could have demonstrated the direct effect on the cells. At the time that was a whole new field of pharmacology. Maybe it was a missed opportunity. Life is full of choices. Even taking the opportunity to gain this research experience was a good choice.

Two other things happened during this period. I was asked to go for a few days to help out giving anaesthetics at the Royal Columbian Hospital in New Westminster because they were short due to illness. I found out that Dr Graves had told them that I was one of his senior residents — it sounded good but I had only done ten months anaesthesia! The experience that I had already gained must have been good as I survived, and so did my patients, even doing some major, challenging cases during the night.

The other event was the first Paediatric Anaesthesia weekend course held at the Hospital for Sick Children in Toronto in November 1964. Some of the anaesthetists, knowing my interest in children, suggested that I should attend. A great idea but the fare to Toronto was a month's salary!

I had developed one of my philosophies in life that one should ask for what one wanted and the worst that could happen would be refusal. When I asked Dr Graves said he did not see why he should support me when I was not even working for him. I pointed out that I had done some research during my times at the Childrens Hospital doing anaesthesia. He paid two thirds of the fare! I went and I heard the legendary paediatric anaesthetists, Digby Leigh, Bob Cope from London and Jackson Rees from Liverpool on a panel. It began with Leigh, in his wild way , informing the audience that the panel were all enemies. They debated, among other topics, how long one could leave a nasotracheal tube in place (a tube inserted into the airway so the patient could breath or be ventilated). Five to seven days, they thought. Then a most dramatic comment was made from the floor by a lady who became one of the leading anaesthetists in Australia and eventually, Dean of the Faculty of Anaesthetists, Tess Brophy. She informed the meeting that one had been left in for 34 days in Australia without problems. It was the most stunning comment that I ever heard at an anaesthetic meeting. The audience was amazed!

I was very impressed with the meeting and what I saw at the 'Sick Kids' so I decided that I should try to procure a job there. On my return to Vancouver I went to see Dr. Graves and told him of my next wish. He successfully negotiated a position for me the following year which led me on to become a paediatric anaesthetist. There was one condition — that I spend two months on the Cardiac anaesthesia rotation with Bill Dodds and Jack Nixon before I went. This experience also proved valuable — I learnt about ventilating patients with a respirator (ventilator) after the operation and how to measure blood gases, which were critical to ensuring that ventilation was adequate and that the free hydrogen ion content of the blood was kept within the narrow range for

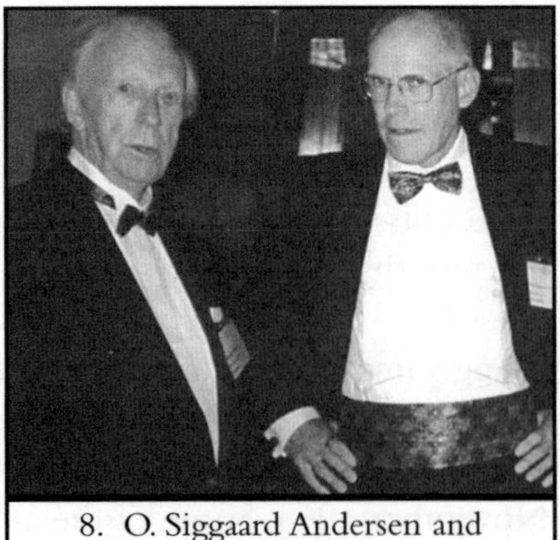

8. O. Siggaard Andersen and Henning Poulsen (Denmark — Chairman of WFSA Executive 1968-76) taken in 1997.

normal bodily function. The Astrup triple pH technique, developed in Denmark by Sigaard Andersen for measuring blood gases, was new at that time. It involved having three blood samples, equilibrating two with high and low levels of CO2, drawing a line between them on the chart and marking where the actual CO2 level was. One could then derive pH, pCO2 and base deficit. It was a tedious method compared to what is available now.

We also had to assess patients in respiratory failure to determine whether inhalation of isoprenaline or "Bird therapy" would benefit them. This was the use of breathing assistance from a Bird ventilator in conjunction with physiotherapy.

One day during cardiac surgery a dramatic event occurred. I noticed all the IV bottles were swinging on their poles — what was happening? I suddenly realized it was an earthquake! Fortunately we were not at the epicentre — it was about 230km away on the Hope — Princeton highway and was of sufficient magnitude for a whole mountain side to cave in and fill the valley below. It is thought that five cars disappeared under the landslide. This occurred about the same time as the Alaska tidal wave and an earthquake up the British Columbia coast which demolished half of the coastal settlement of Ocean Falls in a giant landslide.

We make friends at school, but especially at university and during the early, impecunious years when we are trying to become established in life. Many of the these people become lifelong friends and even if we don't see them for years it is easy to pick up where we left off. I made several such friends during my time in Vancouver.

Ken Leighton (Figure C3) was a Scot, born in Barbados. He had been in General Practice for several years in the Outer Hebrides in Scotland, several places in British Columbia including Smithers, where he finally retired, as well as spending a spell in New Zealand. He joined the anaeshesia training programme shortly after I did when he was already in his forties. He followed an academic career and later became Head of Anaesthesia at the new University Hospital in Vancouver. He developed a great reputation among his peers as an incisive thinker and a very practical man. I had the privilege of attending a meeting, many years later, of the leading researchers from across Canada — at the end of the discussion they asked him for his seal of approval before the decision was finalized — a rare sign of respect. He pursued physical as well as intellectual challenges. He ran four marathons after the age of 59, rowed a boat of Hebridean design that he had specially built, from Vancouver to Prince Rupert, hundreds of miles up the British Columbia coast, and later worked, after he retired, in Honduras, Kimberly in South Africa and in Uganda — all demanding positions. His book, *Oar and Sail*, tells of his rowing adventure and won a literary award. One of the reviewers wrote " Melding a love of language, Gaelic wit, and the sea, Dr. Leighton shares with us the history, personalities and uncountable channels of one of the most beautiful coastlines in the world". It is a wonderful little book with high quality writing. Ken was a great friend and had one of the most challenging intellects I ever came across. His family were also adventuresome. His wife, Nancy, with their three children aged 14, 15 and 16 rode their bicycles from Vancouver to Halifax, about 6500 km, in 58 days — what an achievement!

Another late entry to anaesthesia was Norman Campbell who had also been in General Practice for many years. He was another man with a great sense of humour who became a good friend. I remember him presenting some serious medical information and then referring to his source "Time Magazine"! He visited us twice in Australia. On the first occasion he invited us to dinner with a distant relative he had traced who turned out to be a close friend of my in-laws!

Jim Treloar and Peter Klassen were the first anaesthetists that I know of to set up a day anaesthesia facility in a medical consulting suite building, in 1965. By the 1980s this became very fashionable and now many operations are done on a same day basis.

Dick Jack started after me. Years later I met in England where he had developed a significant reputation as an anaesthesia educator. He has been responsible for many continuing education courses in anaesthesia, particularly in Eastern Europe. Bob Creighton went to the Hospital for Sick Children in Toronto where, after a year in London, he became a member of staff. He was a fairly laid back person who did mainly neuro-anaesthesia. He eventually became Chief of the Department. I maintained some contact with them all over many years and met them all again.

We had had to live frugally as my salary was only $200 per month which was not much when half went on rent and we had two small children. Janet became a very economical shopper and cook! She worked sometimes as a physiotherapist in the evening at the Canadian Arthritis Society clinic which maintained her interest in her work and gave her a break from the house and children. One summer she had a two week holiday with the twins, who were two, at a camp near Narra-matta where the children were looked after and she could have a rest. Ours had grown from babies through the toddler stage to three year olds by mid June 1965 when we set off to drive to Toronto. We had some regrets, as we were leaving some good friends and a city we had come to enjoy but the two and a half years in Vancouver had been wonderful clinical experience and gave me a good grounding for my future career in anaesthesia, teaching and research. I was now on the path to becoming an anaesthetist. I never dreamt where that would lead me. We had also had a wonderful time exploring Vancouver and other parts of British Columbia which is such a beautiful province.

Chapter 4

Anaesthesia and Some History

My decision to go to Toronto indicated that I had decided to try to complete my training in anaesthesia, with a view to hopefully doing paediatric anaesthesia which combined my interest in children and anesthesia. This move was a significant change from my original perception of becoming a country general practitioner based on the fact that I was not keen on cities and I never thought when I qualified that some day I might be able to become a specialist. Now I was heading for a highly specialised interest which necessarily involves living in a big city.

Why did I choose anaesthesia? I thought it was a specialty that I could master — it seemed to be more circumscribed than many others. I was not correct in that but my extra medical training in Vancouver and the way I was taught in Dundee stood me in good stead for the wider requirements of our specialty. In addition I did not like writing case histories and thought working in the operating theatre was more interesting than interviewing and examining patients all day. While that can be interesting there is a lot of hum drum in general practice seeing patients with common complaints.

So what is anaesthesia? It is the administration of drugs to keep the patient pain free during surgery. This may include making them unconscious with general anesthetic agents or by using local anaesthesia making part of the body numb and therefore pain free as is achieved with a spinal, epidural or a nerve block. Essentially one makes the patient comfortable during surgery, a great step forward from the days before 1846 when patients were given alcohol or some other intoxicating potion and, if necessary, held down while they were operated upon. Once, when I visited the London Hospital, I was shown the bell with which they used to summon the orderlies to hold the patients down — a chilling idea. In addition, in those days antisepsis had not been introduced so many patients became infected and often died because they did not have antibiotics. One woman, when asked to consent for her husband's operation replied " and who is going to pay for the funeral". Not an encouraging prospect.

We now recognize that anaesthesia is a process which begins with the preoperative visit by the anesthetist. The aim of this is to meet and gain some rapport with the patient. A good anaesthetist can allay some of the patient's anxiety and provide reassurance. They can tell the patient what to expect. They then have to take a concise history to elucidate any medical or surgical problems that may influence the choice of anaesthetic or warn the anaestheist of potential problems so that he/ she may take steps to avoid them. The drugs the patient may be taking are reviewed to determine whether any of them interact with the anaesthetic. Sometimes adverse effects can result. The anaesthetist therefore needs to be a good doctor and because they usually have to do this more quickly than physicians, I say that a good anaesthetist should be a super-physician.

The next decision is whether the patient needs some preoperative medication to reduce anxiety or to contribute to the pain relief which will be needed. Anxious patients need more anaesthesia because anxiety causes a stress response which makes more blood go to muscles and relatively less to the brain where it is needed to make the patient unconscious. Premedication to reduce anxiety prevents this but may make the patient sleepier afterwards depending on how long the drug works and how long the operation lasts. With the increasing use of day surgery where the patient goes home soon afterwards many anaesthetists prefer not to give premedication and use more short acting anaesthetic drugs so that recovery from anaesthesia is rapid.

Sometimes anaesthesia is induced in an anaesthetic room adjacent to the operating theatre or it may be induced in the theatre. In adults this is usually done with an intravenous injection but that is not the end of the anaesthetist's work as many people think it is. The anaesthetist then stays throughout the operation, monitoring the patients breathing and their cardiovascular system to ensure that the tissues are receiving enough oxygen and that enough anaesthetic is delivered to keep the patient unconscious. Another very important role achieved by monitoring the patients physiological changes and watching the operation is that he/she knows when to give extra fluids or blood, if necessary, when significant bleeding occurs during the operation. *The anaesthetist basically keeps the patient alive while the surgery is performed and takes corrective action if anything goes wrong.* Not all complications can be predicted but an anaesthetist's training teaches him how to react and correct problems. Occasionally unexpected complications occur which are not easy to reverse but fortunately these are uncommon. There have been great advances in patient safety during my career and serious adverse events are much less common — anaesthesia is now probably safer than driving on the roads in most advanced countries.

In the period immediately after surgery the patients usually go to the recovery room where there are specialised nurses to care for them until they are fully conscious and are ready to return to the ward.

Vomiting after surgery has always been a common problem, often occurring only once or twice. It was an accepted side effect of anaesthesia but it can be dangerous if the patient is unconscious and lying on his back. It is more common when opioid drugs are used, and with certain operations such as squint surgery. Some of my early research showed that some old drugs such as promethazine (Phenergan) could reduce the incidence of vomiting. Some of the newer ones are even more effective and hence greater emphasis is now put on prevention, stimulated to a significant degree by the benefits to the drug companies. There are a few people who have a tendency to vomit frequently after anaesthesia. These now usually receive preventative treatment.

Anaesthetists have become increasingly involved in post operative pain management in the past 20-30 years. Now, in many major hospitals there are pain management teams who can visit patients who are having significant discomfort. The major difficulty in setting up such a service is the cost and availability of suitable staff. Anaesthetists may use local anaesthetic blocks to provide pain relief or intravenous infusions of analgesics which can maintain a constant blood level and hence good pain relief. Many patients can control these infusions so that they can give some more analgesic if pain develops — patient controlled analgesia (PCA). Pain management is becoming a specialty in its own right, especially for treating patients with chronic pain. Effective management which enables people to return to work can result in huge savings in the community.

The anaesthetists became involved in the management of very sick people when intensive care units opened. They have been leaders in this field and remain so in many parts of the world. In Australia, Intensive Care has become a separate specialty in which some anaesthetists become involved and this is a trend in some of the most advanced countries. In Australia both these disciplines, Intensive Care and Pain Management have a faculty in the College of Anaesthetists which run organized training programs and examinations leading to a fellowship qualification.

What training do anaesthetists need? In most countries they have three to six years further training after they have completed their internship. In Australia and New Zealand training is organized by the College of Anaesthetists and they have a five year program in which the final examinations are taken in the fourth year. A good grounding in basic science related to the specialty is required and is examined — physiology (how the body works), pharmacology (drugs and how they work) and anatomy (structure of the body). They also have to have a good knowledge of medicine and know about the equipment that is used. They gain a wide variety of experience working with all surgical specialties, obstetrics and radiology (medical imaging). It is a field which attracts people who like to see their drugs working immediately, enjoy the physiology (variations in body functions) and who like some work that requires manual skills. It has periods of stress and intense activity and periods when things just tick along smoothly.

Suitability for the specialty requires someone with a calm temperament who can withstand stressful situations well. People who play musical instruments are often suited because they can read music and use their hands at the same time. Anaesthetists have to be able to watch their patients and monitors while they do other things with their hands. They also have to be good observers and people who are visual learners seem to make better anaesthetists than auditory learners — nearly all of them are visual learners. These three factors are favourable attributes if someone is thinking about joining the specialty. It is not essential to be musical. I am not.

Sometimes it is an interest in aspects of the specialty or maybe exposure to an enthusiastic teacher which leads a student on the path to become an anaesthetist.

What is involved in the anaesthetic? Drugs are either breathed through the lungs or given intravenously so that they are rapidly carried in the blood to the brain where they depress activity and produce unconsciousness.

Comments on the management of patients for surgery go back many centuries. The ancient Egyptians used opium while the Assyrians used a mixture of belladonna, cannabis and mandragora. They also used carotid compression to produce unconsciousness. The soporific sponge containing these concoctions to breathe was an Arabic invention. The Chinese employed cannabis indica for its analgesic properties. Dioscorides, a famous Greek physician of the First Century AD administered mandragora plant boiled in urine before submitting his patients to surgery. Shakespeare mentions the hypnotic effects of mandrgora in *Antony and Cleopatra.*

In 1824 Henry Hill Hickman from Ludlow in the west of England tried to relieve pain with carbon dioxide inhalation. He had the right idea but the wrong gas. Then Horace Wells, a dentist from Hartford, Connecticut found that he felt no pain when he banged his shins while inhaling nitrous oxide. He tried to put on a public demonstration of the use of nitrous oxide in 1844 but unfortunately picked a strong subject who cried out when the tooth was pulled. Wells was shouted out and accused of being a fraud even though the patient felt no pain. He committed suicide.

Forty five years before, Humphrey Davy and his colleagues had observed that they did not have any pain when they injured themselves when they were inhaling nitrous oxide for pleasure. Davy commented in 1799 that "nitrous oxide might be useful to relieve pain in operations where no great effusion of blood took place".

The first modern anaesthetics were vapours and gases which were breathed by the patient. Ether was the mainstay of anaesthesia in many parts of the world for over a hundred years. It was first used by Crawford Long in Georgia in 1842 but he did not realize that he was doing something revolutionary as it also was being used as a recreational drug and was recognised for its analgesic effects. On October 16th 1846 Morton in Boston put on a successful public demonstration of its use for an operation and thereafter the news spread rapidly around the world. He was given the idea by a chemist, Jackson, who unfairly received little credit.

The tale of the spread of the news around the world is fascinating. It was carried to Britain on the Arcadia, a wooden paddle steamer which took fourteen days to cross the Atlantic. It docked in Liverpool on December 16th 1846. The ship's doctor, William Fraser, a graduate of St Andrews University where I trained, traveled to Dumfries in southern Scotland upon arrival. There, on December 19th the first anaesthetic in Britain was given for a surgical operation which was an amputation done by Dr William Scott, an Edinburgh graduate. The intriguing question to which we will probably never know the answer is how did Fraser reach Dumfries. Did he go by the steamship, Royal Victoria which left Liverpool on the 17th, by coach or could he have just possibly have caught the train. The Lancaster to Carlisle line was opened on December 15th.

The first anaesthetic in London was given the same day, December 19th, for a dental extraction. On December 21st Robert Liston amputated Frederick Churchill's leg in London.

The news spread rapidly — to France by 24th December, and to Australia where the first surgical anaesthetic has been credited to William Russ Pugh in Launceston on June 7th 1847. This was remarkable as the journey took about five months by sea at the time and this was less than six months after the first anaesthetic in Britain. There is a statue of Pugh in Launceston, placed walking down some steps on his way to work, in the park opposite the house where he gave the first anaesthetic.(now a famous restaurant — Me and Fee)

There is some debate about Australian priority. John

Belisario in Sydney gave dental anaesthetics on 7 June which were reported in the Sydney Morning Herald on June 8th. One of these patients had had a previous anaesthetic suggesting that Belisario had given an earlier ether anaesthetic which may have been the first in Australia. The first comments on painless surgery appeared in the Sydney Morning Herald appeared on Monday 17th May 1847. The news may have come on the Prince of Wales on the 11th May or on the Niagara on the 15th. It is probable that the news reached Tasmania later than that. It seems that both Pugh and Belisario may have constructed their apparatus from a sketch in the Illustrated London News of 9th January 1847.

The question of priority of the first ether anaesthetic (dental) seemed to have settled on Belisario until Peter Vidler and Owen James in Newcastle found reference to anaesthesia in the Maitland Mercury, the second longest running newspaper in Australia. It carried reference on May 8th to the Boston report of ether anaesthesia. On July 28th the Maitland Mercury referred to a letter written by Dr. Buchanan of Port Stephens written on the 21st (month not quoted) to Captain King and reported in the Sydney Morning Herald of July 6th referring to anaesthesia in the Hunter Valley. If it had been May 21st Dr. Buchanan would have been first but there is no way of knowing whether it was May or June 21st. These reports are both fascinating to historians and frustrating, because they leave doubt.

Chloroform came next the following year, 1847, when J.Y.Simpson, who was Professor of midwifery in Edinburgh, administered it to a boy for removal of a necrotic radius. He was given the idea to try chloroform by a chemist in Liverpool named Waldie, whom he later barely acknowledged. He and some friends had tried inhaling it along with some other chemicals in an attempt to find something better than ether.

John Snow was a remarkable doctor in London, who did some amazing work on ether and then chloroform. He devised an inhaler which took into account many of the physical requirements for vapourizing liquids (baffling to increase surface area and warming to increase the vapour pressure and hence concentration) and he recognized the importance of limiting vapour concentration with chloroform for safe administration and to avoid fatalities. He also stopped a typhoid epidemic by recognizing that Broad Street pump was the source of infected water causing the cases and having it closed.

The art of anaesthesia was to make the patient unconscious and provide the surgeon with the conditions required for operating while not giving an overdose which might kill the patient. This was achieved by varying the concentration of the inhaled anaesthetic being administered. Careful observation of clinical signs in the patient makes it possible for the anaesthetist to achieve this. Now, with many more drugs being given intravenously, in known appropriate doses, and the concentration in the blood often being maintained by syringe pumps which are run with scientifically calculated dose regimes, the depth of anaesthesia can be safely controlled more easily and the chance of overdosage minimized. New monitoring systems are being developed which indicate the depth of anaesthesia. It is part of the anaesthetists on going role to keep monitoring the patient to ensure that the appropriate amount of anaesthetic is being given. This is why they stay throughout the operation. It is not a mat-

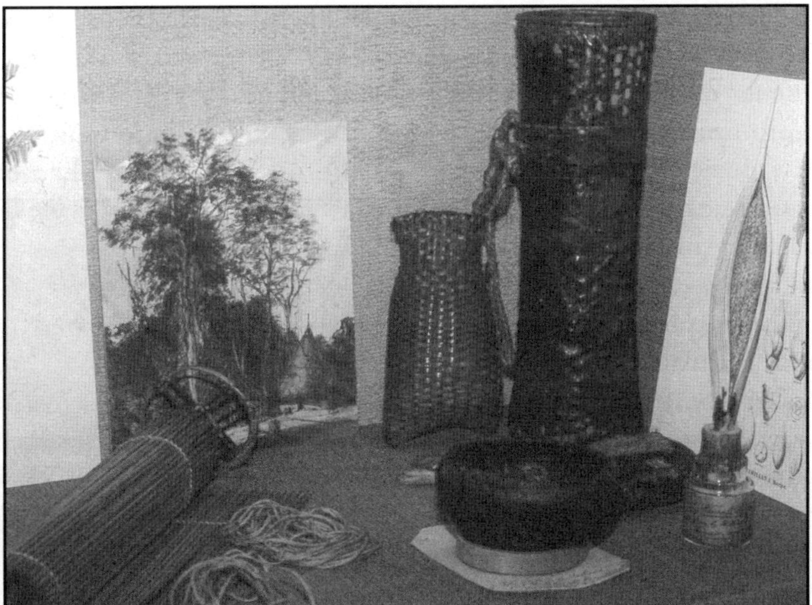

9. An exhibit of items collected by Waterton in 1825, including "wourali" in the dark pot.

ter of one shot in the arm to put you to sleep. That is not all that they do!

The anaesthetist also ensures that the patient breathes adequately and receives enough oxygen. Sometime breathing is taken over by a ventilator and often in this case the patient is paralysed with a muscle relaxant drug. This makes it easier for the surgeon to access the abdomen and chest easily. It is usual then to insert a tube into the airway so that the gas can be delivered to the lungs with certainty.

Muscle relaxants were first used in anaesthesia only in 1942, and yet as far back as 1825 Charles Waterton, the Squire of Walton Hall near Leeds in England, had demonstrated that Indian arrow poison which he obtained on his trips to South America caused paralysis in his donkeys. After two had died following wourali injections he had kept one alive by cutting a hole in its neck and inserting a bellows into the trachea with which he ventilated it for four hours until it recovered. It was from this substance wourali that the first muscle relaxant, tubocurarine, was developed.

Claude Bernard used curare in experimental physiology in the 1870s and Edward Henry Embley, the first anaesthetist at the Royal Melbourne Hospital , used it in his large series of experiments in 1899-1901 when he determined that the cause of death from chloroform was due to cardiac rather than respiratory failure. This amazing work was the first significant piece of basic research in anaesthesia in Australia. Half his animals were anaesthetised with morphine and curare and ventilated through a tracheotomy, more than 40 years before it was used in human anaesthesia. His researches were reported in three papers, which occupied 20 pages of the British Medical Journal in April 1901.

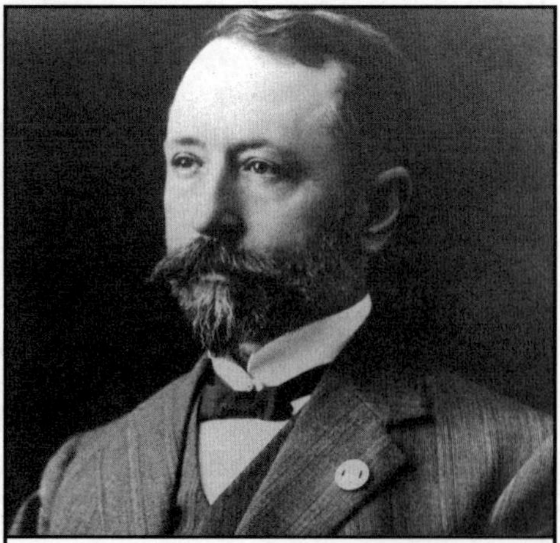

10. Edward Henry Embley.

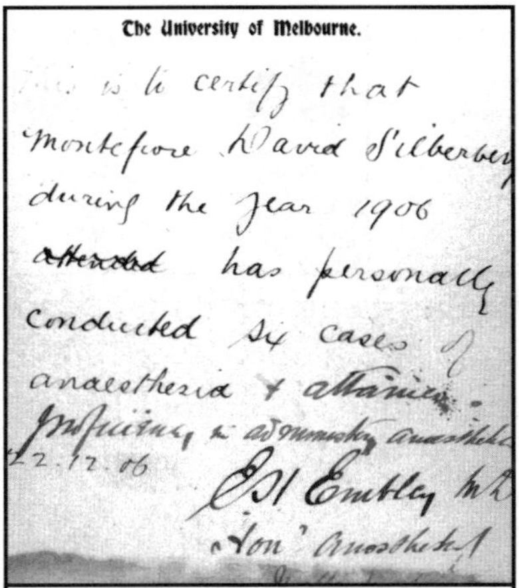

The University of Melbourne.

This is to certify that Montefiore David Silberberg during the year 1906 attended has personally conducted six cases of anaesthesia & attained proficiency in administering anaesthetics

22.12.06

E.H. Embley MD
Hon' Anaesthetist

11. Medical student's certificate of competence to give anaesthesia — signed by Embley.
(Geoffrey Kaye Museum, with permission of the Curator, R Westhorpe)

Eric Webb, one of my best practical teachers, also stimulated my interest in the history of anaesthesia. We had a journal club for the residents in Vancouver. Each year one, which was devoted to historical topics, was held at Eric Webb's home. I continued the idea in Melbourne until we had too many registrars to accommodate in our house. Since then Rod Westhorpe has taken them to visit the Geoffrey Kaye Museum at the College and I have a tutorial session where I show my collection of old drugs.

I met many interesting anaesthetists. Archie Brain developed the laryngeal mask airway which changed anaesthetic practice significantly in the last decade. It has been used instead of endotracheal intubation in many situations that resulted in a great decrease in the number of patients who receive muscle relaxants to paralyse them during anaesthesia, often to facilitate intubation.

When should one retire? I have met some very old anaesthetists who were still very interested in their work. Dr G.S.Ambardeckar from Mumbai in India, who I met when he was 87 years old, was still practicing anaesthesia. He attended one of my lectures and asked pertinent questions. He said he would continue as long as he could insert an intravenous cannula and do a spinal anaesthetic! He retired when he was ninety, probably the oldest person to give anaesthetics. He died about a year later. I

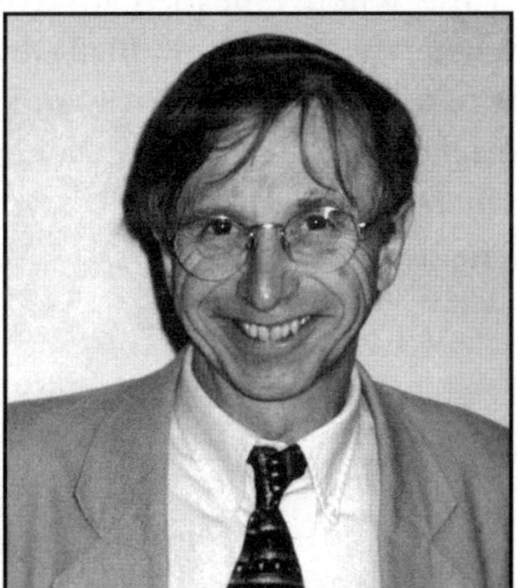

12. Archie Brain, inventor of the laryngeal mask airway.

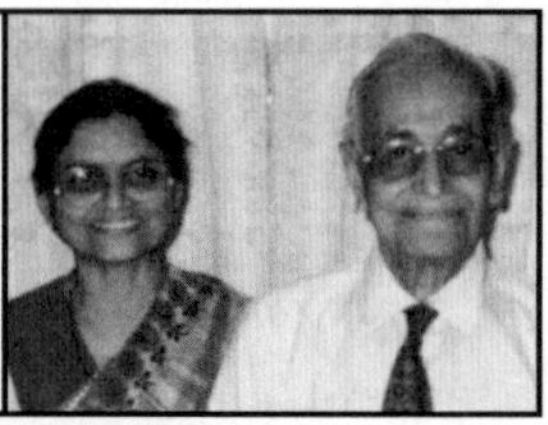

13. Dr.G.S.Ambardeckar, the world's oldest practicing anaesthetist, trained by Macintosh in Oxford, with Professor V. Divekar who developed four anaesthesia departments in Mumbai and was a founder of the South Asian Confederation of Anaesthetists (SACA).

have met several who were still gave anaesthetics until they were eighty such as George Ellis who organized the 1968 World Congress, Carlos Parsloe (76) and Zairo Vieira (85) from Brazil. Torsten Gordh, one of the founders of the WFSA, continued teaching until he was past eighty and attended the World Congress in Sydney in 1996 when he was nearly ninety. (Figure-Colour 24) They were all alert.

When should people retire from anaesthesia? I think that it is probably better for most people to retire from practice much earlier than those I have mentioned above. Many lose interest by the time they are sixty or sixty five. Maintaining an interest is easier if one is still actively teaching at that age. One should certainly not give anaesthetics if one is unsure of managing any complications proficiently. It is advisable to have some colleagues who will advise retirement if the anaesthetist does not realize that the time has come. The saddest situation is when someone cannot afford to retire for financial reasons.

Anaesthesia was the field in which I was beginning to specialise when I headed for Toronto Hospital for Sick Children where my future gradually evolved and became clearer. There was still much to learn and several hurdles to pass before I reached my destination. When one is young one has no idea where life will lead but I have never regretted the choice which I made.

Chapter 5

Toronto Hospital for Sick Children

The Hospital for Sick Children in Toronto was the "Mecca" of paediatric anaesthesia in Canada and one of the best in the world. The opportunity to work there sealed my future direction. I had enjoyed working with children in general practice and was also attracted to anaesthesia so paediatric anaesthesia was a logical combination.

The beginning was not all plain sailing. We were late due to our car breakdown on the Prairies in the small town of Herbert, Saskatchewan. Years later I found out that a Canadian classmate from university, Otto Goertz, practiced there. I began work in Toronto and stayed in the hospital while Janet and the twins stayed in a lakeside cottage in Parry Sound until we took over a townhouse in Don Mills from Eric Furman, one of the fellows who left early. It was 43 years until I met him again. I had to take a bus out to the transit bus and then change to the subway into Toronto. When I was doing cardiac anaesthesia it was winter. As I had to start early, before the local bus started, I had to walk out across the snow covered fields at 6 am to the transit bus — not something I enjoyed. It probably influenced my attitude to early starts for the rest of my life!

"Sick Kids", as it was affectionately called, was the biggest Children's hospital in North America having about 800 beds at that time. It was progressive, even having a day surgery facility in the Emergency Department with its own operating rooms. Patients waiting for tonsillectomy played in the playroom until it was time and then walked into the operating room — that was away ahead of practice in most places but thirty years later it became commonplace.

The work was interesting and varied. To concentrate on children for six months in a hospital that undertook so much highly specialised work was fantastic. The residents had long hours. Our roster involved three of us taking call every third night, or every second night if one of us was on holiday. This would be intolerable nowadays but it did mean that one gained considerable experience, particularly in neonatal anaesthesia.

The Chief of Anaesthesia at the time was Al Conn. He was a stimulating teacher who developed intensive care, at first in the Recovery Room, and went on to become Chief of that Unit. He was succeeded by David Steward.

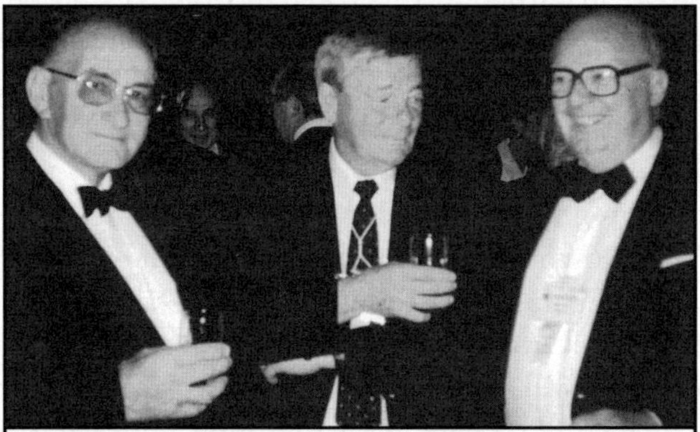

14. Al Conn (R) and his successor David Steward (L) who organized the first two world paediatric anaesthesia meetings at the World Congresses in Manila (1984) and Washington (1988) with Charlie Bryan (Respiratory neonatologist) in 1995.

Several things enhanced my time there. When Eric Furman left shortly after I arrived I had the opportunity to do some intensive care work. Intensive Care was embryonic at the time being housed in part of the recovery room. Al Conn, who was our chief, was a dynamic man who eventually moved into Intensive Care full time as it developed into an independent unit. My work in cardiac anaesthesia and using ventilators post-operatively in Vancouver stood me in good stead when they needed help in the unit. In 1963 prolonged intubation of the trachea was instituted in several centres, including Toronto, to maintain the airway and for use with ventilators when children couldn't breathe adequately themselves.

For the last two months of my time in Toronto I did cardiac anaesthesia working with Bill Mustard, who was the innovative, senior cardiac surgeon and Gordon Trusler who had also worked in the North West Territories before specializing. Mustard developed an operation that was used for many years to overcome the problem of transposition of the great vessels. This is an abnormality resulting from failure of the normal embryonic folding in the heart, which results in the two major blood vessels coming off the wrong sides of the heart. The aorta comes off the right ventricle and the pulmonary artery off the left side, resulting in little blood going through the lungs, where it picks up oxygen and therefore the babies are blue. His operation involved placing a baffle in across the atria and diverting more blood through the lungs. When he completed the first open heart operation it is said that he crawled out of the operating room to meet the press, making out that it was an exhausting experience. It may be a true story, because Mustard was known to arrive at a party on his hands and knees feigning exhaustion because the elevators were not working and he had to climb the stairs!

During this time I was asked to speak to the cardiologists on ventilation of children after heart surgery. I knew very little about it, but read up all the related information and prepared my talk. I had to present this to the Anaesthetic Department first and they were sufficiently impressed with it that Al Conn suggested that I should offer it for publication in the Canadian Anaesthetists Society Journal. After some extra work and the addition of some example cases it was submitted and accepted.

It covered many topics — the types of tubes used and the tests which were carried out to ensure that the poly vinyl chloride (PVC), from which they were made, was not toxic; humidification, because if the gas that was being delivered was not moistened in the nose the secretions would become sticky and the tube could easily become blocked, defeating the purpose of the tube with potentially dire consequences and, in addition the airways would become dry. (The nose normally moistens the air we breathe on its way to the lungs and this mechanism is bypassed by a nasotracheal tube.) Additional problems such as infection and the specific problem of pulmonary hypertension were considered. The latter results from excessive amounts of blood flowing through the lungs in some congenital heart conditions, like a hole between the ventricles in the heart (ventricular septal defect). This causes a rise in the pressure in the pulmonary arteries which, in the long term, can cause damage to the arterial wall and put a strain on the right ventricle which pumps blood through the lungs.

My paper, published in the Canadian Anesthetist's Society Journal in July 1966, *played a significant part in my future* because it helped me to obtain my first position a year later at the Royal Childrens Hospital in Melbourne as Medical Officer to Intensive Care. This was a new position created to help with cardiac surgical post operative care. Many years later, when I visited Toronto, I found out that this was the first paper published on this subject in children.

One of the ventilators which we used was made in Sweden by Engstom. It was a large and very cleverly designed machine. It was driven by a powerful piston pump with an eccentric cam so that it produced a sine wave gas flow. This was used to squeeze a bag in a bottle which contained the gas to be delivered to the patient. The clever part was that when the bag was completely emptied before the top of the sine wave there was a brief period where the pressure in the airways was maintained. When a gas or fluid is passed into tubes of different diameters it will take the line of least resistance — the bigger tube will receive the larger volume. One part of the lung will thus become overventilated and the other underventilated. By holding the pressure briefly on the bag a equilibration occurs so that more gas moves into the underventilated areas thus keeping the lung evenly ventilated. This "sigh"thus overcame the problem which occurred with many other ventilators of having uneven ventilation which necessitated an occasional overexpansion of the whole lung so that the underventilated areas would be reinflated.

Another idea I tried in Toronto, which was ahead of its time, was the use of an infra- red light to warm a baby during surgery. It was not a popular idea, especially with the surgeon who found the conditions too hot. However the concept came into use, especially during the period prior to surgery, years later when it became generally recognized that maintaining infants temperature was important during surgery.

I continued my research into post operative vomiting with a trial of a new drug RP9565. It proved to have similar efficacy to another similar, widely used drug, promethazine. The new drug was not marketed.

I also did a study comparing two anaesthetic agents in common use at the time, halothane and methoxyflurane, to see if one caused more post operative vomiting than the other. The study was done on children having squint surgery which usually has a high incidence of vomiting associated with it. I did the third last case on the morning that I left Toronto. A colleague agreed to finish it but when I returned to visit seven years later he told me that he had recently come across the papers but had never finished it — only two more cases were needed. It was an important lesson which I have told many people that came to work for a limited time — *finish a project before you leave because others cannot always be relied on to do it for you.*

I had many good teachers in that department, each contribbuting something useful to my knowledge. Code Smith, a rather reticent but very thoughtful man, was outstanding. He brought pharmacology (the study of drugs) to life by teaching us how the chemical structure related to drug action and how groups of drugs had similar action with variations which could be explained by variations in chemical structure. It made the whole subject logical and easier to learn. I used this approach with great success throughout my career when teaching pharmacology. He also was a very good practical teacher. One practical point he taught me was that the endotracheal tube can kink if placed in the corner of the mouth because it can bend over the mandible (he had x rays to demonstrate his point) but it will never kink in the midline because it passes over the tongue which is soft. He taught me neurosurgical anaesthesia, a field that has continued to interest me throughout my career.

Norman Parks was one of the older members of the department, a delightful man with whom to work. He had an amazing escape during the war, otherwise he would not have taught me. One afternoon he and some others decided to go to the pictures. When they reached the cinema there were hoards of school children with the same idea so they changed their mind. Half an hour later a bomb landed on the building killing most of the children.

Jack Whelan did most of the anaesthesia for the plastic surgeons while John Relton, an Englishman who impressed me with his open minded attitude to other ideas, did the major orthopaedic work.

Jeremy Sloan, a South African who was fastidious in his preparation, and later contributed for many years to the International Standards Association, Al Johnson and Sharon Nabeta taught me paediatric cardiac anaesthesia.

Malignant Hyperpyrexia was another very serious anaesthetic problem that I saw for the first time while I was in Toronto. It is a condition affecting calcium in the sarcolemic reticulum in muscle causing excessive contraction, heat production, a rapid rise in body temperature, an increased oxygen consumption and production of carbon dioxide due to the rising metabolic rate. If the process is not stopped temperatures are reached where the body can no longer compensate for adverse changes, and the patient dies. It is triggered by some drugs commonly used in anaesthesia, particularly succinyl choline and halothane. The first case was reported in Melbourne in 1962 by a group mainly comprising physicians. Jim Villiers, who later anaesthetised my wife, Janet, was the anaesthetist involved. The patient was a member of a family who had suffered several unexpected deaths during anaesthesia.

There was a probable case in Vancouver while I was there that baffled everyone because we did not know of the condition. She also died.

While in Toronto there was a thirteen-year-old girl who was to have a Harrington rod placed in her back to straighten her scoliosis (curvature of the spine). She indicated that she did not want the operation. One wonders whether she had a premonition because she developed hyperpyrexia (very high temperature) during her operation and died. The condition terrorized anaesthetists at the time because we did not know an effective treatment or how to recognize the condition beforehand. There is nothing worse for an anaesthetist than not to know how to treat a complication.

Fortunately, not too long afterwards, a drug called dantrolene became available which could reverse the changes. In the intravenous form it is a very expensive drug and is claimed by the manufacturer to be stable for only one year. This posed a problem to hospitals that were expected to have a stock on the very slim chance of a case arising as any unused stock should therefore be replaced annually. In Melbourne we overcame the problem by each hospital stocking a starter dose and then if they needed it, they called neighbouring hospitals for their supplies.

I have only had one case in a ten-year-old boy who developed unusual, intermittent E.C.G. changes. Then the patient required increased ventilation to keep the CO2 normal. The temperature was 36.0° C but very slowly rose to 36.8° C. The blood pressure started to drop and the pulse to rise despite being given extra fluids. Then I had to increase ventilation three times to maintain FE CO2 and finally the temperature rose to 37.3° C in a few minutes. A dose of dantrolene had a dramatic effect bring the temperature and pulse down and the blood pressure returned to normal. The operation was abandoned but was done the following week with non triggerring agents, propofol and remifentanil. On the first occasion I was using isoflurane as an inhalational agent which was the most likely trigger. Most reported cases have been triggered by suxamethonium and/or halothane. Probably the most important early sign is having to repeatedly increase ventilation to keep the CO2 at the same level.

Some pigs (Landrace) are also susceptible to the condition. Years later, Dilip Pawar from Delhi was working with me. He was doing a study on pharmacokinetics of suffentanil in piglets as they grew in early life. One of his piglets showed a progression from small E.C.G. irregularities on the first occasion to more marked dysrhythmias and a slight rise in temperature the second time until on the fourth occasion it had a definite temperature rise and developed ventricular fibrillation. This was offered for publication as a report showing the increasing susceptibility to MH with increasing age in the young (first three months — piglets develop more quickly than humans) but it was unfortunately rejected. It was a very interesting and important observation.

The pattern of the disease and its inherited characteristics were also worked out and eventually various tests became available to identify susceptible people, although some, such as the creatine phosphokinase level, was not entirely reliable and could only be used to provide an index of suspicion. Beverly Britt, who was senior resident while I was at "Sick Kids" devoted her life to research into this condition.

There were several other residents with me, including Art Scott who went on to become Professor of Anaesthesia in Toronto. Larry Griffin, a black American, was an amiable fellow whose company I enjoyed — he smoked a pipe and appeared in a very entertaining film that was made for the occasion of the retirement of the chief of Surgery. It was titled "The Last Public patient operated on at HSC". Griffin appeared in the operating room giving the anaesthetic with his pipe stuck through his cardboard mask. This film, produced by the residents, was my first foray into helping with film production. It was very entertaining. Twenty-three years later I met Larry Griffin at a reception at the Smithsonian Institute during the World Congress of Anaesthesia in Washington. It was an amazing coincidence to meet him again. He practiced in Nebraska — I never saw him again.

And so a stimulating and worthwhile six months came to an end. Al Conn, my boss, had been good to me and stimulated my interest further in paediatric anaesthesia.

We had decided that the time had come to move to Australia although I could probably have had jobs in both Vancouver and Toronto and years later I was approached by both places to return. I had applied to both the Royal Melbourne and the Royal Childrens Hospitals. I was told one would offer me a job but both did. I had a predicament, as I really wanted to go to the Childrens but Al Conn wisely advised me to do another year of adult anaesthesia as my training had already been predominantly in paediatric anaesthesia. I took his advice.

It had been a hard six months from a family point of view as I was on duty at night so frequently. Janet had an interesting, part time physiotherapy job and it was easy in the environment in Don Mills to find care for the twins when she worked. They all left in early December for Kenya to have time with my family while I finished off work, packed up — I had to buy three more trunks — and sold our furniture before leaving for Sweden and then a short holiday in Kenya before starting in Melbourne.

Chapter 6

Transit Through Sweden

During my stay in Toronto, Paul Herzog from Stockholm visited the hospital. He was the engineer from Engstrom, a company which made ventilators and anaesthetic equipment. He invited me to visit their factory in Stockholm on my way to Australia in early January 1966.

I left Toronto on a cold winter evening, not to return for 12 years. I had a few days in Britain and then went on to Stockholm to find it covered in snow with the harbour mostly frozen over. I had a busy few days there visiting the Engstom factory to learn more about their ventilators and exploring the city — the narrow streets of the old town, the Royal Palace which was very grand, the changing of the guard — not as well drilled as in London — the City Hall where the Nobel prizes are presented and other interesting sites.

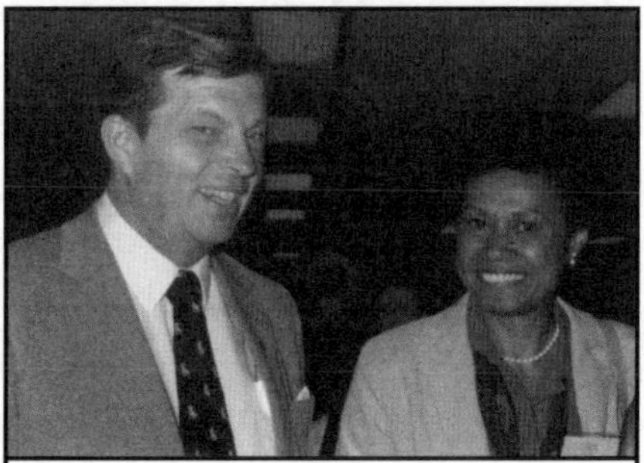

15. Olaf Norlander at the ASA Jubilee meeting in Sydney (1984) with Sereima Bale, senior anaesthetist in Fiji.

Medicine in Sweden is of a high standard and much research is done. At the Karolinska Sjukhuset I visited the Thoracic clinic headed by Olaf Norlander. He was an impressive man who later visited us in Australia. I also met Professor Crafoord, the cardiac surgeon who had developed the first mechanical ventilator in 1937.

Uppsala, north of Stockholm, has a very old university where Professor Martin Holmdahl was Professor of Anaesthesia. He is a wonderful, enthusiastic man with a very warm personality. It was a great privilege for a young man, who had not even finished his training, to meet these outstanding people. Little did I know that our paths were to cross many times. Only nine months later Martin Holmdahl came to Australia as the overseas visitor to the

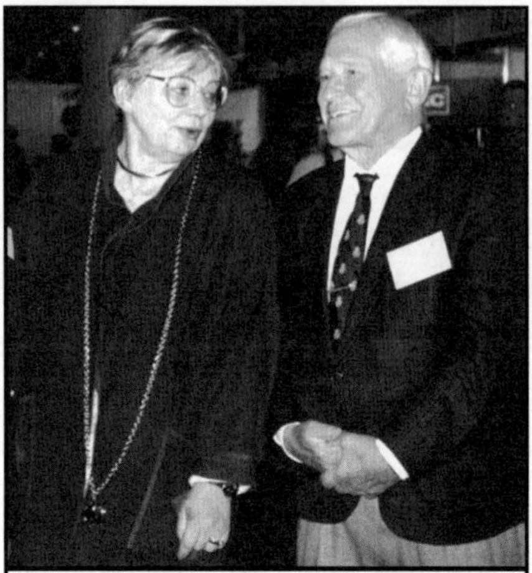
16. Martin Holmdahl, Professor of Anaesthesia and eventually Chancellor of Uppsala University with Barbro Ekstrom-Jodal, chief paediatric anaesthetist in Göteborg, Sweden taken in Stockholm, 1997.

Australian Society of Anaesthetists. In those days, at the end of the period when flying was less prevalent, the visitor had a very strenuous trip visiting all the major cities over a six week period. I think his was the last such trip. As I had met him previously I was sent to the airport to meet him. During his stay I took him to Healesville wildlife sanctuary with my wife, Janet, the day before our oldest son, Fraser, was born!

In 1977 I visited Martin Holmdahl again in Uppsala. In the interval he had been Dean of the Medical School and was now Chancellor of the University. He very kindly showed me some of the interesting parts of the University including the library. It happened that the day I visited was the 500th anniversary of the founding of the University and he invited me to attend a special ceremony in the cathedral in the evening, before I caught my train to Trondheim.

After my visit to Stockholm I traveled to Kenya for two weeks holiday with my family who all still lived there. Sadly my next visit was two years later to see my father on his deathbed at the end of a life devoted to helping others. We went on to Australia via Mauritius where we had nearly a day stopover. We had a warm welcome in Perth — it was about 40° C. We spent one day there before going on to Melbourne.

Years later when I reached positions of prominence I never forgot how important it is to take an interest and encourage young people. Meeting someone eminent in their field is a significant event in a young person's life. They are the future of the specialty. I have stood for hundreds of photographs with them. And as I grow older I appreciate having many of these people as friends.

Chapter 7

Registrar at the Royal Melbourne Hospital

Moving to Australia was a major change in my life — different climate, different lifestyle, sports which I enjoyed and different attitudes at work. And Janet was at home at last. I have never regretted making Australia my home. I was naturalized in 1973 when the Whitlam government decided that it was necessary for even British subjects to go through the process.

It was the first time that I started a job on time, at the beginning of February 1966. Previously, I had been delayed because I was travelling from somewhere else. My director was Russell Cole, an amiable man who played tennis into his eighties. It was basically a service department without much formal teaching or research. The standard of surgery at the hospital was very good and there was plenty interesting work. It was a major teaching hospital in the University of Melbourne. The department had great potential but the academic development did not come until some years later. Intensive Care was also just beginning to develop and could have been taken on by anesthesia as it was in some other hospitals but there was probably a lack of staff and no real interest so it was eventually developed later, by a physician.

The Royal Melbourne Hospital had been situated down town (in Lonsdale Street). When it moved the building was taken over by Queen Victoria Hospital, which was then a women's hospital run by women. The new hospital was built as the Second World War began and was used temporarily by the Americans during the War. It was a six hundred bed hospital with all the medical amenities for adults. The operating theatres were situated on the ninth floor so we had a wonderful view over the city and the dock area to Port Phillip Bay. I didn't enjoy it so much when I watched the sun rise, having worked all night.

My year at the Royal Melbourne Hospital was a mixed bag. I gained very useful clinical experience, became acquainted with some excellent anaesthetists from whom I learnt much but overall it was the least enjoyable year of my professional career. Many of the staff were sessional honorary anaesthetists such as Trevor (Peter) Currie, Noel Cass, Ian Philpott, David Komesaroff, Pat Mackay and Herb Newman; they were in private practice but came to the hospital for one or two sessions a week. I learnt from them all but unfortunately I did not have the chance to work with them as much as I would have liked because I had more experience than the other registrars and therefore was given more anaesthetics to do on my own.

I met Peter Currie on my first day there doing cardiac anaesthesia. I always appreciated his friendliness to me on that and many subsequent occasions. He had done some training in London and had a special interest in cardiac and thoracic anaesthesia and was an expert on endobronchial tubes used to isolate one lung during anaesthesia. He also spent four years on the Board of the Faculty of Anaesthetists. I remember him telling me about the sacrifice in time and income that was to someone in private practice. Later, he became an enthusiastic hiker in Nepal. It was sad that someone who obviously kept fit should suffer a prolonged stroke.

Noel Cass (20) was a wonderful Pharmacology teacher who not long afterwards became Dean of the Faculty of Anaesthetists and was Melbourne's most academic anaesthetist at the time. Later, we worked together at the Childrens Hospital for many years.

Patricia Mackay, an outstanding lady, became one of only two women Presidents of the Australian Society of Anaesthetists and years later successfully headed the Department at the Royal Melbourne Hospital. She managed all this while bringing up five children. She later became Chair of the state anaesthetic morbidity and mortality committee, a position she continued to fill long after she retired.

Ian Philpott was a brilliant young man who had an incredible bent for matters electrical and was an excellent anatomy tutor, although he taught by the method of low tolerance to unprepared students at his tutorials. He did not believe in spoon feeding his students.

David Komesarof had just completed his training and has been an enthusiastic developer of anaesthetic equipment, including a closed circuit machine for delivering the anaesthetic agent, methoxyflurane (Penthrane), years before closed circuit anaesthesia returned to common clinical practice for economic and anti-pollution reasons.

I worked with the most diverse group of registrars that one could put together. Bob Lunt was a gentlemanly, rather reticent Oxford graduate who had begun in General Practice. He eventually practiced in Maffra and Sale in eastern Victoria. Bill Stanisich was an enigmatic man who gave little information away even when questioned directly. He would not even divulge his phone number at the hospital! He was a competent copy artist but I did not discover that until after he retired! The third was Richie Gun, a man with a brilliant mind and a great jazz musician who could play trumpet and piano at the same time. He later went into Federal politics and held the South Australian seat of Kingston several times for the ALP. After some years in Parliament he went into occupational health. Joe Marich joined the registrar group later, when an extra position was created. Joe thrived on lifemanship, had the ability to make outrageous comments and not draw obvious offence. He was fun to work with. He also had a black belt in judo. We played squash together. I remember him saying to me just after our first game together, having won all five games, "Is that all you usually play?" It was his style of gamesmanship. I had my revenge later!

Being accustomed to having tutorials in the departments where I had worked previously I asked for these. Eventually some of the staff took some interest and gave us sporadic tuition. Although we were not taught much in the hospital we were allowed to attend basic science lectures at the University. We had some good lecturers. "Pansy" Wright, Professor of Physiology who later became Vice Chancellor of the University, gave lectures that were designed to make one think. People who had been undergraduates in Melbourne did not appreciate this talent. Another was Sydney Sunderland who was a world renowned neuro-anatomist.

The Royal Melbourne Hospital had many good surgeons. Several of the older ones had been to World War II. Some retired when I was there as, at that time, they could only hold a senior position there for twenty years. One of these was Reg Hooper, an outstanding neurosurgeon who continued to work for several years more at the Royal Childrens Hospital and then became a Radiologist.

Weary (Sir Edward) Dunlop was another surgeon with whom I worked while his regular anaesthetist, Gordon Stanton, was on long service leave. He must be one of the most famous Australians, having made a name for himself while a prisoner of war in Changi and on the Burma railway where many prisoners died from malnutrition and gastrointestinal and other diseases. Weary was a big man. He had been University boxing champion, a rugby player and also an outstanding athlete. He had stood up to the Japanese guards on behalf of his men championing their cause and earned a god-like reputation with them. While Weary had a great reputation he was not the only surgeon who had stood for the men, and operated under the most primitive and trying conditions. There were others, of whom Sir Albert Coates was also outstanding.

Weary was not easy to work with. He never arrived on time. His 8am list often did not begin until 10.30 because he stayed up late and fell asleep in his chair before eventually going to bed. He then operated all day which often meant, with the late start, working into the evening. Once I finished an oesophagectomy (removal of the oesophagus for cancer) at about 10pm and he wanted to proceed to the next patient who was to have the same operation. He was disappointed when I refused, something he was unaccustomed to. He was not a delicate operator but he managed to do major cancer surgery where he removed the tumour and then somehow put back together what had looked like an impossible disruption of the tissues.

About 8pm, if he was still operating, he would start to tell stories of his experiences. One, which illustrates why, even twenty years after the War, his men worshipped him. One of the old soldiers, who was up on a drunk driving charge, phoned him to ask if he would come to court to say a few words on his behalf. Weary went to court and told them how this man had given some of the best years of his youth to fight for his country and pleaded lenience for him for his misdemeanor. He got off with a warning.

In later life Weary's philanthropic and community work continued to make him much revered in the community. He came to be considered a gentle giant. There are at least three statues to him showing how the public perceived this great man. Probably the best is near the Art Gallery in Benalla where, in the rose garden, there is a wonderful sculpture of him, shirtless in the heat, helping a wounded or sick colleague. It is worth stopping to see it.

In January 1967 I was one of twenty who attended the Faculty of Anaesthetists course for candidates sitting the Primary examination. Many were from interstate, some of whom became lifelong friends. We had two outstanding Physiology lecturers, Professors Coates and Kenny. Their diagrams were clear and made it easy to remember the information.

In February I sat the Melbourne University Diploma of Anaesthetics primary examination as a trial run for the Faculty of Anaesthetists Fellowship Examinations. It was a unique experience. I was the only candidate and the second last ever to sit it. We completed the written examinations in Anatomy, Physiology and Pharmacology. I had to do the anatomy oral on a day that was the fifth in a row that the temperature was over 100°F (39°C). I wore a suit, as was customary, which was quite ridiculous in that weather. All did not go well and, although I may not have performed well, I was also prevented from having a chance to recover from a bad situation by being left stuck on a question which had no relevance to anaesthesia. I had defined that the slide showed columnar, ciliated respiratory epithelium but the examiner wanted me to mention basement membrane as well. It was an example of very poor examining in days when assessment was not necessarily related to relevance.

We had visitors the week before the other two orals. I had been told that they usually did them one after the other so when

I read that Physiology was 2.30 on Friday I only read the time for Pharmacology — 3pm. On the Monday evening after my friends had left I decided to check the exam times. To my horror I discovered that Pharmacology was to have been at 3pm that day, Monday, and not following Physiology on Friday! I had a rather sleepless night before going to see Professor Rand in Pharmacology the next day. He said they had concluded that I had made that mistake and I was just to do it after Physiology on Friday. I eventually did very well in that exam but not well enough for the Anatomists to be persuaded to pass me. So I failed the only important exam in my life.

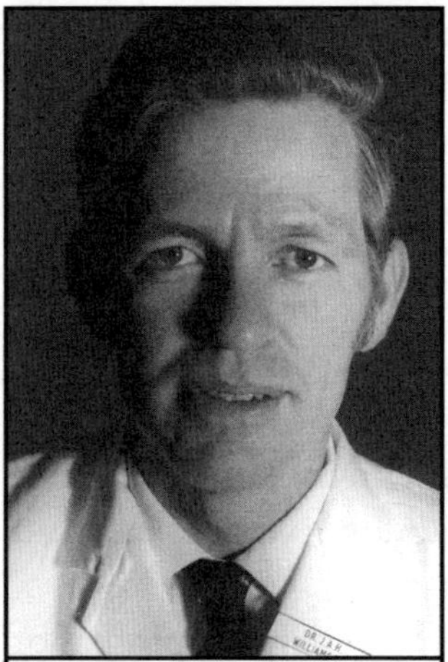

17. John Williamson.

The Diploma was only awarded once more, to John Williamson, a couple of years later. He went on to have a distinguished career in anaesthesia, hyperbaric medicine, and electrical standards in the operating theatre. He was awarded a Member of the Order of Australia (AM).

When I became Director of Anaesthesia at the Royal Childrens Hospital I automatically became an examiner in the final DA. I was never required as there were no candidates. Years later, as a member of the Standing Committee on Anaesthetics at the University I proposed that since nobody had sat the exam for over twenty years it should be taken off the statutes and discontinued. And so it disappeared.

The next month I sat the Faculty of Anaesthetists Primary Examination which, for the second last time, included anatomy. In those days if candidates passed two subjects well and failed the third they could carry the two to the next examination and only repeat the one that they had failed. March 1967 was not a happy occasion for many. Fifty six candidates sat and only ten passed, seven of whom were carrying two subjects. Only three passed all subjects and one of these, who was later to become one of Australia's leading anaesthetists, had sat once before. Peter Thompson won the prize so I obviously came second as only two of us were elligible. Seven others passed two subjects. Having been training for longer than most registrars by then I went on and sat the final exam in September of the same year.

I had been training long enough — four years — which was longer than most people at the time. I had been to see Dr McClelland, the Director at the Childrens Hospital, after I arrived in Melbourne to let her know I was still interested in working there. A new position was advertised at the Royal Childrens Hospital as Medical Officer in Intensive Care. I was encouraged to apply. I was interviewed separately by the Medical Director, L.E.G. Sloan and the cardiologist, Alec Venables. This seemed strange at the time but it was aimed to fill this position with someone who could help with cardiac postoperative care in which I had experience and had published the paper on "Post-operative ventilation in children following cardiac surgery". I was given the position despite not yet having my fellowship.

My final episode at the Royal Melbourne was to attend a dinner for incoming and leaving registrars. I was violently sick the next day — maybe I received my just deserts for being such a stirrer!

I enjoyed living in Melbourne. We had a good year during which Fraser, our oldest son, was born. Our twins went to kindergarten. I played hockey for Kew when I could. We had a trip by car to Sydney and Canberra in August and had seen some of the country.

The year of transition to Australia ended. I had gained some very good clinical experience and prepared for my Primary examinations. I was then about to start the major phase of my working life in paediatric anaesthesia at the Royal Children's Hospital. I did not know that I would still be there 37 years later!

Royal Childrens Hospital

Chapter 8
The Royal Children's Hospital

The Melbourne Childrens Hospital was founded in 1870 by a Mrs. Anderson in a house in Spring Street. It grew and a much bigger hospital was needed. The now "old" hospital was built in distinctive red brick in Pelham Street, Carlton. I had visited it in 1961 when I was putting out feelers for the future. By the time I eventually came to Melbourne it had moved again to a magnificent new site on the corner of Royal Park with views on to it on two sides. This was obtained due to the persuasive powers of Dame Elizabeth Murdoch, President of the Committee of Management, over the dogged Premier, Sir Henry Bolte.

Dame Elizabeth retained her interest in the hospital and in her nineties still attended functions there. Her husband, Keith Murdoch, started the Herald and Weekly Times and his son, Rupert has gone on to become one of the media barons of the world. Her generosity enabled David Danks to set up the Murdoch Institute for Research into Birth Defects at the hospital, now one of the leading medical research institutes in Australia. It was separate from the Royal Childrens Hospital Research Foundation which promoted and funded research within the hospital.

The Queen opened the new ten storey building and granted permission to call it the Royal Childrens Hospital in1963. It is now recognized as one of the great childrens hospitals in the world. People come there to train from everywhere — at one stage 25% of all foreign doctors coming to Australia for postgraduate training worked there. In the Anaesthetic Department alone people from about forty countries have come for post graduate training.

It was one of the biggest hospitals for children, having 499 beds when it opened. The number of beds has decreased to about 320 by 2000. This was due to the trend towards of shorter stay in hospital and the use of Day Surgery. It is also one of the childrens hospitals which covers all specialties and deals with simple to the most complex problems making it an excellent place to train.

The hospital was built with an H shape with the wards and operating theatres on the side facing the park and the administration, laboratories and other departments on the street side facing Flemington Road. The nurses home was a seven storey building to the south-east surrounded by car parks and nicely laid out gardens.

As the years passed more room was needed. First, in 1973-4, an extra building was put up in the north west corner. An additional fourth floor was added to it so that plastic surgery could move from the second floor to make room for an intensive care unit adjacent to the operating theatres. Nurses stopped living in the nurses home in the 1970s and so it was used for other purposes such as the School of Nursing. When the latter closed other departments moved into it.

A major expansion was needed and a fund raising program was instituted in the late 1980s. Unfortunately the economic situation deteriorated and less money was raised than needed. The government was not forthcoming with any funds to support the $25 million project. It was still regarded as a wealthy hospital which was a myth based on the fact that the community contributed to a successful Easter appeal, much of which was used for research, to buy equipment to improve patient care and to provide some scholarships to allowing promising young people to gain extra training (a good investment for the future). For many years it seemed that our annual grant was reduced because of this. The building went ahead in two parts — a much needed expansion of the operating theatres and anaesthetic department and the front building on the street side which included a floor for Day Surgery — an inconvenient location.

Car parking seems to be an ever increasing problem with all hospitals. The hospital was surrounded by beautiful gardens and had two tennis and two squash courts. In 1977 a floor was built over part of the car park and later another floor was built on top of that. Then the gardens were encroached upon and much of them eventually disappeared. The final demise of "civilization" at the hospital came the day the fences round the tennis courts were pulled down, car access was made and the courts were marked out as a car park! This was done in winter when people were not playing but prior to that they were well used , particularly in summer, some staff even playing before work.

I began work in the new position of Medical Officer to the Intensive Care Unit on March 1st 1967. While the position was created to help with cardiac anaesthesia and post-operative care I was also involved in both anaesthesia and intensive care.

My salary was $5000 a year plus accommodation. There was no overtime or on call payments then. We were provided with a house across the road from the hospital which was convenient as I was frequently on call. This meant leaving Janet's family home in Kew, in part of which we had been living, and moving to the back of 22 Gatehouse Street, Parkville. This was an unusual arrangement where we had a double storey part at the back part of the house.

There were two bachelor rooms on the single storey front which had access to their bathroom and kitchenette through our stair well. The nature of our charming neighbours is evident from the story about Maryann, one of our 4 1/2 year old twins who was very observant, asking the lady who cleaned the bachelor rooms, " How many wives can a man have?" about one and " Where does his wife sleep?" about the other who only had a single bed. These were in the days when the nurses lived in across the road in the Nurses Home and were strictly policed about being in at certain times. Many things have changed over the years! One day Maryann came in and told Janet that there was a dead nun in the park behind the house. Actually it was an old drunk covered in a black coat having a sleep!

Later in the year we moved up to a separate house at 64 Gatehouse Street.

In those days there were separate dining rooms for doctors, nurses and other staff. We had waitress service, table clothes and silver cutlery! Another privilege was that our families could come to lunch on Sundays when we were on duty. How it all changed over the years. The first change came with equal pay for women in the 1970s because they had to reduce the number of waitresses. Gradually the other refinements disappeared and by 1983, when there was an economic downturn and money was short, the doctors' and nurses' dining rooms disappeared altogether and everybody shared one large self service room. The valuable asset of having somewhere doctors from all departments could meet and discuss clinical problems and cases over lunch was gone. Increasing isolation of departments developed and much of the old cohesive medical staff spirit was lost. This is one of the unfortunate consequences of so called progress!

The next few years were full of interest with several significant developments occurring at the hospital which will be discussed in following chapters. In addition, I became involved in teaching and research.

Twice during this period I was asked to consider other positions at Monash University and back in Vancouver but I decided that the volume of work and opportunities were greater where I was and I was becoming involved with some exciting research so I stayed on at R.C.H. I never imagined what would happen and that I would still be there 37 years later having become a leader in the field and created what amounted to a worldwide network of paediatric anaesthetists whom we had trained.

The year, 1967, was a very busy as I was studying until October for my final post graduate examinations (FFARACS). This and frequent (one in three) call meant that I did not have as much time with the children as I would have liked. I often felt that I missed a lot of my son, Fraser's first year.

Chapter 9
Early Years at the RCH

My time at the Royal Childrens Hospital can be divided into several phases. The early years when I was Medical Officer in Intensive Care and a Fellow in ICU. I gained valuable experience and became established. During this period I was involved in intensive care, cardiac anaesthesia , perfusion and post operative care, had my initial involvement in burns as well as doing other anaesthesia. I started the department teaching programs and monthly scientific meetings.

During the next phase from 1970-74 I became heavily involved in research and teaching outside the hospital. Then, in 1974, I became Director of the Department (26 years) and of Theatre services (20 years). I began to have administrative responsibilities but continued teaching and research. I always did at least half my time giving anaesthetics in theatre.

After 1980 changes began to occur in the hospital and departments were grouped into divisions for administrative purposes. I became chairman and then Director of our Division of Specialist Services for 17 years so was increasingly involved in administration. My research gradually decreased because of pressure of time but I maintained my interest in teaching and was involved nationally and increasingly internationally.

By the 1990s our work load increased with little increase in staff so life became generally busier. Financial constraints in the hospital added to our difficulties and the government funding system changed to our disadvantage. The government also changed the structures of our Committee, and then Board, of Management. All these changes impacted on our lives. In addition I was involved in preparing the scientific program for the 1996 World Congress of Anaesthesia so it was a very busy time.

When I began at the Royal Childrens Hospital (RCH) our Director, Greta McClelland had restricted the anaesthetics which she did so John Stocks, who was her deputy, Helene Wood and

I constituted the core of the department doing all the supervisory call. We had visiting sessional anaesthetists.

I must have arrived with some sort of reputation. I soon had to anaesthetise for " the Vicar", as our austere, talented, plastic surgeon, Alan Wakefield, was known. He had a low tolerance of any anaesthetist apart from his regular one, John Tucker, or the Director. He seemed to accept me immediately on our first meeting, which was fortunate. No one from Melbourne had ever worked at the prestigious Hospital for Sick Children in Toronto before. Maybe that cast a protective spell for me!

I gained great experience, especially in neonatal anaesthesia, because three of us were involved in nearly all the complex neonatal anaesthetics for a population of about four million. I would have gained as much experience in a year as would take four or five years to gain now because the cases at RCH are shared between so many and there is a second centre doing some of the babies.

We did about 6000 anaesthetics each year then. By 2000 we were doing 16,000. The work in Intensive Care was sporadic with one to six patients looked after in half of the Recovery room by Sister Betty Jaffrey and a small band of nurses including Doris Flett and Louise Blewett, under our supervision. Equipment was scarce and monitoring fairly simple. We had to do our own blood gas analysis by the rather tedious triple pH method devised by Siggaard Andersen, so we became very good at clinical assessment. There was only one ECG monitor for ICU and the other theatres, apart from one in the cardiac theatre. We relied heavily on the stethoscope for in-theatre monitoring. It is amazing how much information can be derived from this simple device. We could detect changes in heart rate, rhythm, and heart sounds as well as the patients breathing. When the blood volume is relatively low following haemorrhage or dehydration less blood is pumped with each beat and the sounds, which are produced by the heart valves closing, become softer. These changes provide a good indication of changes in cardiac output (the amount of blood the heart is pumping each minute) to the trained ear.

I became involved in cardiac anaesthesia and perfusion (running the heart lung machine with the nurse technician, Kevin Curtis) as I had been employed to help improve the cardiac surgical results.

The following year my appointment was Uncle Bobs Fellow in ICU. The Uncle Bobs Club had began with three men in a pub agreeing to put in a shilling (a bob) a week for the hospital's Good Friday appeal. It grew into a major fund raising group. The Good Friday appeal has been a wonderful source of revenue for research and special projects in the hospital for many years. They provided funds to pay me as an Uncle Bobs Fellow for the next two years and then I was given a regular staff anaesthetist appointment. Usually such fellowships were given to promising young doctors to go overseas for further training.

I was lucky in 1968 to be working with Greta McClelland and John Stocks, who agreed to my next proposal that we should establish a half day when the registrars (Trainees) would be free to attend teaching sessions. The operating sessions would be covered by visiting anaesthetists, more of whom would be employed that afternoon. We had had such an arrangement in Vancouver, but no formal teaching was taking place in any hospital in Melbourne at the time except for some early morning pre-exam tutorials run by Max Griffiths at the Alfred Hospital.

The following year I added a departmental meeting one evening a month where most of the staff and trainees gave one 20 minute paper each year. These still continue. There was violent objection by some of the staff against participation but in the end I prevailed and some of them became good speakers. The presentations were aimed to provide the speakers with experience in researching, synthesising and then presenting an allocated topic. The department had become the leading formal teaching department in Victoria.

On the suggestion of Noel Cass, then Dean of the Faculty of Anaesthetists, I was invited by the New Zealand Post Graduate Medical Federation to go on lecture tour of New Zealand. I had just written a paper on the basic principles of drug interactions, a topic which was just beginning to be recognised as a problem at the time. I also lectured on a variety of Paediatric anaesthesia topics. It was a great experience and quite challenging as my audiences often included non anaesthetists. I was in Christchurch on the day when the first men landed on the moon. That was my first overseas teaching trip.

In November 1969 I drove with John Stocks and Brian McKie to Brisbane for the Australian Society of Anaesthetists (ASA) meeting. It was my first trip across the open spaces of inland New South Wales with wheat fields, some of which were contaminated with the colourful blue Patterson's Curse, the grain silos, the huge radio telescope at Parkes and many other features of interest.

It was an interesting meeting in a number of ways. I spoke for the first time on the Refresher Course. At the business meeting the treasurer recommended that the subscription for the next year should be raised to $28. I made a counterproposal that it be $30 so that it could remain the same for two years. Surprisingly, my motion was passed! On Tuesday afternoon the meeting stopped for ten minutes while a television set was brought in so we could watch the running of the Melbourne Cup, the great horse race always run on the first Tuesday in November and for which there is a holiday in Melbourne. I think our American guest speaker, Manny Papper from the USA, was rather stunned by this apparently frivolous behaviour but was compensated by drawing a ticket for the horse which ran second!

John lent me his car to visit Jack McGovern, formerly our neighbour in Yellowknife , who lived at the Gold Coast. I told him how I had sat beside a mining engineer from Weipa in north Queensland at my brother in law, Campbell's wedding. He had been a friend of Murray Pickard, the manager of Giant Mine in Yellowknife, when they were in the Air Force during the War. " Was his name Peter Macleod?" Jack asked because Murray Pickard had told him when he left Giant Mine that if he wanted a job in mining in Australia he just had to find Peter Macleod and tell him Murray Pickard recommended him. An amazing coincidence but the story went on. Twenty five years later I told Campbell this story. He then told me that Peter had died the previous year but his wife was coming to dinner the next night.

Eventually I met her and she told me how these two friends had bumped into each other in Adelaide airport not having seen each other for forty years.

Much of interest happened in 1970. It was the hospital's Centenary and various scientific meetings were held. At the Paediatric one Professor Mary Ellen Avery from Montreal told us how adding positive pressure to the airways of babies with hyaline membrane disease could save their lives. The condition is due to a lack of surfactant which is a substance that prevents the alveoli in the lungs from collapsing when the baby breathes out. In very premature infants there is a lack of surfactant and the lungs develop small areas of collapse and, in severe cases as these increased, the babies died. By putting positive pressure on the airways they were kept open and oxygen could reach the lungs. The idea was simple, but with the introduction of positive pressure ventilation of the lungs in patients who could not breathe adequately, there was concern that an increase in pressure in the chest (mean intrathoracic pressure) would reduce the blood flow back to the heart with detrimental effects on the patient. When PEEP was applied it was found that the body compensated by raising the venous pressure so that the resistance to flow caused by increased intrathoracic pressure was overcome and the normal amount of blood flow reached the heart. The raised venous pressure however, increased the amount of fluid in the tissues causing oedema, and extra fluid had to be given to compensate for this. Another problem arose when PEEP was added which we had not recognized at first. The amount of oxygen reaching the lungs suddenly increased causing toxic damage to the lungs. It was also recognized that high oxygen levels cause damage to the eyes so that the concentration of oxygen administered has to be closely monitored. This development changed the outlook for small premature babies so that they could now survive at a much earlier stage of development. But there was the price to pay of increased incidence of neurological damage in very small babies. This has decreased with improved management. The work of Neonatologists increased greatly with this development.

The next exciting development was the technique of deep

hypothermia, which allowed the cardiac surgeons to perform corrective surgery in babies less than 10 kg, something which they had not been able to do before. We also saw a new problem — an increase in the accidental overdosage with antidepressant drugs. These will be discussed in later chapters.

The Third Asian Australasian Congress of Anaesthesiology was held in Canberra in September 1970. I drove there with Brian McKie and a New Zealand visitor from Gisborne in my VW beetle. The trip was memorable because we had two broken windscreens on the one day. In Victoria it cost $16 to replace but over the border in New South Wales it was $25!

This congress was my introduction to international anaesthesia as I met people from countries as diverse as Japan and Nigeria with whom I am still in contact. Another impressive feature was having the composer, Peter Sculthorpe, present to speak about a piece of his music which was played at the opening ceremony.

The paper which gained most attention was one given to fill in for an absent speaker by Pradit Chareonthaitawe from Thailand on " anaesthetising the King's white elephant." All white elephants belong to the king. This one needed an operation on its eye. He gave some 2 1/2 % thiopentone to the elephant without success. He told the king he was not happy doing something when he had no experience. He was told to practise on some ordinary elephants. Eventually he succeeded in getting it to sleep with a large dose of 5% thiopentone. The problem then was how to keep it unconscious. He could not use a face mask and he did not have a large enough endotracheal tube nor would he have been able to insert one. Eventually he found that by holding a mask over the end of the elephant's trunk and giving 4% halothane he could maintain the anaesthetic for the required 1 1/2 hours. Questions about what would he have done if the elephant had had a cardiac arrest caused much hilarity.

Dr McClelland retired in March 1970 and John Stocks became Director. Helene Wood and I both applied for the deputy position. It was suggested that one of us could be deputy in anaesthesia and the other deputy in intensive care. We both wanted anaesthesia. I knew that John supported Helene but I was still disappointed when I did not get the position as I had developed the best educational program in Melbourne in the department. It was a humbling experience but it taught me one of the best lessons I ever learnt — *out of apparently bad situations some good usually comes*. Soon after this disappointment I was approached to become the first state Education Officer for the Faculty of Anaesthetists. Not having other administrative responsibilities gave me time to do this and pursue my research interests. These expanded during the next few years with a number of collaborative projects outside the hospital. I also became involved with the organization of the scientific program for the Australian Society of Anaesthetists annual meeting. All these topics will be discussed in later chapters.

In 1971 I had a visit from Harold Kester, one of my teachers in Vancouver, who tried to persuade me to return. I was later invited to visit and consider applying for the Chief of Anaesthesia position at the Vancouver Childrens Hospital. It was a miserable week in March when I went to look over the situation. My progressive ideas to develop the then little hospital on 59th Street fell on deaf ears, if they were heard at all. They were good and practical but probably too radical. I was involved at the time in several interesting research projects including work at Monash University so I decided to stay in Melbourne. In the long run it turned out to have been a good decision. A spin off, in an effort to dissuade me from taking up a position that I was offered in Vancouver, was that my title was changed to specialist anaesthetist/ perfusionist which better recognized what I was doing, although I continued to be involved in intensive care until 1974.

The Australian Society of Anaesthetists launched a new journal, Anaesthesia and Intensive Care, in 1972. I was asked to join the Editorial Board. My major contribution to it was to sub edit the first three symposia issues. I chose Paediatric Anaesthesia, Education in Anaesthesia and Toxicology as the topics. Later, when we discussed a new cover for the journal I suggested the use of photographs of items in the Geoffrey Kaye anaesthetic museum as a way of bringing this valuable collection to the wider anaesthetic community. This has now been done for about 20 years. Rod Westhorpe and Christine Ball have written short, informative commentaries on each item bringing the interesting history of anaesthesia to the readers. I did not expect to remain on the Board for 23 years but when I suggested withdrawing the Editor kept persuading me to stay on to provide advice and ideas. After finally retiring in 1995 I was awarded the Ben Barry medal. He was the first Editor and a medal was stuck in his honour to be given to those who had given outstanding service to the journal.

Helene Wood had meantime decided to get married in Sydney in 1975. John Stocks died in March 1974 and I succeeded him as Director of the department in July 1974. The freedom I had during the previous few years had allowed me to accomplish much in research and teaching that laid the foundations for the future.

Chapter 10

Dr Margaret McCelland and Trilene

Dr. Margaret McClelland, commonly called Gretta by her friends, was a wonderful woman. She was the first Director of Anaesthesia at the Royal Childrens Hospital, appointed half time in 1952 and full time in 1956. We became lifelong friends and I delivered the eulogy at her funeral.

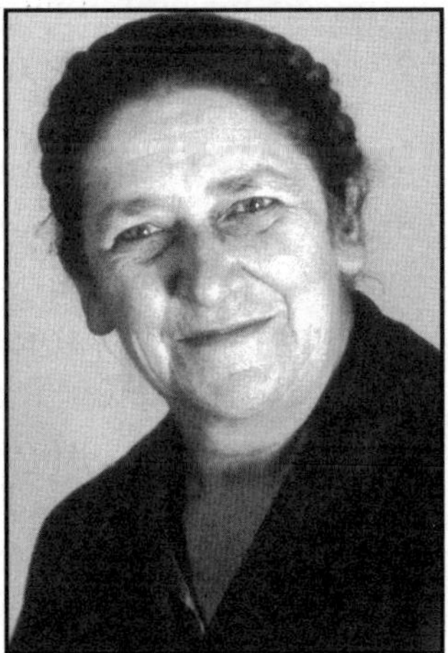

18. Dr Margaret (Gretta) McClelland

She was born in a little country town called Berriwillock, out on the flat open plains in North Western Victoria. The main street is called McClelland Street. Her father was the Country Party member in the Federal Government for that constituency for some years. She was educated at Presbyterian Ladies College, one of the leading schools in Melbourne where she became head girl. She was a keen hockey player. I remember her telling me about her trip to Perth by train to play intervarsity hockey and how they had practiced on the station platforms when they stopped. She studied medicine at Melbourne University, graduated in 1931 and became a resident at the Queen Victoria Hospital, which was run by women for women in those days. For the next two years she was Medical Superintendent — the staff was small. In 1936 she moved to Sydney where she worked at the Coast Hospital (now Prince Henry's).It was not a busy job and the hospital had a golf course next to it. On quiet afternoons she played golf. This was long before beepers and mobile telephones so they arranged with the nurses that if she was needed urgently the nurses would hang a sheet over the balcony which could be seen from the golf course! For two years she was medical director before she went to London where she took up anaesthetics at the Central Middlesex Hospital. She was there throughout the War, at times alternating between being on night duty for anaesthetics with fire watching during the air raids.

In 1946 she returned to Australia as an anaesthetist with great skill with children and in thoracic anaesthesia . Soon she was in demand by the surgeons. She was the first person in Australia to use the new muscle relaxant drug, tubocurarine, in children to paralyse them for surgery.

In 1952 she was persuaded to become the first Director of Anaesthesia, half time, at the Childrens Hospital. She was already distressed by children crying before surgery and being in pain postoperatively. She was determined to improve the situation.

It was a paid position. Paying consultants to work at the hospital was the idea of Vernon Collins, who was Medical Superintendent and later became the first Professor of Paediatrics at Melbourne University. He was an outstanding man who realized that parents of young children did not have much money and therefore it would be difficult for doctors to specialize in paediatric work because they would not earn enough. He thus insisted on the staff being paid at a time when most doctors worked part time in public hospitals on an honorary basis. It was his foresight that led to many outstanding people specializing in various fields solely caring for children. The consequence of this was that strong teaching, training and research developed in the hospital and it became a place of international repute.

In 1956 Dr McClelland became full time director. She was assisted by Ian Mcdonald, who was the first registrar with anaesthetic duties in1953. He went overseas for further training in Oxford. On his return he continued as a sessional anaesthetist until he retired in1988.

Greta was a strong personality but achieved her objectives by rational discussion. She was a kind person with wide interests. As well as carrying a big clinical load she became involved in research in the early days of cardiac surgery. She developed anaesthesia and the use of cooling the patients (hypothermia) for open heart surgery, helped Harry Adams at CIG to develop appropriate equipment for paediatric anaesthesia (Figure — Colour 12) and facilitated the early development of intensive care. She was the first woman president of the Australian Society of Anaesthetists and became an examiner when the Faculty of Anaesthetists was founded in the Royal Australasian College of Surgeons in 1952. Her outstanding contributions were recognized with the award of the Orton Medal by the Faculty of Anaesthetists and by being made an Officer of the British Empire (OBE).

She retired in 1970. Unfortunately she broke her pelvis the week before. She then had problems which eventually led to her being unable to walk which was sad as she had developed an interest in geology which she wanted to pursue in retirement. She spent her last years rather frustrated in a nursing home until her death in 1990. She had been a great leader in the early development of paediatric anaesthesia and a good friend to many.

She had achieved what she set out to do — to improve the care of children when they needed anaesthesia and she had established a good department. As well as the above achievements she contributed the following important investigative work on *trichlorethylene* (Trilene) during the war in London.

St Bartholomew's Hospital (Bart's) is the oldest in London. In 1941 Trilene was re-introduced there as an anaesthetic agent by Langton Hewer. There had been an isolated report of three hundred cases from the United States in 1934. Its advantages were that it was a good analgesic (pain reliever), and it was not flammable like ether and cyclopropane, the two commonly used anaesthetic agents at that time, and so was safely transportable. It was used at Central Middlesex Hospital where curious cases appeared with blisters on the face over the distribution of the trigeminal nerve. Dr McClelland made the astute observation that all the cases were anaesthetised in one of the two operating theatres. What was the difference? The theatre in question had a soda lime canister on the anaesthetic machine and the other did not.

Soda lime is used in the anaesthetic circuit carrying the gases to remove the carbon dioxide breathed out by the patient. In this way much lower flows of the gas mixture — usually nitrous oxide, a weak anaesthetic gas, and oxygen which is essential for survival, could be used. The Trilene vapour is picked up by the gas passing through the bottle over the liquid Trilene. Sodalime nowadays is usually a mixture of sodium hydroxide and calcium or barium hydroxide. These react less vigorously with the carbon dioxide than the soda lime in the 1940s which contained some potassium hydroxide. The latter produced considerable heat when the reaction took place.

The next step in the detective work which she organised was to have the contents of the canister analysed. The chemists found phosgene and dichloracetylene, both of which are toxic. These were formed when Trilene was heated. One interesting aspect was that sometimes it was the following patients who were not having Trilene who developed the symptoms. This resulted from the remaining Trilene continuing to react with the soda lime in the canister after the conclusion of the previous anaesthetic. The cause of the problem had been found but then some dirty work occurred. She told someone who had a similar case what they had found and he wrote up the information and had it published before Dr McClelland and her colleagues had their original report published. The consolation is that her story is well known and the other author, who pirated her work, is long forgotten!

Trilene was an interesting inhalational anaesthetic. The same chemical is also used in the dry cleaning industry. It was cheap to make and therefore ideal for the Third World. It could be used in a draw over system or as a supplement to thiopentone — muscle relaxant anaesthesia instead of nitrous oxide. I sometimes used it in this way for tonsillectomy. On one occasion after a tonsillectomy, I reversed the paralysis, took the endotracheal tube out and the child opened her eyes and said "Thank you". It has very good pain relieving properties which last into the period following recovery of consciousness, hence the child could wake up without pain. Another feature was that only low concentrations were needed for anaesthesia (MAC 0.17 %). This is the amount which one can just smell.

It had another feature which made it different to all other inhalation anaesthetics (ones which are breathed). It increases muscle tone, thought to be due to activating muscle spindles. When patients breathed spontaneously they tended to breathe more rapidly and shallow. Sometimes small doses of pethidine were used, as it is a respiratory depressant, to slow breathing. Another trick was to use very small doses of a muscle relaxant called gallamine, which helped, probably by reducing the muscle spindle activity. I probably did the last studies on this drug . I demonstrated that rather than decreasing the dose of non depolarizing muscle relaxant needed, as happens when other inhalational anaesthetics are used, Trilene often increases the requirement. My interpretation of the rapid breathing is that by increasing muscle spindle tone it reduces the chest wall compliance and the chest wall becomes stiffer. This is similar to what happens in patients with pulmonary fibrosis (stiff lungs). The bigger the breath they take the more energy they use. The body is very clever at making adjustments to make it work most efficiently. It reduces the volume of each breathe but compensates by increasing the rate of breathing so that the amount of gas reaching the lungs for gas exchange is achieved with the least effort or work of breathing. I was able to do these studies because we had computer controlled electromyography (EMG) which I will discuss more later. It measures the degree of muscle paralysis.

Trilene is now almost unavailable as an anaesthetic agent because it was not profitable for the company manufacturing it. It has been widely used to provide analgesia (pain relief) in labour and in ambulances in South Australia. It is now just another anaesthetic of only historical interest. It was a cheap, potent and useful agent when used intelligently.

Chapter 11
John Stocks and Other Colleagues

Many of those with whom we work in the earlier part of our lives develop some special significance to us as teachers, colleagues or contemporaries, who have become friends as we went through the developmental years together. I would like to introduce you to some of them.

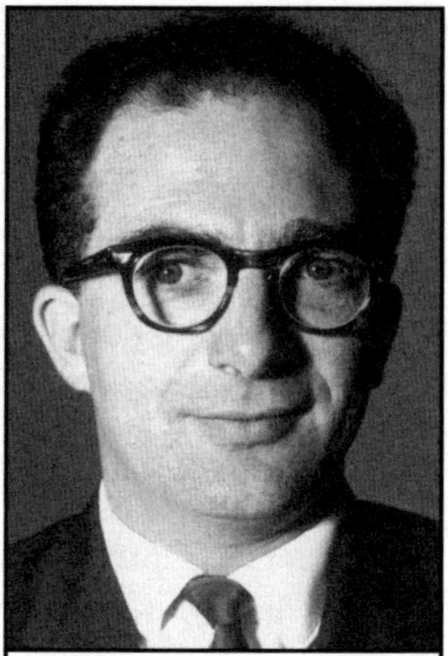
19. John Stocks.

John Stocks came from Sydney to train in anaesthesia. He became assistant, then Deputy to Dr. McClelland and eventually became Director of Intensive Care in 1969 and succeeded her as Director of Anaesthesia as well, in 1970. John was a diligent, dedicated, quiet man who devoted himself to the care of his patients and his family. Those who worked with him knew little of his past until his funeral. John originally came from Young in southern New South Wales. He graduated from Sydney University. He was University and New South Wales country chess champion. He was a small man who did not play sport but was a fanatical Australian Rules football (Carlton) and cricket fan.

John was a quiet, rather introspective person who was quite brilliant. He smoked endlessly. He would teach on request and offer valuable information if asked but he did not readily impart information spontaneously. I always felt it was a pity that he did not pass on his considerable knowledge more freely.

He made several important contributions. He developed Intensive Care at the hospital, using prolonged nasotracheal intubation and ventilation. His early paper with Ian McDonald was one of the first on this technique (1965). He also played an important part in paediatric anaesthesia carrying much of the clinical load of difficult cases. His "Notes on Paediatric

Anaesthesia" were read across the country and even overseas. They filled a gap because there was a lack of books on the subject. His last paper on "Respiratory Failure in Infants" became a classic on the subject.

In 1973 he suggested that the paediatric anaesthetists, of whom there were only about a dozen in Australia at the time, should form a section in the Australian Paediatric Association to which both paediatricians and paediatric surgeons belonged. He felt we should have a closer association with them. He gained support from his colleagues out of loyalty to him and we met in Canberra to discuss the idea once before he died, but it never came to fruition. This was probably fortunate because it would have created divided loyalties for paediatric anaesthetists. Instead we held our own meetings.

As a department head John Stocks achieved much, not through political manoeuvring, but because he was so highly regarded as a clinician by his peers, particularly the surgeons. They often acknowledged that they could not have made their advances in paediatric surgery without the support that John and other anaesthetists gave them. It is a pity that the older generation of surgeons did not pass this attitude on to some of their younger colleagues who do not seem to appreciate how difficult it was before these advances were made.

John had ulcerative colitis for many years and eventually died following complications of surgery for cancer when he was only 43, in March 1974. It was distressing to see someone who did so much for sick children suffer as much as he did.

A quarter of a century after his death his contribution was recognized posthumously, at a World Paediatric Intensive Care Congress, as the greatest to Paediatric Intensive Care in Australia.

Helene Wood had been an anaesthetic registrar at the Childrens in 1965 and returned as a staff anaesthetist at the same time as I arrived. She was a very competent, practical clinical anaesthetist. She was brought up and trained in Melbourne. The three of us shared the on call at nights and weekends for both anaesthetics and intensive care which was still evolving and not nearly as busy as it is today. In 1967 we had 750 patients for over

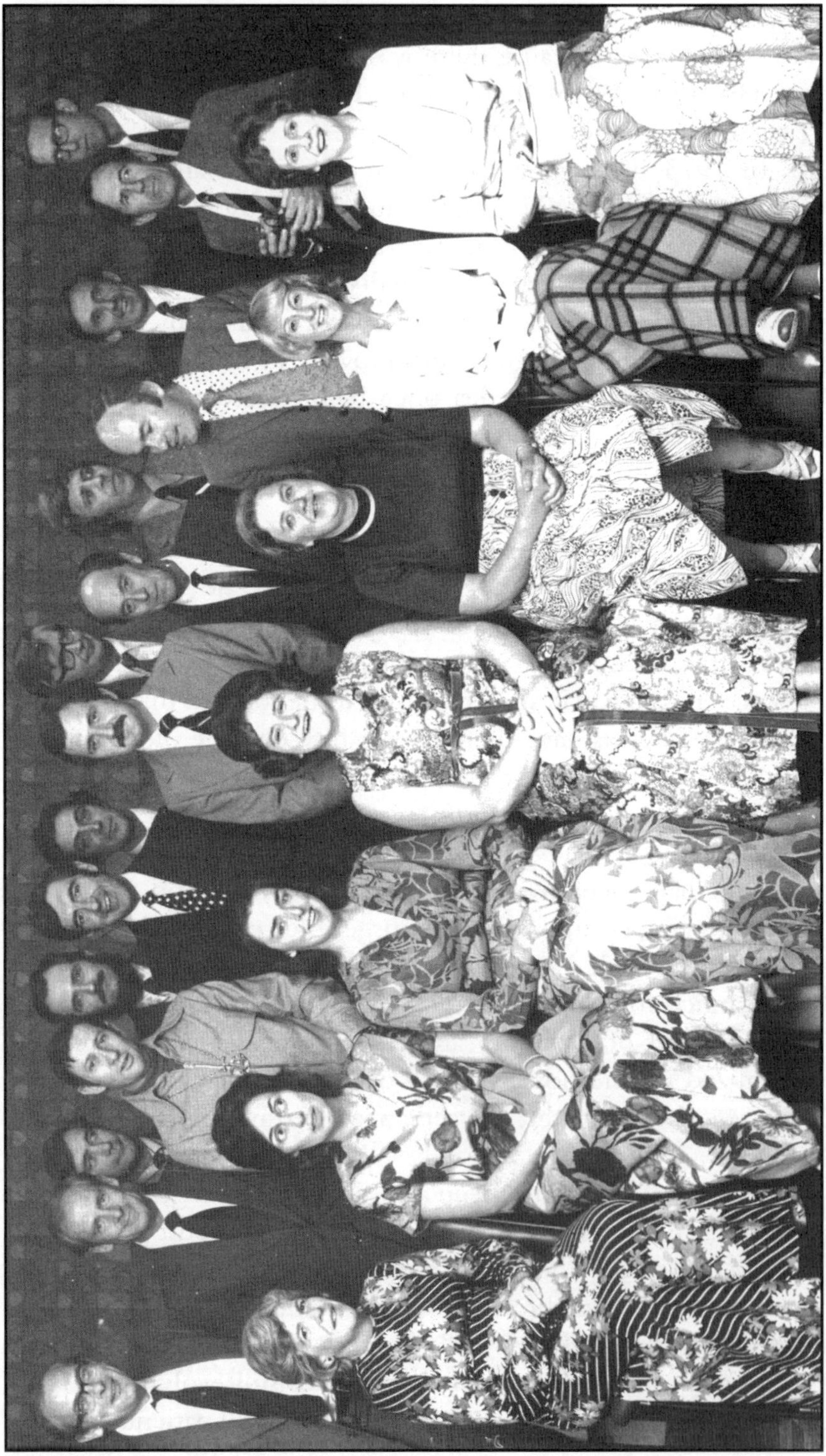

24 hours in ICU.

Much of the routine anaesthesia was done by visiting anaesthetists, who were predominantly in private practice, and our registrars. One of us was in charge to organize the theatre and supervise where necessary.

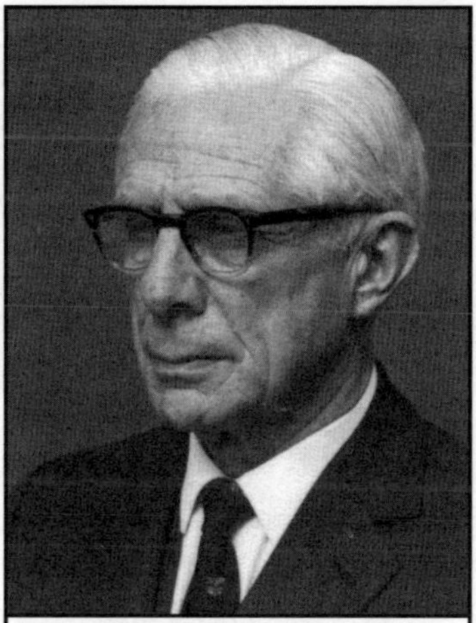

21. Laurie Morton (1946-72)

The visiting anaesthetists who had already been there for about twenty years were Laurie Morton and W.H.J. (Bill) Cole (1949-83). The latter came from Perth to do medicine as Perth did not have a medical school then. He was an enthusiastic clinical researcher and during nearly every anaesthetic some aspect was studied. He did many studies on new drugs which were important at the time because the rigor of clinical trials had not reached what is demanded today. He also had an imaginative mind and was awarded a MSc. in 1965, when he was 52.

His thesis included a study on the uptake of methoxyflurane (Penthrane) when administered with a weak anaesthetic, ethylene. The blood:gas solubility coefficient determines the rate of uptake of an inhalation anaesthetic. Penthrane's was 12 which is high compared to other agents, except ether. This results in a slow uptake and onset of effect. Ethylene, on the other hand is very low at 0.14. Its uptake is very rapid and this study showed that it enhanced the uptake of Penthrane so that it behaved more

20 Opposite. The full time and sessional anaesthetists at RCH on the occasion of Helene Wood's farewell in 1975.
Standing from left: Kester Brown*, Noel Cass*, Robert Gillies*, Stewart Bath (went to Launceston), Brian McKie (went to Geelong)*, Bill Stanisich (worked at St Vincents Hospital), Frank Whan, Geoff Mullins (went to Toronto and Perth), Brian Jordan, Bill Grey, Geoff Barker (went to ICU in Toronto), Robin Smallwood (Austin Hospital and Dean of Faculty of Anaesthetists), ian Sutherland (went to Sydney), Ian McDonald*, and Richard (Dick) Cohen (went to Penrith, N.S.W.)
Sitting: Janice Gillies*, Janice Peeler*, Mary Dwyer*, Helene Wood (went to Sydney), Beryl Jack*, Dawn Giltinan*, Anne Thorp*.
(* 25 or more years service to RCH)

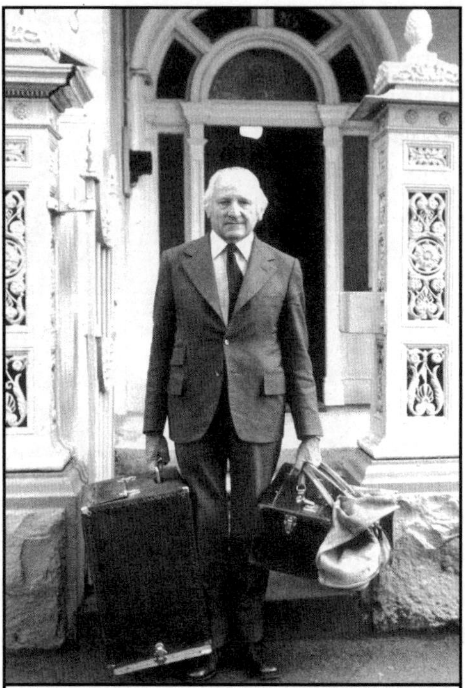

22. Bill Cole with his transportable anaesthetic apparatus with decorative Victorian gates in the background.

like the commonly used agent, halothane (blood:gas 2.3). Ethylene is a weak anaesthetic like nitrous oxide but it is flammable and it is lighter than air. This made it hazardous to use in theatre as the electrical outlets are set high so that explosions with ether, which is denser than air, are avoided. One of the stories about how the anaesthetic property of ethylene was discovered is interesting. It was used in the transportation of carnations to stop the buds opening too soon. In 1923, Luckhardt and Thompson wondered if it a similar effect in humans might cause unconsciousness.

Another of Bill Cole's studies used a 100ml thiopentone bottle as a halothane vaporizer and then the vapour was passed through an ordinary flowmeter on the anaesthetic machine to assess how much was being delivered. This was a very novel concept but it never came into general use.

Ian McDonald (20) was the first registrar with anaesthetic duties at the Childrens Hospital during 1949-50. He then went to Oxford where he worked with some of the great anaesthetists of the time such as Macintosh and Bryce Smith. For many years he was assistant to Gretta McClelland on a part time basis. He was one of the first (with Evan Watts from New Zealand) to use caudal anaesthesia at the hospital. He was also well known locally as the Victorian state cricket team's wicketkeeper. A keen sportsman, he continued playing cricket and hockey until he was in his 50s. He retired in 1988.

Among the sessional anaesthetists were Bill Grey (20) who

was a very good neuro- and plastic surgery anaesthetist. He was very helpful to me during my preparation for the final FFA examinations. I heard him present a brilliant paper on nerve blocks where he used cut down, shortened needles and placed them so that they looked as if the tip was in the patient. This paper stood out against a bevy of international speakers. Beryl Jack (18) was part time director at Queen Victoria Hospital came for one session a week. Her interest was a farm to which she retired. Noel Cass was on the staff but Dr. McClelland allowed him to use his session to pursue research on neuromuscular monitoring at the University.

The registrars in 1967 were my near contemporaries. They came from Brisbane, Perth , Wellington in New Zealand and the Philippines as well as the locals. Mary Dwyer (20) was registrar for the full year and after a further year at St Vincents hospital came back on staff in 1969.

Ken Williams, when he left us, went to work at the Royal North Shore Hospital before returning to Brisbane. He was somewhat hostile about the interview with a large panel which he had for that job. Later he found out that he was the first interstate registrar to apply to that hospital and they wondered if there was something strange about him!

John Marum came from Perth by ship. He had to go through customs. The customs officer was not amused when he said that "the West were thinking of seceding but hadn't done so yet"! John remained a visiting anaesthetist for many years. He was a good raconteur and sang in the Victorian Opera.

Ash Bishop from New Zealand went on to become a leading paediatric anaesthetist in Brisbane.

Alfonso Doloroso returned to Manila and eventually made a significant contribution to obstetric anaesthesia. He became President of the Phillipine Society of Anaesthesiologists.

Ian Sutherland (20), a keen tennis player and sportsman who spent some years in General Practice, was my study companion when we were preparing for our final examinations. He eventually moved to Sydney.

The paediatric anaesthetist community in Australia at that time I arrived in 1967 was small and remained a close knit group for many years. They made an extraordinary contribution to anaesthesia generally in Australia.

Mary Burnell, who became Dean of the Faculty of Anaesthetists, was nearing the end of her career when I started. She and Gilbert Brown, who was the first President of the Australian Society of Anaesthetists (ASA), worked at the Adelaide Childrens Hospital; Andrew Distin Morgan was the first paediatric anaesthetist in Sydney, being appointed to the Royal Alexandra Hospital for Children in 1940. Douglas Wilson (1906-70) began anaesthesia after World War II in Perth. With some help from Gilbert Troup he became the first full time anaesthetist in Western Australia. He was honorary part time director at Princess Margaret Hospital for Children from 1945 to 1956. He made a wide variety of his own equipment for infants.

Tom Allen and Ian Steven became well known names for their early work and publication on prolonged nasal intubation in children with respiratory problems. Tom had worked in Fiji and told me how they had some premature infants survive there without all the modern treatment. Ian Steven was Treasurer of the ASA and later became President. He received an Officer of

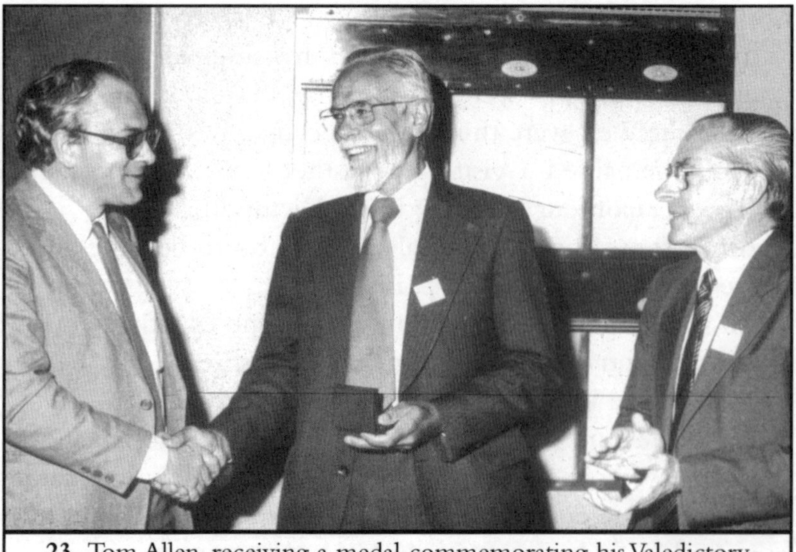

23. Tom Allen, receiving a medal commemorating his Valedictory address at an RCH meeting in Melbourne, with Ian Steven.

the Order of Australia — AO. They were, in turn, Director of Anaesthesia at the Adelaide Childrens Hospital.

At Princess Alexandra Hospital for Children in Sydney George Lomaz was appointed Director in 1959, followed later by John Overton (26) and then John Keneally (26). Charles Sara did some good work on humidification and on neonatal resuscitation, which was very controversial when he started. Verlie Lines, a lovely gentle lady , was well known for her great experience on airway problems.

Graham Fisk (25) moved to the Prince of Wales Hospital at its inception as a second paediatric centre. He became a leader in research, paediatric intensive care and education in Australia. He helped develop the Objectives of Training for the Faculty of

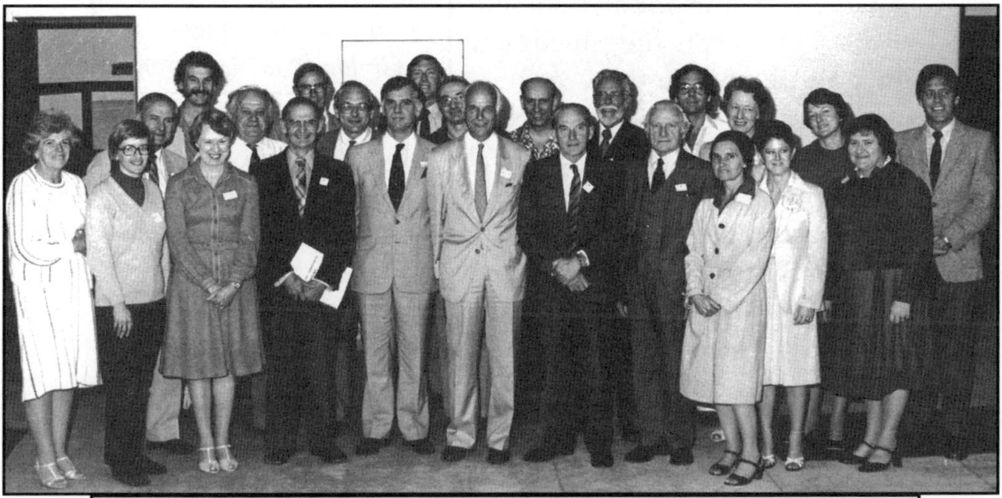

24. Paediatric Anaesthetic meeting at RCH, 1982 speakers and leading interstate participants.
Front: Janice Gillies (RCH), Geraldine Hill (Prince of Wales Hospital, Sydney), Verlie Lines (Sydney), Tom Voss (Capetown > Brisbane > Westmead, Sydney), Peter Morris* (Manchester, UK), Ottheinz Schulte Steinberg*(Starnberg, Germany), Ian Steven (Adelaide), WHJ (Bill) Cole (RCH), Jeanette Thirlwell (Sydney), Jill Robertson (RCH), Helene Wood (former RCH)
Behind: Noel Cass (RCH), Rod Westhorpe (RCH), Des Dineen (Adelaide), Graham Fisk (PoW, Sydney), KB, John Overton (Sydney), Neil Abrahams (PoW, Sydney), Tom Lambert (Queen Victoria Hospital, Melbourne), Tom Allen (Adelaide), Rob Eyres (RCH), Nerida Dilworth (Perth), Barabara Main (RCH), Geoff Barker (HSC, Toronto, Formerly RCH — John Stocks Memorial Lecturer). * Overseas visitors.

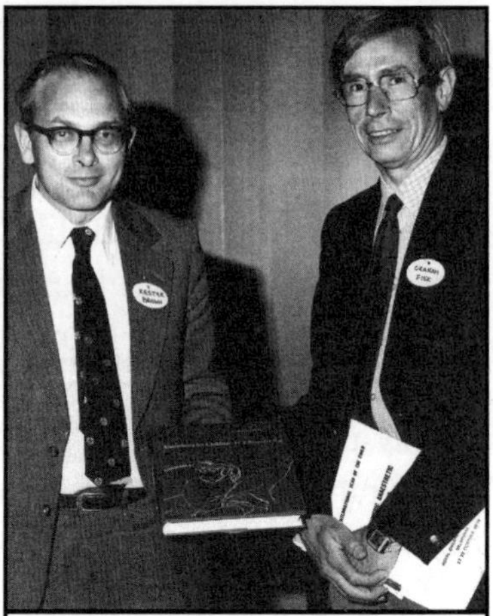

25. Graham Fisk and Kester Brown at the launch of their textbook "*Anaesthesia for Children*" in Nov. 1979.

Anaesthetists and was chief examiner; he was on the original Board of Anaesthesia and Intensive Care and organized some ASA meetings. He helped me produce the textbook, *Anesthesia for Children.* John Stocks had planned to write a book so after he died we decided to carry out the project. Graham was also an incredible chairman for scientific meetings. I recall an occasion where there were only two 10 minute papers on membrane oxygenators for a 90 minute session. He kept the discussion going for the whole time.

Later John Vonwiller and Neil Abrahams (26) joined him at the Prince of Wales Hospital. The three Johns, Overton, Keneally and Vonwiller all had active roles as examiners and contributors to the Faculty and were on the Editorial Board of *Anaesthesia and Intensive Care.*

Nerida Dilworth (26) was Director at Princess Margaret Childrens Hospital in Perth for 30 years. She was an outstanding lady who was on the Board of the Faculty of Anaesthetists for many years and became Assessor. She received a national honour — AM. Peter Brine who worked with her part time became President of the ASA. I remember meeting them on my first day in Australia in 1966 when we passed through Perth.

Tess Brophy , whom I met in Toronto in 1964, was the leading person in paediatric anaesthesia in Brisbane until she was joined by Ash Bishop. She was outstanding, becoming the second lady Dean of the Faculty of Anaesthetists, an examiner, organizer of the ASA scientific program, and eventually Professor of Anaesthesia. When she retired she became involved in Palliative care. She received several honours, including AO.

This incredible group of outstanding people welcomed me into the paediatric anaesthesia fraternity. Anaesthetists are generally congenial and less aggressive people; paediatric anaesthetists tend to be even more caring and gentle because they look after children all the time.

I have made friends with paediatric anaesthetists all over the world at various meetings. On occasion we have travelled together which is a way to become even better acquainted. Many of these people appear in the photographs (24,26) but there are too many to write about them all.

There were many outstanding surgeons at the hospital. The following were the leading ones when I arrived there. Russell Howard was the senior surgeon. He liked to be punctual and was a fairly domineering figure. His special interest was sternochondroplasty — correcting chest wall deformities. Douglas Stephens was head of surgical research and has remained interested in the field, even at 90. He also painted watercolours. One required patience when working with him. Peter Jones was an entertaining man with a fund of knowledge on all sorts of topics including heraldry, history, publishing and many others. He designed the hospital crest. He was involved in early cardiac surgery as was Nate Myers whose special interest was oesphageal atresia. The latter presented a Hunterian Oration on the subject in London. Durham Smith, later President of the Royal Australasian College of Surgeons, was technically the most organized surgeon with whom I ever worked. He had his operations worked out ergonomically so that they were done smoothly in the least time. It is a pity that he was never filmed operating. Alan Wakefield, plastic surgeon was a champion rose grower and breeder of Murray Grey cattle. Murray Clarke was a kind, unassuming man who made a great contribution, particularly in the important field of prevention of burns and childhood accidents. George Westlake, who was ambidextrous, was the cheerful cardiac surgeon with whom I worked in the early years.

There were many other great doctors around the hospital with whom I came in contact and, in many cases, wrote papers. It was a privilege and usually a pleasure to work with them.

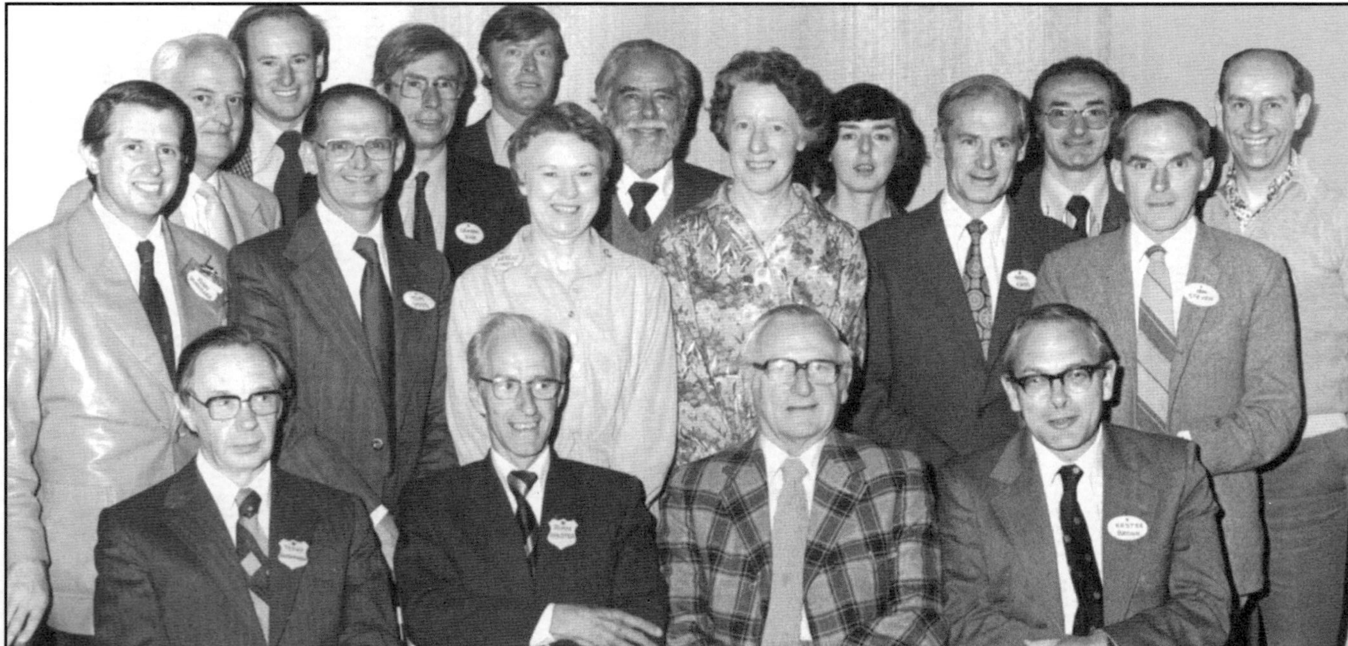

26. 1979 Paediatric Anaesthetic Meeting. Standing — from Left : John Vonwiller (Sydney POW), Peter Brine (Perth), John Keneally (Sydney), Tom Voss (Capetown > Sydney), Graham Fisk (Sydney POW), John Overton (Sydney), Verlie Lines (Sydney), Tom Allen (Adelaide), Nerida Dilworth (Perth), Mary Dwyer (RCH), Noel Cass (RCH), Neil Abrahams (Sydney POW), Ian Steven (Adelaide), Tom Lambert (Melbourne , Queen Victoria Hospital). Sitting : Toivo Suutarinen (Helsinki, Finland), John Inkster (Newcastle, UK), Bill Cole Melbourne — RCH — John Stocks lecturer), Kester Brown.

Chapter 12
Paediatric Anaesthesia

You may wonder why paediatric anaesthesia has developed as a subspecialty. There are psychological, anatomical and physiological changes during development which all have some relevance to paediatric anaesthesia. Infants and small children are not miniature adults. Babies have relatively larger heads and smaller limbs. This results in more blood going to the head and the large surface area of the head allowing greater heat loss when exposed to a cool environment. Babies generally cool more easily so that efforts are made to avoid cold environments or the babies are wrapped up.

They have double the oxygen consumption per kg and so require to breathe more rapidly and to have a higher heart rate so that the blood carrying the oxygen reaches the tissues in double the amount. The cardiac output — the amount of blood pumped by the heart each minute — is double.

The kidneys are immature so that they cannot concentrate urine as well, so infants require larger amounts of fluids. Even the amount of water in the body and its distribution differs. Babies have less inside the cells and more extracellular. This has important consequences when a baby becomes dehydrated because it loses more from the extracellular space and the intracellular space, being smaller, cannot redistribute as much to make up the extracellular loss effectively as in an adult. Thus dehydration has much more serious consequences in a baby.

The blood volume is 80-85 ml/kg compared to an adult with about 70ml/kg. Newborns have different haemoglobin (F), which takes up oxygen more readily from the placenta before birth. During the first year this is replaced gradually by adult haemoglobin (A) which more readily releases oxygen to the tissues. Between three and six months babies have a physiological anaemia while this transition is taking place.

Drug responses vary because of some of these differences in physiology. Neonates are often more sensitive and doses relative to body weight have to be adjusted. Infants and small children may need relatively bigger doses and then the dose may decrease towards adult levels on a per kilogram basis. It is not satisfactory just to divide the child's weight by the average adult weight and multiply by the adult dose.

The baby also has anatomical differences which affect anaesthesia. The ribs are more horizontal than in an adult and thus they cannot increase the chest volume as much by rib movement. The diaphragm (muscle between the chest and abdomen) which moves down when we breath in, is therefore relatively more important in an infant. Anything that splints it, like a large bubble of air in the stomach, pushes it up and reduces the volume of air that can be taken into the lungs. Too vigorous ventilation with a bag and mask may inflate the stomach — it must be done gently.

There are other differences in the airway — the level of the larynx (voice-box) is higher in relation to the vertebrae, its shape and the fact that the first part of the trachea inclines forwards require modification of the technique for intubation. The way the mask and laryngoscope are held is different.

Babies have very small veins which makes cannulation more challenging. Much finer cannulae are used.

Various sizes of equipment to suit different sizes of children must be available and the anaesthetist must know which size to use. Often the delivery system for the gases differs so that there is less resistance in the breathing system. The first simple system was devised by Philip Ayre (29) in Newcastle, UK. It was a metal tube with a another tube coming in at a right angle for gas delivery which became known as Ayre's T piece. (30) (see below) Another anaesthetist, the famous Jackson Rees (Figure C 9) from Liverpool, added a bag on the expiratory limb to act as a reservoir so that ventilation could be controlled easily and so that spontaneous breathing could be easily monitored.

Regional and local anaesthesia can also be used in children but the layers of fascia, aponeurosis, ligaments and muscle which the needle has to pass through are thinner. The anaesthetist can locate these with a short beveled needle because fascia and aponeuroses offers some resistance. In muscle, there is resistance to injection, when gentle pressure is applied to the plunger of the syringe, until the needle has passed through the muscle when injection becomes easy. I spent many years working on the anatomy related to nerve blocks, making dissections to demonstrate which tissues the needle passed through and using these to make teaching videos to demonstrate this work.

In 1993, I had the good fortune to meet Dr Curwen in Durban. He was an old man who had presented a paper in 1950 on 99 caudal anaesthetics (injection of local anaesthetic into the lower end of the spinal canal) in neonates (babies under 28 days old). When I expressed interest in this work he gave me a typed carbon copy of it. He concluded that he did not know whether his idea would be used or just considered a funny concept! It became a very useful technique to provide analgesia in the lower half of the body. Our department was one of the early ones to popularise the use of the technique in children, beginning in 1968.

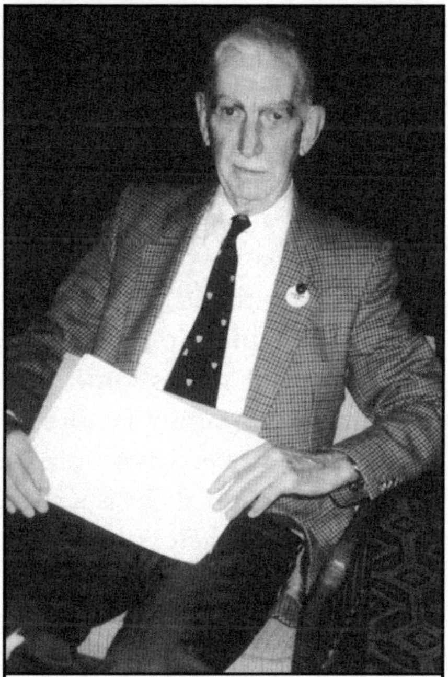

27. Dr Curwen in Durban holding a copy of his original paper on caudal anaesthesia in neonates. (1993)

As well as the differences outlined, the stage of psychological development is important in how the infant or child is handled. The anaesthetist is not only dealing with the patient but also with the parents or guardian. I usually introduce myself to the parents and then turn my attention to gaining rapport with the child if he/she is old enough. I think that if I can achieve this or at least show kindly concern towards the child the parents relax because they can see that I will look after their child well. I then consult the parents about their child's health and any problems before examining the patient. Some children, especially up to age six may be frightened. It may be advisable to give these children some tranquilizing premedication so that they are sleepy or calm when they reach the induction room. In older children one can try to explain what will happen. I tell them that I will look after them while they are asleep and that their mother and /or father will be waiting for them when they wake up. I always tell them that they will wake up otherwise they might feel that the situation is like the dog being taken to the vet to put to sleep for ever.

Sometimes, when the child has a complex or unusual condition, the parents are very well informed about it. Their comments may be very useful. One day I started to tell the mother that the anaesthetic for her child was a very difficult one with potential complications. She responded "I know. I have read your paper about it!" I was somewhat taken aback.

Sometimes family factors have to be considered in deciding whether to proceed with an anaesthetic when a child has, for instance, a cold. If there is a slight added risk but the anaesthetic could be given factors such as how far the family has traveled, has father taken a day off work, are there problems organizing baby sitters for the other children, can all come into consideration when making the decision.

How does the stage of development affect us? A baby under six to seven months can usually be separated from the mother easily but after that the maternal or paternal bonding is strong and it is better if a parent can accompany them until they go to sleep. In todlers who do not understand what is happening premedication may be needed. As well in school age children the presence of a parent may be enough to calm and reassure them. Older children of nine or ten may appear calm when visited preoperatively but are really nervous. This becomes apparent to the anaesthetist when they arrive in theatre with very constricted veins making venepuncture more difficult.

One of the great advances of the past thirty years has been the increasing acceptance of parents coming to the induction of anaesthesia. At first anaesthetists had to overcome their apprehension about the parent being there. To some this was an added stress which they did not feel was to the child's advantage. Gradually they came to realize that this was far outweighed by the reassurance that the parent could give the child. The parents leave as soon as the patient is unconscious. Sometimes the child can even be anaesthetised sitting on the parents lap. During an inhalation induction, stroking the child's cheek often has a calming effect.

It is important to explain to the parent what is going to happen. It is a stressful and emotional moment when their child suddenly becomes unconscious and relaxed in front of them. Parents also need reassurance — I tell them that I will look after their child throughout the procedure. If a parent doesn't want to come or is very nervous it may be better for the child if they do not come into the induction room. The child senses the mother's apprehension and may become difficult to handle. In such a situation the anaesthetist needs to make it clear that there is no obligation to come.

While the child is being anaesthetised some form of distraction is often helpful — telling a story or singing to the child or asking questions often takes their mind off the immediate activity.

It is because of all these differences in babies and infants that they are better anaesthetised by someone who is specially trained, both technically and theoretically, in paediatric anaesthesia. They have to be careful, gentle in their work and know how to deal with children.

What is a paediatric anaesthetist (or anesthesiologist)? My definition is "*a paediatric anaesthetist is someone who can safely handle and anaesthetise neonates and infants and any paediatric patients who have congenital anomalies and syndromes which have anaesthetic implications*" (such as airway problems and difficult intubation).

According to this definition there are highly specialized anaesthetists who can fulfil these criteria and who work in specialist childrens hospitals or large paediatric units but there are many more who regularly anaesthetise children and who would only occasionally, if ever, anaesthetise babies. The first group obviously need extra intensive training in a childrens hospital or major paediatric unit. This usually varies from one to two years and should ideally include some paediatric and/or neonatal intensive care, preferably where there are surgical patients, some acute pain management experience as well as at least a year doing a full range of paediatric anaesthesia.

It is desirable that the second group have some, but preferably six to twelve months, extra training in paediatric anaesthesia after their basic training which should have included some paediatric anaesthesia. The amount during basic training varies, depending on the number of trainees and the availablity of training positions, but four to six months in a paediatric centre is ideal.

How old should the children be, before an anaesthetist who looks after children occasionally or part time, anaesthetises them? It depends on training, experience and how often the person does small children. Opinions vary from one to two years old. However, between those ages the infants often have fat limbs which make insertion of an intravenous cannula difficult. In the end, the person giving the anaesthetic should be comfortable that they can do it. If they are not it is neither good for the patient nor for the individual, who will be stressed by the experience. There is no room for a cavalier approach.

The first chloroform anaesthetic and the first reported death from chloroform anaesthesia were in children. They have always constituted part of anaesthetic practice. How much varies in different countries and depends on the age to population ratio. It is far lower in developed countries than in some less affluent countries where large families still exist, because it is acknowledged that some will die and the parents want someone to look after them in their old age, or there is a lack of birth control and some religions do not encourage it. In some African countries over 50% of the population is under 15 years of age. AIDS has aggravated this situation because many of the parents have died with the disease leaving huge numbers of orphans for the grandparents to look after.

Why did paediatric anaesthesia develop? The main reason was the existence of childrens hospitals and that some anaesthetists were appointed to these hospitals and became experts by devoting much of their practice to children. In the early days anyone gave the anaesthetics. I remember Vernon Collins, the first Professor of Paediatrics at Melbourne University telling me how , as a junior resident, he had to "pour ether" for tonsillectomies without adequate training. These were done as outpatients! That was just before the World War II. One of Margaret McClelland's great desires in improving the lot of children at R.C.H. was to reduce deaths due to anaesthesia. Her archives have much material on this subject. It is reassuring that with better conditions and *improved training* the mortality is now very low. In one study in Uruguay the infant anaesthetic mortality, which had been the highest age group, was reduced by having a second anaesthetist to help. Having people who have had some paediatric anaesthesia training designated to do it will improve the situation. We are fortunate in Melbourne that most of the trainees have the chance to come to the Royal Childrens Hospital for four months during their training.

Courses, meetings or parts thereof, have been run in many parts of the world for years because many anaesthetists are involved with children to some degree in their practice. When the numbers of paediatric anaesthetists was small, meetings have been fairly informal. From 1975 to 2000 our department ran a meeting every three to four years which was open to all anaesthetists. Part of the program was general and part catered for the specialists. Between these there were occasional meetings in Sydney or Adelaide. In this way the paediatric anesthesia fraternity kept in touch and this seemed to satisfy our needs. With increasing numbers of anaesthetists and a trend to establish more and more formal specialist groups, a Society was proposed in 1996 by Johan van der Walt, who was the Director in Adelaide. When this organization was formed in Australia and New Zealand — SPANZA — there was much debate about who could be members. Was it aimed at the specialized people with the idea that anyone could attend the meetings or should anyone with an interest be allowed to join. The latter held sway as our national discrimination laws would prevent the former. To me this made it more of a special interest group than the society, which was proposed. After much debate it was agreed to try to become a special interest group within the College/ASA system. Agreement could not be reached with the College about some aspects of the group's independence, so the Society was formed separately, creating another fragmentation of anaesthetists. Now most members belong to three organizations — the College, the ASA and SPANZA. The interesting thing about this organization was that subscriptions were collected before the Society was formally established!

The Association of Paediatric Anaesthetists of Great Britain (APA) was formed in the 1970s. It was open to specialist paediatric anaesthetists and could have overseas members elected, the number not exceeding the home membership. I was one of the early overseas members.

In Europe, the Board of the European Federation of Associations of Paediatric Anaesthesia has representatives of each country. They hold a Congress every four years.

The Society of Paediatric Anaesthesia in USA developed later and is open to anyone with an interest.

An Asian Society was also formed at a meeting organized by Agnes Ng in Singapore. The meeting was organized first rather than after a large meeting where a wide view could be obtained of how to go. The Asian group generates its funds from its meetings and is open to individuals. This creates difficulty with countries which have their own societies — some members belong to the Asian Society, many don't.

When setting up an organization its *aims and objectives need to be defined* by a steering group. The main aim is usually to bring people with a common interest together. They will also have to formulate a draft constitution. It will often involve organizing meetings and this requires deciding where to hold the first one. It is probably better if the proposal is first discussed at an open meeting which then gives the people a chance to comment and decide if the aims are worthwhile and the organization is necessary. Usually those proposing the organization are given the job of setting it up, if the idea is approved, or else the group elects a steering committee.

In 1984 David Steward (14), from Toronto, organized a very good paediatric meeting concurrently during the World Congress in Manila which he called the First World Paediatric Anaesthetic Meeting. These have continued with or after each World Congress since.

At the conclusion of the first meeting David Steward opened discussion about formalizing a paediatric group, possibly as a WFSA Committee. I asked what the aims were because without any I felt it was inappropriate. No conclusion was reached. In the evening there was a dinner which most of us attended. John Zorab, then secretary of WFSA appeared and said that if we wanted a paediatric committee we would have to decide as there was a meeting where an application could be discussed the following day. I still opposed it on the grounds that we had no aims. The APA had a nominated representative who was not asked for his views. Jackson Rees asked for an informal show of hands where he obtained a positive response. I abstained and was attacked by Jack about it afterwards. I told him that as a matter of principle I would not support an organization which did not have defined aims. A committee was set up to which I was appointed for four years — I gather I was the only person on two WFSA committees at once, the other being Education and Scientific affairs. Aims and objectives were not defined. After some years a paediatric manual was produced, after many delays, when Anneke Meursing took over the editorship. More recently its chair, Charlie Coté, established a paediatric anaesthesia training fellowship in Calvo McKenna Hospital in Santiago, Chile to provide specialty training for less affluent South American countries. This committee lacked direction for many years.

With this background one can see why I think it is vitally important to clearly enunciate the aims and objectives before starting a committee or organization. I would like to see the World Federation of Societies of Anaesthesiologists (WFSA) provide a focal point for regional group representatives to meet at the World Congresses. This would help to maintain some unity in our specialty of anaesthesia, while allowing the subspecialties to retain their autonomy, under this single umbrella.

There have been many outstanding paediatric anaesthetists, some of whom will be mentioned later or whose photographs are included. Jackson Rees (Figure C 10), who modified the T piece by adding the bag, was one of these. He and his colleagues in Liverpool formed a group which influenced anesthesia all over the world. Jack, as he was called by his friends, was an inspiring person who was always coming up with interesting ideas. In his early retirement he worked part time in Rotterdam helping guide and drive their research. They instituted a named lecture after him, which I had the privilege of presenting once before he died. It was disappointing that he wrote and published very little because he had so much to offer. All the same he was a great inspiration to many.

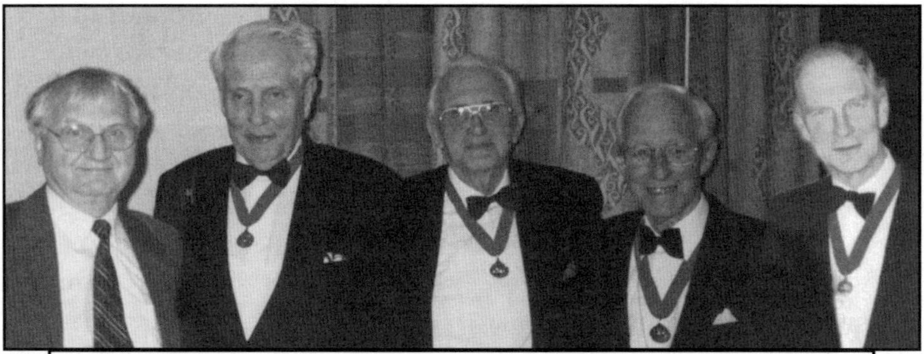

28. From left: Gunnar Bö (Norway), Gerry Black (Belfast), Harold Love (Belfast), John Inkster (Newcastle) and Gordon Bush (Liverpool) wearing past presidents medals, at the Association of Paediatric Anaesthetists meeting, Liverpool, 2001.

Another leader in the British scene was my good friend, John Inkster (28) from Newcastle. He was an outstanding neonatal anaesthetist who had the most organized neonatal anaesthesia set up I have ever seen. He promoted special neonatal low dead space connections and made an oesophageal stethoscope with and ECG and temperature probe attached. John has written the following segment on Philip Ayre, with whom he trained, which is of special interest to paediatric anaesthetists because he devised the much used T piece.

"Very soon after I arrived in Newcastle in 1950 I met and, for ever more, was influenced by Philip Ayre. He was a truly charismatic person, transmitting an enthusiasm for anaesthesia which was very infectious. This is, in part, why he was such a good teacher and why he was sought out by most of us during his sessions at the Infirmary. His teaching was always of great practical value and the product of immense experience but it was made even more valuable because he included many accounts of his adventures.

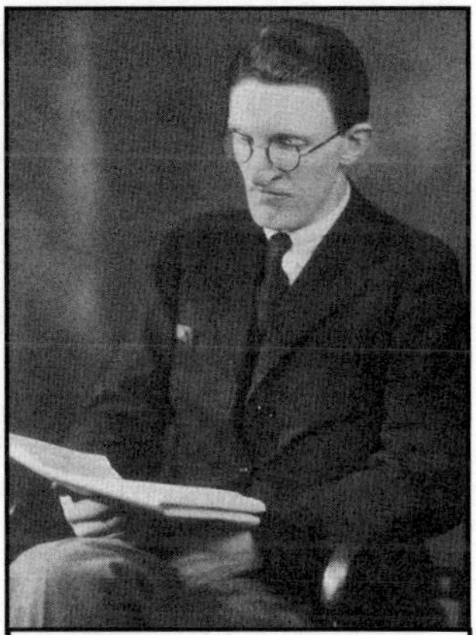

29. Philip Ayre, who popularised the T piece for paediatric anaesthesia.

He had an acute sense of humour so that he could see amusing aspects in the events which surrounded us and he was endowed with that rare quality, spontaneous wit. For example, on one occasion he was walking down the main corridor when he passed the open doors of an operating theatre where they were mending the terrazzo flooring. There was a pneumatic drill stuck in the centre of the floor and as he passed Philip said to his companion " What do you think that they are doing in there — do you think that they have lost a swab or something ?" His accounts of domiciliary anaesthetic practice included advice regarding the administration of open drop ether with one hand whilst beating off the family dog with the other.

Because of a very badly repaired hare lip and cleft palate his speech was often difficult to understand and he spoke with a 'honking' sound. He turned even this to advantage. Small children, to whom he spoke during induction became mesmerised by this sound and were unaware of the administration of various vapours."

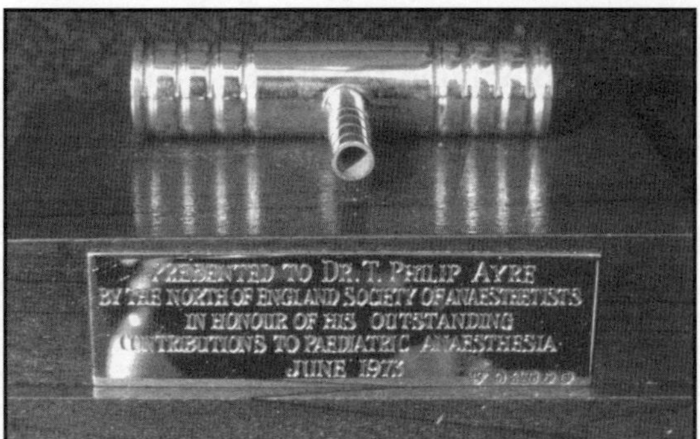

30. Golden T piece presented to Ayre upon his retirement.

Ayre was interested in anaesthesia as a student. He watched Dr. H. E. Boyle at Barts use a Clausen-Evans oropharyngeal airway in ENT surgery. This airway incorporated a T piece. Later, when he was having difficulty with infants having hair lip and cleft palate repairs, who were intubated, he realised that if he removed the T piece attachment he could use it to solve his problem. Originally the side arm had a tube bent inside the T piece to direct the gas flow towards the patient without causing increased dead space in the circuit. Although he didn't realise its significance at the time the gas flowing against the patients expiration was applying slight positive pressure throughout the respiratory cycle. He observed that his patients did better when it was attached in this way but unfortunately allowed the bent part to be discarded for ease of manufacture.

Ayre's respiration monitor was a piece of cotton stuck over the end of the T Piece. It waved to and fro with respiration. In my early years we sometimes placed a piece of cotton wool over the patient's nostril for the same purpose."

John Inkster made a valve in the mid 60s called a *residual positive pressure valve* which was aimed to allow free expiration down to a specific pressure and to prevent the adverse effects of negative pressure which was used at the time. Unwittingly, he had created PEEP (positive end expiratory pressure), which was formally defined some years afterwards (1969).

Many years later my small contribution was to persuade Portex to make plastic Y connectors (53) instead of T pieces so that the inflowing gas created a slight positive pressure. An alternative approach could have been to deliver the gases directly towards the patient and to have the expiratory limb attached to the side arm of the T piece. Jackson Rees by controlling ventilation manually with his bag, also applied some PEEP. Such simple ideas but they required some lateral thinking to develop.

Chapter 13
Evolution of the RCH Anaesthetic Department

Two years before she retired Dr. McClelland had drawn up a five year plan. It had been fulfilled in two years. When I took over the department in 1974 it was running smoothly. Plans to build an Intensive Care Unit on the second floor next to the recovery room were being considered. We were doing about 8000 cases a year and had a reasonable staff to cope with that workload as well as providing cover for intensive care. The staff had increased gradually with the addition of Mary Dwyer, Brian McKie, Stewart Bath and Anne Thorp. There were also several new sessional anaesthetists who had done extra training with us, such as Janice Peeler who took on a special interest in scoliosis surgery, or returned on completion of their training, such as Bob Gillies, Janice Gillies and Dawn Giltinan who continued on staff for over 25 years. (20)

The Director's role in those days was to provide an efficient service, to have enough staff, to ensure that the rosters were organized and to see that equipment was available and functional. We had to justify expenditure on things we needed but the hospital looked after the finances. It was only much later that departmental and, later , divisional heads became responsible for budgets.

I was fortunate to have the opportunity and the ability to fulfil the four components of running a department — clinical, teaching, research and administration. Nowadays it is almost impossible to do all four mainly because the administrative function takes too much time. I always believed that it was important to spend at least half my time giving anaesthetics so that my teaching and research was based on practical clinical experience.

When I took over, the anaesthetists played a role in organizing the theatres, but it was only after an independent, outside review that the Director of Anaesthesia became responsible. This was shortly after I took over but the Director of Nursing did not want me to have a title. So for a year I ran the theatres without the staff being notified except the chief surgeon who tried to prevent me taking on this role effectively. The Director of Nursing wanted to be sure that I would not suppress the nurses! Anyway after a year, she and the Medical Director agreed that the Director of Anaesthesia would be given the title of Director of Theatre Services as well. It was a logical step as the anaesthetists were most available, did much of the organizing anyway and were unbiased, whereas some surgeons would have found it difficult not to take advantage of the position for their own benefit. An amicable working relationship developed with the surgeons when they realized that I only wanted to help them by running an efficient theatre suite. The personal problem with the senior surgeon disappeared when we were respectively chairman of the state committee of the College of Surgeons and regional committee and Faculty of Anesthetists at the same time. I continued as Director of Theatre Services for about twenty years when it was decided that a separate position should be created because the business management side of the job, budgets and the keeping the statistics was an excessive workload on top of running a department, and by then, a division.

We always had one anaesthetist *in charge* for each session. This person had to help when there were complex cases or when somebody needed help, and also organized emergencies, any other cases that needed to be done and dealt with rostering problems. I had difficulty with those who worked at the two ends of the spectrum. At one end someone who was trying to be helpful would accept cases and then find out that they could not be done as planned because there was no staff or theatre, while at the other end they would say cases couldn't be done when sometimes , with a little co-operation they could be done. Both aggravated the surgeons. The solution is to say that one will try to work it out and then make the necessary enquiries. Then, if it cannot be done, at least you have tried to help and the surgeons will appreciate your efforts.

By 1976 we had computerised records of the theatre cases,

times and throughput by units. I could also obtain the anaesthetic workload of any anaesthetist with all their cases. This was probably the most advanced hospital in the country in relation to computer usage at the time. Unfortunately the man who had done a good job of starting all this was eased out of the position a few years later.

I always believed that good rostering of staff was important. People like to have some constancy in their work and anaesthetists develop working relationships with surgeons which are beneficial to the patients. I considered registrar rosters very important in ensuring that they received a balanced, well rounded training through all the surgical specialties while they were with us. They also rotated to intensive care until it had so much staff of its own and the complexity of the work increased to the point that our people could not function effectively unless they were there for six months. We arranged this for senior registrars for many years.

Each year I personally went through all the rosters to ensure these principles were maintained and to accommodate any new staff. For over twenty years, Mary Dwyer was responsible for making these master plans work each week, making adjustments where necessary when people were away or sick or when special surgical requests had to be accommodated.

My first important task was to look out for good potential staff to replace John Stocks, and the following year, Helene Wood, when she left. I needed a new deputy. I decided to delay that appointment until I found the right person. I was allowed to appoint an extra registrar for six months to cover the work but the hospital made an error and appointed Rob Eyres (31) for 12 months. I had interviewed him in London where he had done his training in anaesthesia. He achieved remarkable success winning the prize in the final fellowship examinations there while working at Whipps Cross Hospital. The mistake was fortuitous and Rob proved to be an outstanding, although somewhat unconventional registrar. At the end of that year there was a position available in the department. I never regretted appointing him to it. The following year I recognized the need for research on blood levels of local anaesthetics in children and he took that on as a long term interest. He also became leader of our cardiac anaesthesia team and oversaw our monthly department meetings as his contribution to helping me run the department. He eventually took over from me as Director in 2000.

One day, while I was wondering about my deputy, Noel Cass (31) was chatting to me and happened to ask if I had a job for him. He had been Dean of the Faculty of Anaesthetists and was one of the most active teachers and researchers in anaesthesia in Melbourne at the time when I became Director of the department. He had done much to give me a start, particularly in teaching and education in Victoria, and had organized for me to lecture in New Zealand in 1969 and to teach the Primary course in Malaysia in 1973. After some discussion, he solved my problem by agreeing to become my deputy. It was an unusual situation but we were friends and respected each other so it turned out to be a very harmonious and fruitful partnership for twelve years. He helped to stimulate research and teaching which made the department more attractive for some other bright people to join it. Noel had many talents — he became president of the RCH Ski Club, commodore of Mt. Martha Yacht Club, he had a jazz band which played at many functions for us and he played and organized early morning tennis at the hospital. He was heavily involved with medical defence and was Vice President of the Medical Defence association of Victoria for many years. He has been involved with our journal *Anaesthesia and Intensive Care* since its inception over 30 years ago. He is a remarkable man and a good friend.

Staff selection was important in building a good, cohesive department. We were fortunate that the best trainees in Melbourne nearly all came through the department. I was able to encourage good people to come back as senior registrars, during which year they also did some intensive care and so were well trained if any openings came up, either because people left or when new positions were created. I was caught short once when two people left for practice elsewhere at the same time.

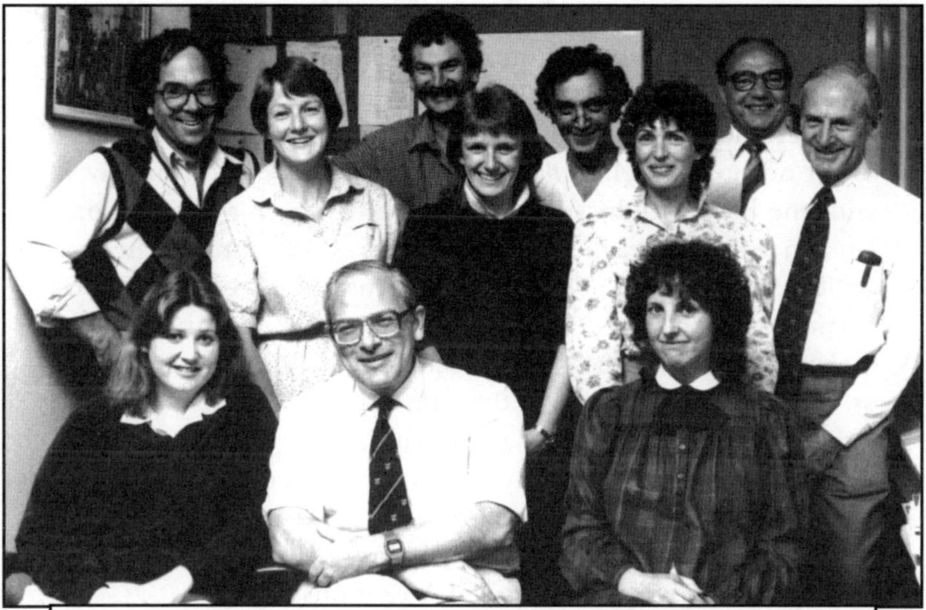

31. RCH Anaesthetic Department members involved in research, 1981
Standing: Rob Eyres, Barbara Main, Rod Westhorpe, Cathy Hastings (Pharmacy Masters student), Frank Whan, Corinne de Moerloose (Geneva), George Cauchi (Animal Laboratory Supervisor), Noel Cass (Deputy Director). *Sitting*: Brenda Bell (Research Technician),Kester Brown, Josianne Edwards (Research chemist)

Rod Westhorpe (31) came late in 1976 for three months as a registrar, when he came back from London where he had been working at Hammersmith, the Post-Graduate Medical School. It was soon obvious that he was an excellent organizer and I was glad the following year to be able to keep him on. He had a special flair for equipment so I gave him responsibility in this area. He helped to design an ergonomic anaesthetic machine which, unfortunately, only reached the prototype stage. He participated on several Australian Standards committees and was often consulted on, and tested gas supplies to new anaesthetising areas. He developed a keen interest in history of anaesthesia and, at my instigation, became involved in, and later became Curator of the Geoffrey Kaye Museum at the College. He became one of the leaders in anaesthesia political affairs, President of the Australian Society of Anaesthetists, as well as holding many other important positions, including being a College Councilor.

I liked to have people with different talents — teachers,

researchers and administrators so that we had a balanced department. Steve Robinson, who came from Newcastle, proved to be an unruffable organizer and excellent and efficient anaesthetist. Ian McKenzie is a great lateral thinker who became assistant editor of our journal, *Anaesthesia and Intensive Care*, and is involved with the hospital ethics committee. Phil Ragg is a great raconteur, anaesthetist, teacher and sportsman. As a youngster he was skilled enough to play in the Australian Open Tennis Championships. Karl Alexander, whose career with us was cut short by a serious illness, was outstanding during his time with us. He undertook a study on the adsorption of halothane by activated charcoal as a possible anti-pollution measure. Fortunately he recovered and eventually returned to anaesthesia. Barbara Main (31) developed a special interest in cranio-facial surgery and fibreoptic intubation when this first became available. She was a prize winner in the final FFA examinations.

There were too many to mention all those who have worked on our staff but they all played their part in making a happy, cohesive department which has been a pleasant place to work. Some stayed while others moved on, particularly some of the outstanding ladies such as Judy Kermode, Suellen Walker and Janette Low. Stewart Bath and Brian McKie were involved with cardiac anaesthesia and intensive care early on, but moved to Lauceston and Geelong respectively, after some years at the hospital. Most of the staff continued in the department for many years.(20)

It was *my philosophy* that the best way to have a good department was to encourage outstanding people to join it and then to give them responsibilities in the department and the chance to use their talents. I tried to arrange for them to have some area of clinical work in which they could become experts. In that way one could attract the best people to join the team.

The director is the administrator and should be a coordinator who encourages and trusts those to whom he or she has given responsibility. At the other end of the spectrum directors who want to be dictators do not usually tolerate people who are more able than they are. They usually employ mediocre, non-threatening people. This results in a mediocre department, often with friction between the members, especially if the Director does not command respect.

New directors usually have the opportunity to upgrade something in the department. When I took over I was able to replace our anaesthetic machines which were at least 12 years old. The new ones cost $10,000 each but lasted for 20 years so that they cost less than a dollar per case. We gradually gained offices but never had enough until we moved to our new department in 1990. They soon became inadequate for the number of staff.

The teaching program, which I have already mentioned, was running and has continued to do so. We aimed to cover all topics related to paediatric anaesthesia including the child in hospital and, as well, topics such as how to teach, administration , disasters and history of anaesthesia, which are not generally covered anywhere else. In addition, Rod Westhorpe takes all the registrars for a visit to the Geoffrey Kaye Museum at the College. This has multiple benefits — it uses the museum for teaching and it stimulates an interest in history among the trainees, some of whom later help with the museum. It is one of the best collections of anaesthetic equipment in the world.

In addition to the monthly scientific meetings there are now early morning meetings once a week for clinical review, Quality Assurance and other topics.

Research was almost non existent when I arrived but by 1974 we had several projects going in the animal laboratory and at Monash University. We continued to expand our research in collaboration with departments outside and within the hospital. They had the facilities while we had the projects so much worthwhile work was done, benefiting both sides.

By 1971 I was doing research at the Electrical Engineering Department at Monash University on hypothermia.(51) I was a research associate in that department for eight years. In the animal research laboratory at the hospital I had done a project on controlled ventilation during bronchoscopy. When the former chief of surgical research, Douglas Stephens, retired in 1973, I was asked to take over the responsibility of overseeing the animal Research Laboratory. It was run by George Cauchi (31) for over 30 years. He maintained very high standards of cleanliness and animal care.

In 1976 we began another association with the Richard Oppenheim at the Pharmacy College to study blood levels of local anaesthetics after various blocks had been performed. I realized at a meeting on local anaesthesia which I attended in Sydney that no work had been done blood levels in children. I asked Rob Eyres who had recently joined our staff to take on this project. Three Master of Pharmacy students (Wilma Bishop, Jenny Kidd and Cathy Hastings (31) measured the blood levels.

Our next association developed with Bert Hoveling who worked in the Applied Chemistry Department at Royal Melbourne Institute of Technology. He had a mass spectrometer attached to a gas chromatograph and was looking for projects for it. Not many people had such equipment then in the late 1970s. We received a National Heart Foundation grant to study amitriptyline metabolites to determine whether they changed during early development. I was working on antidepressant overdosage at the time.

Another project followed with one of Bert Hoveling's colleagues, Keith Phillips, measuring fluoride during methoxyflurane anaesthesia. This was a metabolite thought to cause high output kidney failure in adults if too much methoxyflurane was given for too long. It had not been reported in children so Rod Westhorpe and I did a study using a mass spectrometer to measure the amount given. We demonstrated that the fluoride blood levels were about half those obtained for the same dose in adults. Probably some was taken up in bones and teeth. One patient who had it many times never needed any fillings, so we were probably giving free preventative dental care with our anaesthetics! A side benefit of this project was that they refined their measurement technique which they were using to measure fluoride in krill.

My next association was with the Anatomy Departments at the Royal Australasian College of Surgeons and Melbourne University. Several people (Alex Babarczy, Khoo Siew Tuan (36) from Singapore and Corinne de Moerloose (31) from Switzerland) helped me with dissections done for anaesthetists with windows cut to show the layers needles pass through when nerve blocks are being performed. These have been used as the basis for a series of videos on anatomy and nerve blocks which are now available in English, Spanish, Japanese and Arabic. Various trainees and fellows have helped me with the translation.

Our success in research at the time was because we had these very fruitful associations with outside departments who had equipment and were looking for projects, which we could supply. Later, we acquired some research assistants. Brenda Bell (31) came first as an applied science student. She returned and helped me for seven years with electromyography and studies on muscle relaxants. The equipment was built by the Electrical Engineers at Monash University and included the first computer controller for the electromyograph.(60) Some of the studies are mentioned elsewhere but the main thrust of my work was to show situations when an unusual response occurred so that we could adjust the dose in those circumstances.

When Brenda left we were joined by Denis Clare (Figure C14), who had done the same course. He was a brilliant builder of equipment. When we couldn't afford to buy ventilators he built us some which we thought were better than comparable ones on the market (Figure C15). We went into a joint venture with David Komesarof who was an anaesthetist, inventor and entrepreneur, to produce them but hold ups with the hospital solicitors lost our chance for significant success before the new generation of anaesthetic workstations arrived. Denis also helped to design an ergonomic anesthetic machine with Rod Westhorpe. A company made a couple of prototypes but then decided not to proceed probably because they already had established equipment on the market. It had interesting features like a sloping front with LED flowmeters, it could be raised and lowered to suit the individual, the gases could be delivered from either side and it was relatively compact which was an advantage over the other giant machines which were being produced.

Josianne Edwards (31) worked with us as a chemist for some time doing drug assays but then our work in this area declined and she found other work. She had been sent to me to see if I had any ideas of what she could do. I never dreamt that I would find her work with me when she came!

The period from 1970 to the mid-80s was an exciting research time but after that time became scarce as our workloads increased without more staff. The department now has a new lease on research with people who have time to devote to it, which is allowing some really good work to be accomplished.

We had other non-anaesthetists in the department — our technicians and secretaries as well as our research helpers. Although our first Director, Margaret McClelland, instigated technicians as anaesthetic assistants they were originally under nursing. It took many years to have them shifted to the Anaesthetic Department. The nursing establishment in Victoria has always resented their existence, which is unfortunate as they provide dedicated, stable assistance to the anaesthetists. They are experts at looking after our equipment and helping us in our work, without being distracted by other duties. This is an important factor in making anaesthesia safer. They should be accepted by everyone as part of the team. The fact that at least eight of them have given the hospital more than 25 years service, some even 33 or 34 years, shows their dedication and stability as a group. Some of them, with Rod Westhorpe's help, have been involved in improving their training through educational courses.

We had only four secretaries during my time as Director. Elaine Saccardo was a very fast typist and typed the many drafts of the first edition of our book. She was also very active in the hospital auxiliary. She was followed by Pam Corden who told me that she never stayed more than two years in job but stayed four years with us and only left when she married. Pam had a novel filing system. She kept copies of letters in a drawer and from time to time came and asked me which ones needed to be kept and filed! It saved a lot of filing and unnecessary storage. Fiona was a country girl from Ouyen who had been at school with my daughter, Maryann. She developed into a good organizer helping with two of our meetings. When she went overseas she helped Anneke Meursing organize the first European Paediatric Anaesthesia congress in Rotterdam. When she left we were lucky to get Cathy Taylor who had been working in the Executive office. She has been many years in the department and has been valuable in helping with many of the administrative tasks which have to be done in an ever increasing department. I appreciated her help with masses of typing associated with my many roles before the advent of email through which we now do most of our own correspondence. To have a good secretary or personal assistant is invaluable when one holds busy administrative positions — we were fortunate with the ones we have had.

Chapter 14

Trainees and Overseas Fellows

Trainees are the future of the specialty. As I have already indicated, I tried to optimise their training by working out their rosters carefully and providing the best tutorials that I could arrange. I enjoyed training the young Melbourne anaesthetic registrars, usually in their third year of training. We have had many outstanding people through the department who have gone on to be major contributors and hold high office. Many became directors of departments. I would like to have employed many of them but there were too few positions available. A few preferred to work with adults rather than with children. In all, about five hundred local and overseas trainees came through the department while I was Director.

At first we had nine per year gradually increasing up to 23 as the years went by. That number has since increased further. How long should they spend in paediatric anaesthesia during their training? They used to have six months and usually after four months they said they were beginning to feel comfortable with children and after six months they were confident anaesthetising them. Their time with us was reduced to four months to allow a greater proportion of the trainees to rotate through the department.

Working hours have also declined due to changes in their industrial awards. Some in other hospitals used to work excessive hours but often ours were on duty for about 50 hours a week, which included night call, when they were often able to sleep part of the time. Our department was fairly progressive being one of the first to give registrars a half day off after they had worked a night. This was then increased to the full day off. The usual working week negotiated by unions in Victoria became 38 hours. A pay award for hospital resident medical officers was argued on industrial lines in the early 1990s whereby they work 43 hours, which includes five hours training time. Beyond that they receive time and a half for the next two hours and then double time. The situation changed so that it was as cheap to employ another registrar as pay four for working fifty hours or more. I and many of the registrars could see the disadvantage of this as far as gaining experience went, particularly at night when they could sometimes sleep. It also meant that many of their incomes dropped as the amount of overtime decreased. As time has passed the young anaesthetists have adapted to the shorter hours and probably have a better home life-style but gain less experience. I did not mind working long hours when I was young provided that I was gaining good experience. In Toronto I averaged over eighty hours a week in the hospital. Some of the trainees now have second part-time jobs to supplement their incomes which really defeats the purpose of the award.

The reduction in time at the hospital and in working hours means, I believe, that they have reached the minimum time for useful general training for later, unless they take further specific training in the field. Their exposure to paediatric anaesthesia is now about half what it was for registrars when I started at the hospital.

When longer hours were acceptable and when training time was introduced and we had enough registrars to cover the clinical workload I tried to broaden their experience by sending them on ward rounds in cardiology, neurosurgery and in the burn unit so that they developed an appreciation of the total care of patients. I also sent them to the Dental Hospital where many of them were taught by a very skillful anaesthetist called Mary Morland. They frequently commented on how much they enjoyed this session. One day she asked me to help with a difficult case. I then found out why she was such a popular teacher. One simple thing she did, which was not common, was to hold the mask on the face and at the same time keep one finger on the temporal pulse so that she was continuous-

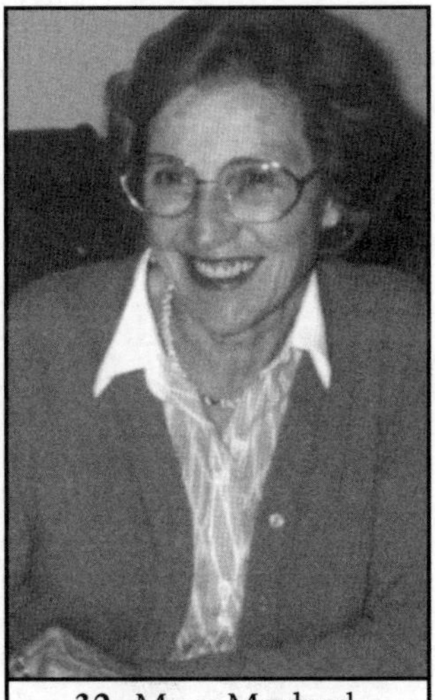

32. Mary Morland, one of the first registrars at RCH.

ly monitoring the patient by the simplest means. For a few years I was also able to send them to visit an anesthetist, Alan Belcher, who only did dental anaesthesia in dental surgeries, each of which he had equipped with suction and the essentials for an anaesthetising location. He had a machine which turned on the radio when the halothane (anaesthetic) was turned on. These were the only opportunities during their training for our registrars to gain experience in outpatient dental anaesthesia.

I had a funny experience with a registrar who was known for his unusual antics. He had already been involved in giving anaesthetics in some out of the way places such as Eritrea. He had not worked with me and was due to leave in a couple of weeks so I arranged for him to be rostered with me. When I told him that I had done this he "Oh! You haven't have you." I replied " Didn't you want to work with me?" " I was hoping I wouldn't have to", he said. I was on the spot but decided to play his game. " It wasn't for your benefit, but for mine." I replied. It turned out to be an interesting experience because he monitored the patient with his hand on the abdomen where he could feel the aortic pulse and the patient breathing. He had learnt this on one of his trips when there wasn't any fancy monitoring equipment.

Another, having had some good sessions where I taught him several things asked "What are you going to teach me today?" After his last list with me he said that he would be happy to give me an anaesthetic when he had finished his training, and he wouldn't charge me for it! I wonder if I will need to call on his generosity!

Many people from interstate and about a hundred others, from forty countries overseas, came for training and further experience. (Figure C4, C6)

The first ones came to do their total training in Melbourne in the late 1960s. They were Alfonso Doloroso from Manila who later became an eminent anaesthetist in the Philippines. Lee Choong Keet was from Malaysia. He went back for a few years but returned to Australia later. He was a very bright fellow and shared the prize in the Final Fellowship examinations with Michael Cousins who later became the Foundation Professor of

Anaesthesia at Flinders University in Adelaide before returning to Sydney to run a major Pain Unit at Royal North Shore Hospital. He recently became President of the ANZ College of Anaesthetists.

Radha Krishna came on a WHO fellowship in 1976 and was the first of a long line of people who came from overseas while I was director. He returned to Malaysia where he became chief government anaesthetist, a post he held for many years. He went into private practice when he retired compulsorily from Government service at age 55.

Later, another Malaysian who worked with us, Ng Siew Huan, climbed through the government service ranks from Penang to Ipoh to the senior government job in Kuala Lumpur. Karis bin Misrahi did his training in Melbourne and returned, eventually becoming the head of department at the National University in Kuala Lumpur.

During a trip overseas in 1977 I had met Frank Wagner working in Starnberg in Bavaria with Ottheinz Schulte Steinberg. He had impressed me during our brief encounter so he came for a year with us as a senior registrar, our first from overseas. He had tremendous powers of concentration and was very industrious. He eventually obtained a state grant to develop

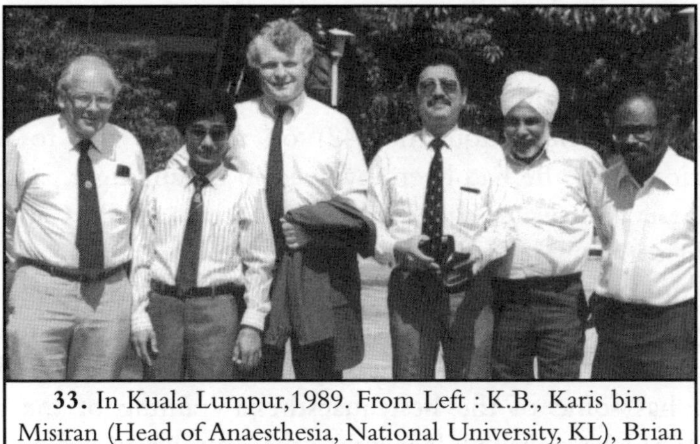

33. In Kuala Lumpur,1989. From Left : K.B., Karis bin Misiran (Head of Anaesthesia, National University, KL), Brian Horan, Sydney (second Editor of Anaesthesia and Intensive Care), Lim Say Wan (President WFSA1992-96), Karpal Singh (Surgeon who trained at RCH about 1970), Radha Krishna (Chief Government Anaesthetist in Malaysia).

computerised monitoring in the operating theatre when it was in its infancy. He became an examiner in the European Diploma examinations. Many years later I asked him what he gained from his year with us. He told me he learnt (a) to anaesthetise neonates so that they did not worry him, (b) to think about why he did what he did when giving anaesthetics — previously he had been told what to do without necessarily understanding the reason, and (c) that one does not need to be tense while giving anaesthetics. I felt his time had been well spent.

Khoo Siew Tuan (36) wrote from Singapore asking to work with us when her husband came on a Research Fellowship at the Royal Melbourne Hospital. We had no position but she came anyway and had a very fruitful year. As well as gaining practical experience she helped me with anatomical studies of where we do nerve blocks, some of which were later used to make teaching videos. She delineated the fact that doing a femoral nerve block there are two layers of fascia which can be felt with a short beveled needle is passing through the tissues to the nerve thereby making the technique much more precise.

Two Swiss ladies came next, Corinne de Moerloose (31) and Doris Suter. Both worked part time while their husbands undertook research fellowships. Corinne had a variety of experience in paediatrics and related fields and began her anaesthesia with us — the last person to do so at RCH. Eventually she went back to paediatrics because it was too hard doing anaesthesia training in Switzerland with children.

I met Carlos Riquelme (42) on my first visit to South America where he had been involved in organising a paediatric anesthesia course at which I spoke in Santiago, Chile. Carlos had sought somewhere in USA to go for further training. He had been offered a three year basic training position followed by a two year paediatric anaestheisa fellowship — five years in all. It seemed ridiculous to me as he was already trained. I found that Chile has some of the best anaesthesia training of the many countries I have visited. It is either the only, or one of very few countries where the candidates have to give an anaesthetic in their final assessment. I found a position for him and he came in 1985 with his wife and three little boys. Carlos proved to be an outstanding anaesthetist from whom I learnt many practical tips. He was well read, thoughtful and always had a reason for what he did. He spent two years with us, the second one doing research. We have met and traveled together many times over the years and I considered him one of the best paediatric anaesthetists that I have known.

Susana Cueva (Figure C4) came from Ecuador in similar circumstances. She was my translator when I spoke at a meeting there. She had a severe limp from polio. She had written fifty hospitals in various countries seeking the opportunity of going for further training. Only one, from Sweden, replied, regretting that they could not take her. She was obviously worth helping and so she came for a year. I persuaded the department members to fund her from our private practice fund. She has since contributed a great deal to anaesthesia in Quito and has taught Primary Trauma Care courses there and in at least one other country. She is a wonderful lady who has not let her disability hinder her progress. Susana and Carlos were both at the World Congress in The Hague in 1992. I tried to organize a meeting but failed. Then Carlos went to Paris and one day visited the Palace at Versailles. He heard Spanish being spoken behind him and turned round to talk to the two girls. Amazingly, it was Susana and her friend Nellie Castro.

We had other Chileans. Italo Zamudio (Figure C4) who was a thoughtful and intelligent man and went on to teach on Primary Trauma Care courses and had an interest in blood conservation. Margarit Calderon stimulated an interest in poetry when she gave me a book of poems by Pablo Neruda who won a Nobel Prize in Literature. Maximo Sepulveda from Osorno, who was also a pilot. He took his family by car to the centre of Australia and back by Queensland in three weeks, much to our amazement. Guillermo Galeoti came from Cordoba, Argentina. He was a body building champion and a great character. On one occasion he took a group to a night club in Melbourne and when he was refused entry he said "But Dr. Brown from the Childrens Hospital arranged for us to come." They were allowed in at half price. I had never heard of the night club so he was obviously a good bluffer!

Sergei Rajev (Figure C5) from Moscow was a wonderful and very promising man who spent a year with us. He had translated for me and showed me around when I visited Moscow just after Perestroyka in 1990. Life was very hard for them then. I gave him a copy of the proceedings of a European Congress which I had just attended. I was stunned when he looked at it and said to me "This is like giving me diamonds." He had been selected to go to England for a year but the plan fell through and he wrote to ask if he could come and train with us. Again, I was able to persuade our department to fund him from our private practice fund,and so he came with his wife and lovely six year old daughter, Anastasia. She did not speak English when she arrived but left speaking fluently with a beautiful international accent derived from the variety of people she met. She is now a medical student. Unfortunately, Sergei died from leukaemia in his early 40s. I became aware of the impact he had already made when two young Russian anaesthetists who had trained with him came up to me at separate congresses and thanked me for training him, as he had trained them. I was very moved.

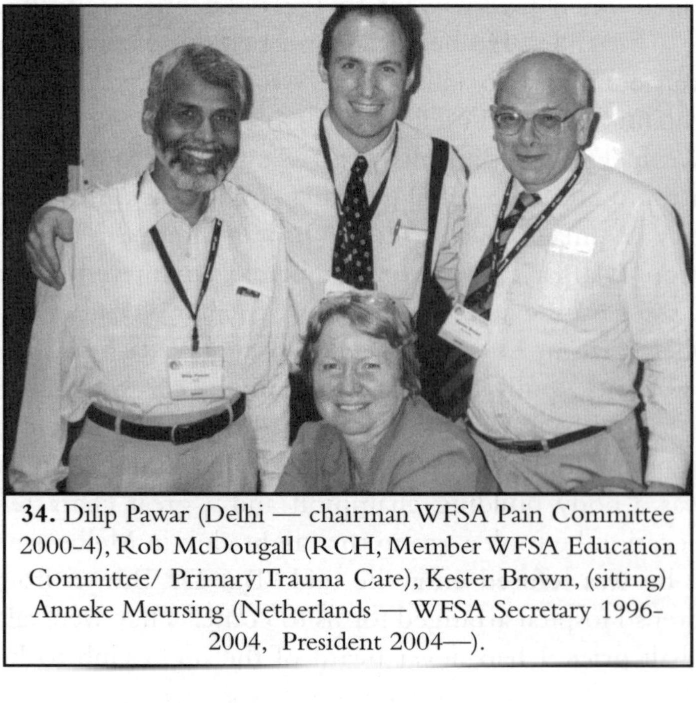

34. Dilip Pawar (Delhi — chairman WFSA Pain Committee 2000-4), Rob McDougall (RCH, Member WFSA Education Committee/ Primary Trauma Care), Kester Brown, (sitting) Anneke Meursing (Netherlands — WFSA Secretary 1996-2004, President 2004—).

Dilip Pawar (34) wrote from Delhi asking to come. His reason, I found out later, was that he had found while reading my book on paediatric anaesthesia that we had similar ideas, which differed from most of his colleagues. He proved to be an outstanding person who has taught widely since his return to India. I have done several workshops around India with him when I have been visiting. He became chairman of the WFSA pain committee and introduced a modular teaching program to take to other countries with a view to improving the management of post-operative pain.

I met Victor Mwafongo (Figure C4) in Dar es Salaam, Tanzania when I was visiting in 1985. He asked to come and work with me and fortunately I was able to find a position which enabled him to come for eight months. During the same visit I had the interesting experience of seeing a wonderful American surgeon, Glenn Gordon, working with a Russian anaesthetist. It was still during the time of the cold war when we were supposed to think that we should avoid everyone from Russia. What a pathetic attitude. The more that I have travelled the more I realize that there are good people all over the world. It is largely politicians and power hungry individuals who create the animosities.

Victor was a wonderful, round-faced, cheerful man who made a great impression in our department. After he returned home, he became chief anaesthetist in Dar–es-Salaam, dealt with the disaster following the bombing of the US embassy there and later became President of the East African Society of Anaesthetists. He has been on the Board of the African Regional Section of WFSA and on some WFSA committees. He named one of his sons after me! I wondered when I took him whether the contrast would be too great and that he might find it difficult to return to Tanzania, which was in poor circumstances at the time. It was hard for him to return but I think his time with us made it possible for him to benefit more easily from chances of international travel and involvement which came later.

Anneke Meursing (34) was already head of the department at Sophia Childrens Hospital in Rotterdam when I visited her after meeting at the World Congress in Manila in 1984. She told me that she was thinking of going somewhere for further experience. I persuaded her that she should do an exchange with someone in our department, which she did later that year for six months. She learnt about organizing meetings while with us and went on to organize the first two European Paediatric Anaesthesia congresses, was secretary for the World Congress in the Hague in 1992. She became Secretary of the World Federation of Societies of Anaesthesiologists and in 2004 became the first lady President. She was one of those who were already in responsible positions who came to broaden their experience with us.

Others who were already heads of their units included Olli Meretoja (36) from Helsinki who worked on muscle relaxants with me. We wrote eight papers between us, in the last two months he was in Melbourne, on our research. That was an exhausting experience!

Gerry Goresky (Figure C27) from Calgary was a good stimulus and gave us some refreshing ideas, Gunnar Bo (28) from Oslo, Gunnar Olsson and Stefan Lundeberg from Stockholm, came and contributed to exchange of ideas. (35)

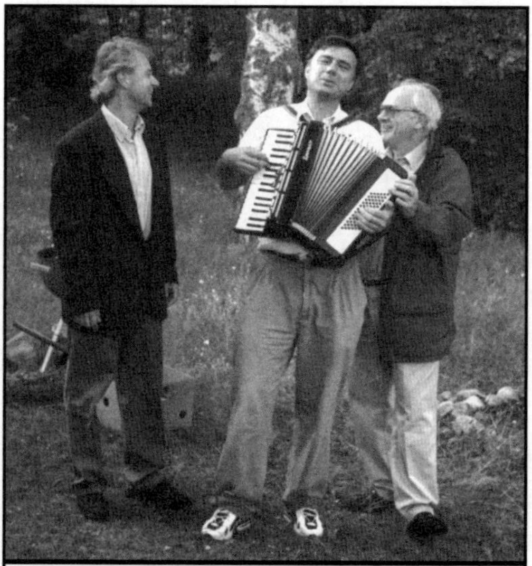

35. Gunnar Olsson playing the accordian and Stefan Lundeberg from Stockholm with the author in his well travelled green parka which has been all over the world — at the Archipelago near Stockholm. 1999.

We have also had several from Thailand who are an enthusiatic group to visit (Figure C6). Thitima came to me before going home to ask my views on operating suite design. I told her my views and then found out that they were planning 75 theatres on three floors. I was stunned! They built eight blocks of eight and she was responsible for moving into them and equipping them! It is at the 4000 bed Sriraj hospital.

Angie Gapay (Figure C4)) came from the Philippines for six months. She has worked in Tacloban, the former home of Imelda Marcos, for many years. Recently she went on a WFSA teaching trip to Micronesia.

The forty countries from which people came to work or visit included : New Zealand, England, Scotland, Ireland, Wales, France, Netherlands, Belgium, Germany, Switzerland, Italy, Norway, Sweden, Finland, Denmark, Poland, Russia, Ukraine, Canada, USA, Ecuador, Chile, Argentina, Costa Rica, Brazil, Tanzania, Kenya, India, Malaysia, Thailand, Singapore, Hong Kong, Philippines, Japan, Sri Lanka, Pakistan, Myanmar, Tonga, Soloman Islands and Fiji. Sadly, the young lady from Myanmar died of fulminating hepatitis not long after her return home. Many of these people appear in some of the photographs, particularly Figures C4, 5 and 6, and 34 which were taken when I retired as Director and from full time work.

A few of these came for short periods but most spent six months or a year and occasionally longer. Many of them became like members of a big, adopted family and continue to have regular contact with me. I tried to ensure that they received more than just training in paediatric anaesthesia, and also learnt about teaching and organizing training programs. I tried to broaden their outlook generally. I sometimes took them to meetings or for trips around the country or to the National Gallery of Victoria to view paintings and the stained-glass ceiling in the Great Hall.

They had the opportunity of meeting people from many other countries at the hospital because many departments took overseas fellows. Many international friendships were made. Nearly all our fellows returned home and many have made significant contributions in anaesthesia in their countries, and some at an international level. This program was a most exciting aspect of the department and it certainly made it well known around the world.

The friendship of all these people is one of the things I value most. They may not have worked together but when they meet they immediately have something in common which can create a bond of friendship. It is wonderful to know that most of them have gone home and passed on what they have learned to others, creating a great ripple effect.

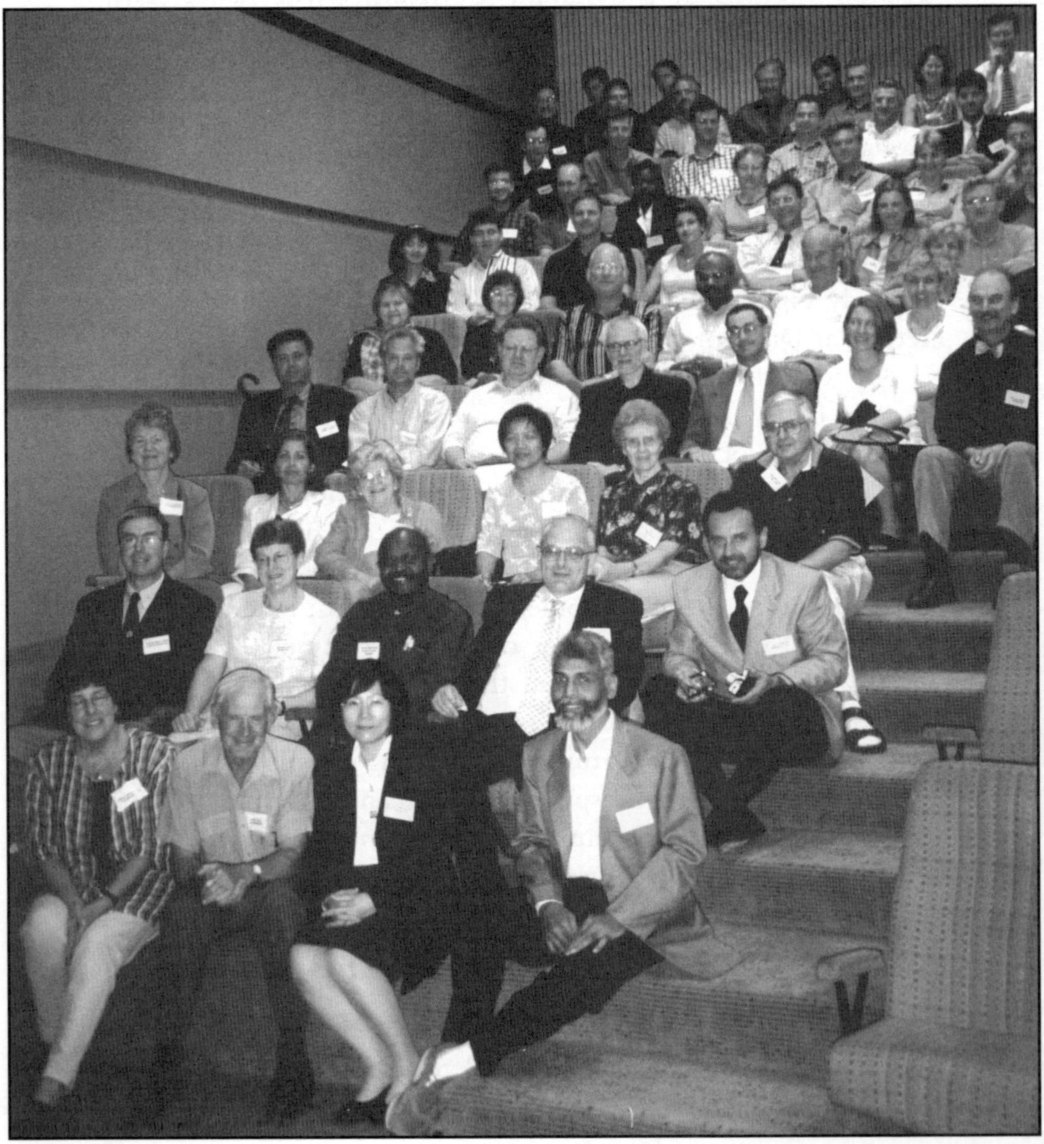

36 Opposite. Present and former members and fellows of the RCH Department at Kester Brown's Retirement Meeting, November 2000. *Front row:* Nancy Bouwmeester (Netherlands), Noel Cass (RCH retired), Khoo Siew Tuan (Singapore), Dilp Pawar (India). *2nd row:* Peter Kempthorne (New Zealand), Barbara Main (RCH), Victor Mwafongo (Tanzania), Kester Brown (RCH), Italo Zamudio (Chile). *3rd row:* Anneke Meursing (Netherlands), Susana Cueva (Ecuador), Janice Gillies (RCH), Angie Gapay (Philipines), Anne Thorp (RCH), John Newstead (New Zealand, Saudi Arabia). *4th row:* Gunnar Olsson (Sweden), Stefan Lundeberg (Sweden), David Murrell (Sydney — born in Kenya), Olli Meretoja (Finland), Chris Johnson (Perth), Janette Low (RCH), Rod Westhorpe (RCH — Deputy Director). *5th row:* Helene Wood (Sydney), Agnes Ng (Singapore), Michael Claxton (Hobart), Radha Krishna (Malaysia), Chris Evans (New Zealand), Antoinette Brennan (Melbourne), Penny Hall (RCH). *6th row:* Jirawat (Pia) Limprayoon (Bangkok, Thailand), Alvaro Brilla (Costa Rica), Norbert Weidner (USA), Robin Amerena (RCH), Ian McKenzie (RCH), Cathie Hill (New Zealand), Steve Brazenor (Canberra). *7th row:* David Allen (Geelong), Andrew Sharples (UK>New Zealand), Praxy Okutoyi (Kenya), Ruth Matters (Hobart), Malcolm Anderson (Hobart), Yasmine Layher (Victoria), Lindy Cass, Andrew Davidson. *8th row:* Jeff Rowlands (Shepparton), Rob Ray (Ballarat), Bruce Christie (Ballarat), Tom Mohler (Hobart), Joe Novella (Melbourne), Phil Ragg (RCH). *9th row:* Ken Brownhill (Melbourne/RCH), Andrew Jeffries (Melbourne/RCH), David Meyers (Mackay, Queensland), Barney Cresswell (Perth), Robert Gillies (RCH), Jill Robertson (RCH), Chris Bolton (RCH). *10th row:* Ian Chapman (New Zealand), Brian Anderson (New Zealand), Petra Schaeffler (Germany)

Present but not pictured: Noel Hosking (New Zealand), Geoff Mullins (Perth), Mary Dwyer (RCH), Guillermo Galeotti (Argentina), Sylvie Herbeau (France), Brian Spain(Darwin, NT), Rob McDougall (RCH), Geoff Frawley (RCH), Christian Herbeau (France), Rob Eyres (RCH — Director of Anaesthesia).

Chapter 15
Teaching

I am including this topic here because it is an important one in which I have had a special interest for many years. It has been a regular one on our registrar teaching program as I believe that if we can teach even a few points about how to improve presentation and teaching, the benefits will be great and standards will improve. It is also a topic which I have presented around the world. The essence of my lectures is presented later in this chapter.

My first foray into teaching was giving some classes to my father's trainee nurses when I was back in Kenya as a fourth year medical student.

The next I remember was giving a lunchtime lecture to the nurses on treatment of cancer when I was an intern. How I dared to take on such an assignment now leaves me wondering. I was not an expert but I had been exposed to some exciting new work that was going on in Nairobi. People from the Sloan Kettering Cancer Institute in New York had been out doing some trials shortly before I visited. They had inserted catheters into the carotid artery in the neck and infused methotrexate, an anti cancer drug, so that very high concentrations reached the tumour. These awful growths in the mouth and face had melted away leaving a hole. Who could not be impressed that these Burkitt's lymphomas could respond so well? I had obviously learned a bit about radiotherapy as well. I made the most of an opportunity to share my knowledge, something I have done ever since.

One does not have to have encyclopaedic knowledge to teach. One just has to understand something well and pass it on clearly. Although some brilliant people are excellent lecturers, many are not. Sometimes they know too much and cannot simplify the information for the ordinary person to understand. Some people who have struggled to learn can see where the problems lie and analyse the subject to see how it can be simplified and better explained, thus making them better teachers.

Looking back over life I had many teachers, both theoretical and practical, good, mediocre and bad. One can learn much about teaching by analysing what made one person a good teacher and another not so good. I am a visual and practical learner so good diagrams, seeing examples and being shown how to do practical things helped me the most.

I have learnt to teach by accumulating key ideas from many people. Al Cox (7) with whom I did research in Vancouver, was a major stimulus to my interest in medical education particularly after he returned from a six week course in Chicago where many concepts on medical education were revolutionized. He went on to become Professor of Medicine and later Dean and Vice President of Memorial University in Newfoundland. One of the highlights of my teaching career was nearly thirty years later when he visited Melbourne on sabbatical leave. He visited our department on the day when I was due to teach about how to teach and we did the session together. What a thrill it was for me to share this with him.

Don Kinsey took over public relations at the hospital after years as a newsreader on the Melbourne radio station, 3DB. He also taught public speaking to businessmen. He passed on many useful tips about vocal presentation over lunchtime conversations with me. He has a wonderful speaking voice and I was very grateful to him for doing many of the commentaries on my videos and films.

John Paull was one of the outstanding teachers in anesthesia. He did a Diploma of Tertiary Education which was unusual for an anaesthetist then. He was a clear conceptual thinker and I learnt much from discussions with him, including many of the principles of making good slides. Some of my colleagues at work were lateral thinkers which stimulated me to think in different ways.

Written presentation has been helped by my daughter, Maryann, who is an English teacher and educationalist. She proof read my second book, corrected the English and made sure it was easy to understand. Editing our major book, Anaesthesia for Children, with Graham Fisk (25) was an educational experience as he was strong on grammar as well as critically reviewing content.

An invaluable part of my learning to teach came when I was asked to teach the nurses anatomy and physiology when they were just out of their preliminary training school. It was a challenge because the course had to be covered in ten lectures! I had to simplify the subjects down to basics which then had to be presented simply so that they could understand and acquire the key information. Many of them had not done chemistry or physics at school. I taught this course for four years so near the end I had taught all the student nurses in the hospital.

Learning how to learn is the other important aspect of the process. Auditory learners may read aloud to themselves while visual learners may draw diagrams and write notes. My mother was certainly an effective teacher as I advanced rapidly when I reached school at the age of nine. She was also a strong disciplinarian who taught me to study and learn by diligent effort. That diligence stayed with me through school, university and on to later life. At university I adhered to the principle that I should do at least twenty hours study each week outside classes regardless of what sporting and social activities I also pursued — and pursue them I did. I also learnt the art of taking short naps to overcome fatigue so that I could study or socialize more effectively.

Teaching can be accomplished in many ways. Lectures and tutorials are widely used. Interactive teaching is more interesting and maintains attention more easily, particularly when the students have some basic knowledge of the topic. Films and videos or CDs can be useful when teaching practical methods. Self-learning by reading, computer programs and the internet provide other important ways of learning. Practical training in the operating theatre is very important.

Anaesthesia simulators are being used more and more but are expensive to set up and run. Computer programmes are a simpler way to work through a series of choices in problem solving exercises.

There are certain key points in *lecturing*. Most peoples' concentration span may be limited to as little as 15 to 20 minutes unless the lecturer does something to maintain it. It may be even less after a good meal when it is sometimes difficult not to fall asleep!

A lecture should be built up from *basics to more complex* information. It should try to highlight the important points and any basic principles. In the same way as an anaesthetist gives extra boluses of drugs when the drug concentration falls, the lecturer has to give a "bolus" to raise the level of concentration. This can be achieved by an illustrative example, a relevant but not too funny anecdote, asking questions, showing a different slide or a segment of video. Very funny stories or pictures of a beautiful girl and handsome man sitting on a tropical beach with palm trees are distracting because they can cause the audience to think about them rather than listen to the following part of the lecture! An alternative is to divide the lecture into shorter sections so that questions or discussion can take place when arousal is needed. As drugs which are given by a constant infusion maintain the drug concentration in the blood so there are a few people who are "infusion lecturers". These people are so fascinating that they can maintain the audiences concentration for long periods. Lecturing therefore has similarities to anaesthesia.

It does not seem rational at congresses and refresher courses to have long 50 to 60 minute lectures — they are very hard to concentrate and listen to one after another for hours. A good lecturer who has the ability to pick out the important points can usually convey them in 20 to 30 minutes.

Visual aids are useful especially for people who are visual learners, which includes most the vast majority of anaesthetists. Slides should have key points only and NOT long sentences. The information on a slide should not exceed five or six lines and should be presented in large clear letters using appropriate colour combinations. White or yellow on plain blue or green backgrounds are usually clear. Red and purple tend not to show up well. Computer generated slides can fall into traps — bad colour combinations, fancy backgrounds which may look nice but do not make the message any clearer, and too much information. Centre the information on the slide and use the whole space. Check for misteaks! It is easy to miss spelling mistakes when making slides.

Complex tables and diagrams, which cannot be absorbed in the short time they are displayed, should be avoided. Often the writing is too small to read. The most essential information can be extracted and stated simply. There is nothing worse than the speaker putting up a complex table and then saying that this is a rather busy slide. It means that he has been too lazy or not bothered to extract the essential information and present it separately. He should be removed from the podium!

Dual projection is often badly used. Fortunately it is becoming less commonly used since the advent of computer presentations. There is no point in having two slides so that more information can be projected at the same time. It can be very distracting to have a fancy title slide on one side and the information on the other. The distracter will do just that. Dual projection is useful when one side has the explanation of an illustration on the other.

The laser pointer is often badly used. A shaking hand with the laser point wobbling all over the slide is very distracting. It is insulting to intelligent people to point to all the words in a long text as if the audience is in Grade 1, just learning to read. There shouldn't be long texts anyway. Keep the pointer still and use it to highlight the point under discussion or to show something in a diagram and then turn it off.

Delivery is extremely important in making a good presentation. The speaker should speak clearly, vary the tone and pitch and, most importantly, PAUSE after making an important point so that the audience has time to think about the point and absorb it. If there is no pause when an important or new point is made the audience has to make a choice. They have to continue listening and possibly forget the point, or think about the information and absorb it but lose track of the lecture. The rate of presentation can be crucial. If it is too fast, without pauses or any punctuation, the audience may absorb very little of it. *So many lectures with good content are ruined by failing to follow these guidelines.* Too slow can be boring. It is very important to SPEAK SLOWLY when talking to a mixed language audience and where the lecture is being simultaneously translated. Many people can follow another language if it is presented slowly but not if it is spoken too fast. Translators need time to translate especially when the second language takes longer to say the same thing, which is often the case in relation to English.

Tutorials are a very useful form teaching, especially when the students already have some knowledge of the subject. There are some important points about running them.

There are usually some people who want to dominate the discussion. They have to be gently suppressed. Often they are knowledgeable and are useful when the more complex or detailed information is being sought. They can be held back to provide that. On the other hand some are reserved and try not to be noticed. They need to be encouraged to contribute. One method of encouraging participation is to ask a question with a numerical answer. If several answers are given the group is asked to vote on the numbers. When the students realize that the tutor does not mind if they don't know the correct answer as long as they know it by the end they will become involved in the discussion more easily. Shy students usually take a seat at the back while the talker usually sits right in front of the teacher. In big groups the tutor can move back and forth to overcome this situation. A small group can sit in a semicircle.

When asking questions it is important not to point to someone and then ask the question. They immediately become stressed and have a sympathetic nervous response. This includes a rise in pulse rate and blood pressure, proportionately more blood goes to the muscles, which don't think, and less to the brain and then the person cannot easily come up with the answer. Meanwhile everyone else is relaxed because they have not been asked the question. *It is better to ask the question, let everyone think and then indicate who should answer.*

Don't go round the group in regular sequence asking questions because the person being questioned and the next one will be stressed and the others can virtually go to sleep! *Ask the questions in a random order* and then they all have to remain attentive.

The *summary answer tutorial* was a method I devised about 1970. The students are given a question on a topic related to the tutorial. They are given 5 minutes to prepare a summary answer. The headings can then be presented by several of the students so all aspects can be covered and then more questioning can elucidate the extra detail. The advantages of this method are that all the students have to activate their brains and work to full capacity for the first five minutes. They then all have something to refer to for answers and so are not stressed when questioned. The students also provide most of the subject matter for the tutorial and the tutor only has to act as a catalyst and add detail or clarify points. In the end they have a logical answer which could be useful in a written or oral examination or could be used later when they become teachers. Everybody is involved and because they have had to think they also benefit more from the discussion. The extension of the process is that the students can use the method to run their own group discussions, because they are contributing most of the material anyway.

While running a two-week full time course on physiology and pharmacology I developed another important concept for teaching people who are preparing for non competitive examinations. It is the *seventy per cent principle.* The important point is for the students to comfortably reach the pass mark with some to spare. This requires a good understanding of the basic principles and how to apply them. It then requires some extra knowledge but not an immense amount of detail. Too much detail often confuses the student, Particularly if he/she cannot see the wood for the trees. The bright people will probably be able to learn the extra detail by themselves, although one's teaching may give them fresh insights. The aim should then be to concentrate on lifting the 40 to 50 per cent candidates up to 60 to 70 per cent.

When I was a student, Willy Tulloch was our Professor of Bacteriology. He was already old and regaled us with tales of how he had worked with Bruce of brucellosis fame. Tulloch smoked like a chimney, coughed and huffed and puffed but seemed indestructible. He understood people. One day, during a lecture he told us "not to believe everything that (stop for a breath) books say." During his pause I muttered "that Professors say." My neighbours laughed and he asked what the joke was. I had to tell him what I said. He thumped the desk and said "You are quite right, you are quite right." Years later, when I learnt to appraise information more critically, I realized that his comments might have been the most useful thing I learnt at university. How often do we read or are we taught things which critical analysis and commonsense would show us are nonsense?

For instance, many paediatric anaesthesia books about infants tell anaesthetists that babies are obligatory nose breathers. For years I could not understand what this had to do with anaesthesia. It seemed as if it affected how we ventilated them. Of course babies are obligatory nose breathers because they have to breathe through their nose when they are breast feeding. It isn't really of any importance in anaesthesia because it is actually easier to ventilate them when their mouths are open. I try to provoke my students to think and challenge concepts. Some facts are untrue, others vary depending on circumstances. The human body with which we deal in our work is very finely modulated by various feedback loops governing its function but these can vary with circumstances. Facts often need some plasticity because the values given as facts can vary with certain factors. We have to know these variations if they have clinical relevance.

When planning a teaching or training programme the *aims and objectives* should be defined first. What is to be taught and how is it to be taught and learned? When this has been defined there should be an assessment to determine whether the student has accomplished the task satisfactorily. This may take the form of an examination or maybe a practical or oral assessment. Failure indicates that the student has not achieved the standard but it may also result from the examination not assessing the content of the Aims and Objectives, or that the course has been poorly taught. The latter points should be considered if many candidates fail.

The Australasian Faculty of Anaesthetists was the forerunner in our specialty when they produced an Aim and Objectives of Training in 1976. Don Harrison and Graham Fisk with an educationalist, Max Dunstan, in Sydney did the bulk of the writing and a number of others, including myself, reviewed this important document. It laid out in some detail all that had to be covered during training.

Practical training is vitally important in anaesthesia. Ideally trainees should work under direct supervision until they reach a reasonable level of competence. As training progresses they can be allowed to work on their own but should have expert assistance readily available in case there are any difficult or complicated cases. The progress should be a gradual progression towards working independently and becoming self reliant.

Practical training can occur by observation but being actively shown how to do procedures is better. I gradually developed methods to teach which depended on analysing the technique into steps so that the most ergonomically efficient way is demonstrated. Using these methods some fairly complex manoeuvres can be taught to relatively inexperienced people in a few minutes. These can also be shown on films, videos or CDs.

Discussion can occur while the operation progresses but it is important that the patient and monitors are always being observed. This means that one cannot look at the other person all the time while talking as usually happens during conversation. Teaching cannot occur if the teacher is absent from the operating theatre.

I had several people sent for training on setting up teaching programmes. I now teach all the fellows coming through the department. My approach with them was to discuss this under six headings.

1. Aims and Objectives

2. How to teach — tutorials and lectures, etc.

3. How to organize the training program — content, timing including freedom from clinical duties during teaching sessions. This requires rostering of other staff to do the work.

4. Learning and modalities which can be used — books, computers, internet etc, videos, CDs.

5. In-theatre teaching, including practical procedures. Careful rostering can enhance this by giving trainees blocks in different specialties.

6. Assessment — ongoing, in theatre, and examinations — methods — written, multiple choice (which I do not like), oral and clinical.

Another important point is to train the trainers so that the teaching is more effective.

The feedback from one department was that it had changed from having difficulty attracting enough residents to one where many people wanted to train. That was very gratifying.

The choice of topic for a lecture or what to teach at a course requires thought about who you are teaching. When the audience has a wide range from beginners to knowledgeable people it is wise to begin simply and gradually develop the more complex ideas. High powered research is best presented to high powered researchers who can provide stimulating feedback and discussion.

When one is preparing a course for anaesthetists in a less advanced country the content must be relevant to their practice and not what is done in some very academic department. Teaching basic science in relation to practical anaesthesia provides a good basis for understanding. Teaching practical procedures — how to do it — is useful. Regional and local anaesthesia with the related anatomy fits this category well. Case discussions, particularly ones with which they have had problems, are very helpful. I remember an islander, describing a problem with a caesarean section, concluding with "the patient died". He didn't know why. Another time in Africa the anaesthetist told me how a patient had died in the corridor because they had no recovery room. "What could she do?" was her anguished question. Discussion of the problems and how they might be avoided or overcome is always very worthwhile. I always try to present something of practical value in my lectures.

Film, video or CDs can be useful teaching tools, which should be used more often in teaching sessions and anaesthetic meetings for this purpose, because so much of our work is practical. Film and video production for teaching purposes has been one of my special interests, as photography is one of my hobbies.

First one needs to decide what is to be demonstrated and then how it is to be done. A script should be written so that the correct material is filmed. Usually much more is taken than needed so that a choice of the best illustration can be used. I personally had about 3 to 5 times what is needed while professionals tend to be much more extravagant. I think wastage can be minimized if the shots are carefully planned. This takes experience. During the editing various points may need to be highlighted with, for example, arrows or dots. Titles need to be consistent. Imaginative presentation and quality photographic shots enhance films greatly. Some humour draws the audience in to listen. The video should be kept concise and not long winded because the audience will lose concentration — the same problem as arises in long lectures. Another advantage with video is that the commentary can be recorded in several languages. With DVD it will be possible to switch from one to another.

Editing is time consuming, taking about an hour for each minute of the final production, but is immensely satisfying if a good production results. My first films were 16mm, which required tedious cutting to the length of the script and joining each segment. The end result was a high quality image which is not achieved with video. The introduction of video with computer editing has simplified the process, just as word processing made manuscript typing more efficient. Advances continue so that now the video can be transferred to CD or DVD, which are much easier to transport than the old, heavy 16 mm film or even video. This should make them much more accessible as a teaching aid around the world. If they are put on web sites their availability increases immensely.

I made four 16mm films with the Photographic Department in the Hospital. The last one was *Lives can be saved*. A representative from the Laerdal company brought one of their self inflating resuscitation bags to show me. I suggested a film would be useful and when he agreed I offered to make it for him. When I thought about it I realized that a film just about the bag and how it worked would be very boring. So I decided to show it in situations where it would be used. The first was a little child in a drowning scene. The pool gate had been fixed open. We then showed a gate being carefully shut. Then my nine year old son rode his bicycle down the footpath beside our house. My daughter backed our VW Kombi out. On the first take he reached within 30 cm of the Kombi which had just stopped. He fell sideways on to the ground as if he had been hit and lay as if seriously injured. At the time he played war games in the street and frequently fell "dead". Minutes later the Director of Intensive Care (Alan Duncan) arrived in his big red Mercedes and just happened to have a Laerdal resuscitator in the back of his car. There are scenes showing cardiopulmonary resuscitation with Ken as the subject. After showing one rather washed out video copy someone asked me where I got the cadaver to film! He managed to act well and keep very still! In the final scene I collapsed while jogging round the park. Two people (Cathy and Fraser) appeared. One went to the road nearby to get help. The big red Mercedes arrived again. (laughter) Alan leapt out and rushed over with his resuscitator. While the commentary is saying that 'the outlook is bad if resuscitation is not begun soon' the camera zoomed up with the telephoto lens to the tombstones in the cemetery next door. For musical background I recorded the bird song in the early morning which is intense in October and November in Melbourne.

I scripted, supervised the filming and did all the cutting and pasting myself. It was a much more time consuming and difficult job with dozens of strips of film hanging on the wall than video editing which came in soon after.

When a video unit was set up I was asked to be on the selection panel. We interviewed 12 out of 50 applicants. I gave them the resuscitator and asked then how they would make a film to demonstrate it. Only half said they would show it in use in the introduction.

I made many teaching videos. Several were on nerve blocks which showed the anatomy with the dissections which we had done. Some were on paediatric anaesthesia and one was how to intubate infants. Another classic was on fire training in the operating theatres. It is a potentially boring subject which we managed to make very funny using shots taken of staff being randomly asked questions on fire topics — where were the fire extinguishers, the alarms, how would you organize the training. It was amazing how few had noticed fire extinguishers which they walked past every day. As the morning went on staff realized that questions were being asked about fire equipment and so they went round looking to see where it was, many for the first time. By the end of our morning of random questioning and filming of the responses, the staff's knowledge had increased about 500%! It helped us to pass hospital accreditation.

Good videos, films or action CD's should show the message clearly, have some fun in them to keep the audience's attention, not be too long and have good photographic shots. In fact the principles are similar to good lecturing.

John Stocks had some notes which he hoped to convert into a book but he died before he accomplished the task. Graham Fisk (25) from Sydney and I decided we would continue with the plan, so with great help from Graham and many colleagues, we produced the first paediatric anaesthetic textbook in Australia in 1979 — *Anaesthesia for Children.* The result was somewhat different to John's notes, but we achieved what we set out to do — to produce a comprehensive book which was easy to read, not too long winded and illustrated to show how to perform many of the practical procedures used in anaesthesia. It took three years to write. For some years it was the main text on the subject. It was translated into Spanish and German.

I am sure it helped me to become better known around the world. In Argentina a young lady approached me as I was going up some stairs at a congress. She asked, "Are you Dr Brown who wrote the book?" "Yes," I said. She went on and said that she had studied it during her training and that it was her ambition to meet me. I was rather taken aback and could only reply that she had achieved her ambition that day. She came from Resistencia in far north Argentina. The book was used all over the world. Someone else came to work with me because the ideas expressed coincided with his much more than those of his colleagues.

Writing a book is a challenge. One has to agree with a co-author that complete frankness is necessary and that offence must not be taken on any comment even if it is that a chapter is no good! Graham was an excellent co-author because he was critical, knowledgeable and grammatically good. His comments were all dictated as the manuscript was typed — there were no computers and word processors then. What a difference they have made. I noticed that his comments were more benign when he was sitting on the verandah with birds singing than when he was inside with music in the background!

We wrote a second edition which was published in 1992, but by then several other books on the subject had become available. Elsewhere I have mentioned my small book written for students and nurses called "*Anaesthesia and Patient Care*". I contributed to "*A manual of acute pain management in children*" which our department produced jointly with Adelaide Childrens Hospital and to chapters in many other books. I wrote a chapter in a prominent textbook (2nd edition) and was rather amused, but disappointed, to receive a letter later on saying that a third edition was going to be produced but that only people in full time practice were going to be asked to contribute so I would not be asked. I was still in full time practice and probably spent more time giving anaesthetics than many of the other contributors. I had a suggestion for a colleague who could take over my chapter but an American had already been selected. Such is life. An unfortunate mistake had been made because he wrote too much. This chapter eventually held publication up for a year.

Some other aspects of teaching are mentioned in other chapters of this book. The ideas presented here are the distillation of many years' experience. It has been exciting to help other to teach better. When two professors came up to me at a conference asking for comments on their lectures because they had tried to incorporate some of my ideas, I had a sense of fulfillment. On another occasion I was rather stunned when a lady who had spoken before me at a meeting where I spoke on this subject, came up and tossed all her slides in a bag and said "Now I will start again!" Another, who had heard the lecture told me years later that she had made her slides according to my suggestions. The message was getting through. The problem is that many famous speakers do not attend this talk. Many of them think they know it all because they are famous but spoil a very informative lecture by breaking basic rules.

One of the most fulfilling aspects of my career has been having the chance to teach and inspire others, particularly the younger generation. I have always been happy to spend time talking and encouraging them as they are the future practitioners and teachers. At some congresses, where the local trainees have been helping with tasks necessary for running the meeting, I have offered to run a teaching session for them as a way of showing my appreciation and as reward for their work, which may have prevented them attending sessions. I received very enthusiastic feedback from some of these, such as once in Florence at the European Congress, because they had never been taught my way before. Hopefully having exposed them to forms of teaching where there is more interaction they will try these methods when their turn comes to be the teachers.

Chapter 16

Overseas Visits and Paediatric Anaesthetic Meetings

In this chapter I will tell about some of my trips and conferences where I met many paediatric anaesthetists — it will tell something about some of the mainly older ones now or have some of their photographs.

I was fortunate to have worked in Vancouver and Toronto before I came to Melbourne so that I had developed a wider view of paediatric anaesthesia than those who had only worked in one place. After six years at the Childrens Hospital in Melbourne I was entitled to some sabbatical leave. I had decided before John Stocks died, to go to Britain and Europe and visit some other centres. The Hospital thought that I should go anyway even though I had just taken over the department.

During this trip in 1974 I attended the European Congress of Anesthesiology in Madrid. It was my first big congress and I had a problem because I knew the names of people who I wanted to meet but did not know who they were and had nobody to introduce me. One day I decided I would just introduce myself to the three people sitting on the only bench in the large foyer. The older man turned out to be Toivo (known to his friends as Topi) Suutarinen who was the father of paediatric anaesthesia in Finland. He immediately invited me to visit him but I was not able to do so until my next trip in 1977. We became good friends and he later came to one of our meetings in Melbourne. He had two young ladies with him. Twenty years later I met one of them again in Iceland. I told her how I had visited Finland several times and how this had come about. She then told me that she was with Topi in Madrid in 1974! It is amazing how one can discover things if the conversation is directed in a certain way and yet many conversations between the same people might not have elucidated the information.

Before going to Madrid I asked to meet a paediatric anaesthetist. Manuel de Luna Infante, befriended me and looked after me, taking me to see his hospital and visit his home. I found out that he also painted — he liked to copy Goya. Later I invited him to write the foreward for the Spanish edition of our book *Anaesthesia for Children*. I was sorry to hear that he died young, from a massive heart attack.

My colleague, Helene Wood, and I went to Madrid early so we had two days to tour around before the Congress. We visited El Escorial with its magnificent tapestries and paintings, including several magnificent portraits by Ribera; the great underground sanctuary at Valle de los Caidos, Segovia with its great Roman aqueduct, and the walled town of Avilla where we spent the night. Our large rooms cost $2 each — how prices have risen!

The next day was hot. We were driving across country and eventually stopped for some refreshment. Our lack of Spanish resulted in us being given anchovy sandwiches! We continued to Toledo, a most interesting city where we saw some of the famous El Greco paintings. I developed a special interest in Spanish art. I had read up about the great Spanish painters before going on this trip. Some of Ribera's portraits are among my favorites. I also had two visits to the Prado, Madrid's famous art gallery where I saw Velazquez' *Las Meninas*, one of the world's most famous paintings. There were also two by David Teniers which attracted my attention — an operation being performed on the head and 'the monkeys tea party' where monkeys were imitating humans! He must have had a sense of humour.

I travelled extensively on that trip. I visited Peter Dangel in Zurich. He was interested in intensive care and flew helicopters on retrievals. I persuaded him to do a study relating to PEEP on one of his patients. Later I found out that he had other interests — flowers and fishing.

Hans Feychting in Stockholm was well known for his intensive care work. He always had a thoughtful look about him as he puffed on his pipe. He became involved in the international standards for anaesthetic equipment. The father of Swedish paediatric anaesthesia was Alvar Swenson who had visited Melbourne in 1970. I found him to be a very thoughtful, gentle man who had great concern about how children were handled.

In Paris I visited the toxicology clinic at Hôpital Fernand Widal in St. Denis. I was impressed by its size and activity. It was the biggest such clinic that I ever came across. I went there to discuss my antidepressant work with Dr C.Bismuth and Professor Gaultier. They seemed to think that the reversion of arrhythmias caused by the tricyclic antidepressant group of drugs was due to the sodium rather than lactate or bicarbonate when these were given. My work demonstrated to the contrary. It was clearly the bicarbonate.

I was looked after by Pierre Carlo who had visited us in Melbourne. He introduced me to the concept that parenteral nutrition, which contained the essential nutritional requirements for intravenous use in very sick patients, can be economically justified. It was very expensive but because the patients had fewer days in intensive care and hospital the overall costs were reduced. He took me to visit the makers of gammahydroxybutyrate as I had made a film about its use in microlaryngeal surgery and wanted to encourage them to get it into Australia. Afterwards he took me to see one of the most dynamic men I ever met — Laborit. He introduced chlorpromazine in 1960 to suppress the stress response to surgery. He was a personal friend of Hans Selye from Montreal who had written extensively on the stress response. Laborit had a large laboratory and even produced his own journal (37). I often thought he deserved to be considered

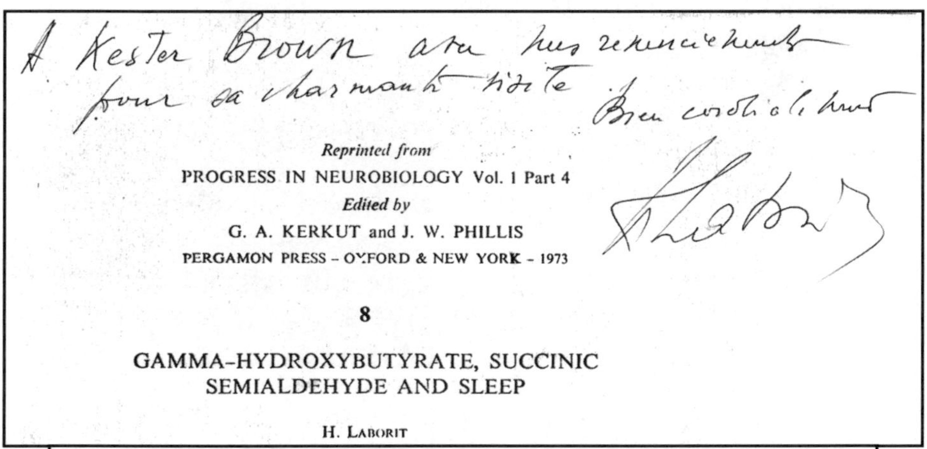

Reprinted from
PROGRESS IN NEUROBIOLOGY Vol. 1 Part 4
Edited by
G. A. KERKUT and J. W. PHILLIS
PERGAMON PRESS – OXFORD & NEW YORK – 1973

8

GAMMA-HYDROXYBUTYRATE, SUCCINIC SEMIALDEHYDE AND SLEEP

H. LABORIT

37. Paper autographed by Laborit in 1974.

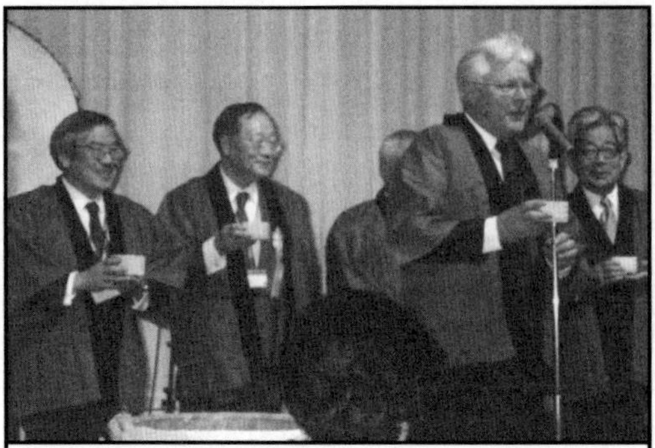

38. Sten Lindahl, Professor in Stockholm and former chairman of the Nobel prize in Medicine and Physiology committee. He is seen here at the Japanese Society of Anaesthesiologists Congress in Fukuoka, 2002, at the saki opening ceremony. Behind left : Kazuo Hanaoka (WFSA Executive), Ryo Ogawa (former treasurer , Asian Australasiann Region of WFSA) and right a Nobel Prize winner in Literature.

for the Nobel Prize, having introduced the first of the huge family of drugs which became the basis of psychopharmacology, chlorpromazine. I met Sten Lindahl from Stockholm (38), in Iceland at a Scandinavian Congress and was telling him this but that I did not know how people were nominated. He was on the committee so said I should write to them. I left him and as I walked across the hall I met a French lady anaesthetist who came from Paris. I asked her if she knew of Laborit? "Yes" she said, " He died last year." So I was too late.

I found Paris to be a wonderful city during my visit there. The highlight was attending a Bach cello recital in Sainte Chapelle (39) and then returning in daylight to see the beautiful windows between the soaring Gothic arches. I think it is one of the most beautiful buildings that I have seen. I walked many kilometres absorbing the sights and visiting places like the Louvre and the Rodin museum with all his wonderful sculptures.

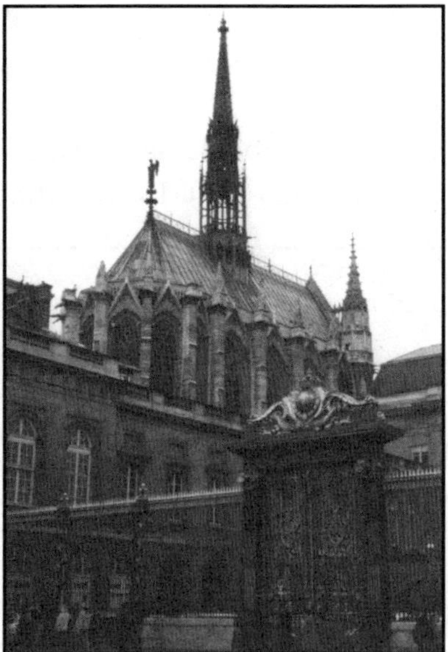

39. Sainte Chapelle in Paris with the gates of Palais de Justice in the foreground.

In Britain I visited Great Ormond Street Hospital for Sick Children where I met Bob Cope again and was introduced to such eminent paediatric anaesthetists as Bill Glover (41), David Hatch (40) and Ted Battersby. Liverpool was a sort of Mecca in those days with Jackson Rees (Figure C9), Gordon Bush (28), Allan Stead, Tony Nightingale and others all there. Jack spent the first day assessing me and on the second morning when he picked me up he asked if I could write a chapter for a book he was editing, *Current trends in paediatric anaesthesia.* He had asked John Stocks to write on prolonged intubation and tracheotomy, but John had died so I agreed, but then he wanted it in a month. I said I wouldn't be home in time to do that but would let him have it in 2 months as I had some experience in the area and had all John's papers to refer to. After a while I learnt that Jack was a great man, an inspiration to many people but he was not strong on writing. The book was finally published seven years later, and only after Professor Cecil Grey had come in to help.

I recognised Gordon Bush as one of the leaders, and it was he who had written the article on suxamethonium in burns which had stimulated my interest in that subject. I invited him to be the first overseas visitor to a paediatric anaesthetic meeting I was organizing the following year. Years later I was asked to be Editor of Paediatric Anaesthesia but I was not suited to such a position and did not have time anyway so Gordon took it on and gave it a great start.

I had met Gordon McDowell in Madrid and arranged to visit Leeds. I told him my interests and I think he was surprised that I had so many. I had a very interesting time there. Denis Smith (62) took me to an exhibition of the 200th anniversary of the manufacture of oxygen by Priestley. Now it is thought that Scheele in Sweden preceded him. He also took me to see Walton Hall, the home of Charles Waterton whom I discussed in Chapter 4. Denis Smith and Richard Ellis ran a very good teaching program. Richard was also interested in Malignant Hyperpyrexia (a potentially lethal condition with high temperatures during anaesthesia). Later both he and Gordon McDowell came to Australia as ASA visitors.

Several years later I did a paediatric workshop in Leeds with John Inkster and Peter Morris. Afterwards Richard took me hiking on the Yorkshire Dales. He had a farmhouse up there. We climbed Ingleborough on a cold March day. On the top the snow lying packed on the ground was fluted by the wind. It was a great outing as I loved hill walking when I was young. In his younger days he had been a keen on exploring caves. Later Richard became a member of the Royal College of Anaesthetists Council in London.

I visited John Inkster (28) at the little Fleming Hospital in Newcastle where he did a lot of neonatal work. The morning I was there they did an oesophageal atresia repair. John was an obsessive and very good anaesthetist who was recognised as one of the top in the country With the biomedical engineers they had made a neonatal ventilator based on fluid logic and what was essentially a PEEP valve. He had also developed an oesophageal stethoscope with an ECG electrode on attached to it. His equipment was organized exactly as he wanted because there were only two anaesthetists at the hospital, unlike our large department where things had to be standardised to cater for a large number of anaesthetists working in seven theatres. We became very good friends. He too visited Australia. In later years he sent me a diet which said that I should encourage my friends to eat more so that they would get fatter and that would make me look thinner!

In Edinburgh I met David Grubb, who told me that they intubated their patients with epiglottitis sometimes for as short a time as 2-3 hours, which was much less than anyone else at the time. Of course he was right to advocate a shorter time than the 12-24 hours most people used, if the swelling has started to reduce by then. They had to re-intubate one patient. In my view something in between was a sensible compromise.

These visits were invaluable, as I was meeting anaesthetists, especially some of the paediatric fraternity. I made some very good friends among them. Later, I invited several of them to come to Australia to visit and lecture. They provided me with many useful ideas, making the visits worthwhile interchanges.

My next trip was in 1977 when my daughters, Catherine and Maryann, who were fifteen, accompanied me for part of the trip. We went to Kenya, Rome and Munich.

I then visited Ottheinz Schulte Steinberg (24) who was a leader in caudal anaesthesia in children in nearby Starnberg, south of Munich. It is an attractive town situated on a lake of the same name. It was there that I met Frank Wagner, who later came to work with me. Ottheinz, a tall, balding, fit looking man and I had remarkable similarities in our lives. We both spent years of our youth in East Africa and after graduation in medicine both went to Canada to intern, then did country general practice in the north before beginning anaesthesia, he in Montreal and me in Vancouver. Then we found that we had both done a similar study injecting radio-opaque dye in the caudal canal to see how far it spread. The only other similar study was done in Auckland by Cedric Hoskins.

On this trip I spent a most enjoyable six days in Helsinki with Topi Suutarinen (26, Figure C7) whom I had met in Madrid in 1974. I visited hospitals. I think the Childrens Hospital there was one of the most impressive I came across in Europe. They had an excellent surgeon then named Lohimo. Topi took me to sauna where I experienced the change from 109° in the sauna to 4° when we entered the sea immediately afterwards. He had an artificial leg from a war injury so had to change to a wooden one which would not become so hot in the sauna. I saw a film on blood pressure telemetry once which showed the blood pressure rising to over 300 mmHg when entering the cold pool after sauna. Finns with weak arteries must succumb early! I was also taken to the studio of their most famous artist, Akseli Gallen Kallela, where I found myself looking at a painting of Mt Kenya painted not far from where I was brought up. I was amazed when I found out that he had spent a year painting in Kenya in 1909, which was very early in the period of white settlement.

On this trip I also visited North America. I attended the Paediatric Anaesthetic meeting in Toronto. It was my first visit back for 12 years. In Toronto up to that time they had treated epiglottitis by passing a brochoscope and then doing a tracheotomy over it. This seemed to me, after my experience in Melbourne, an unnecessary approach when passing an endotracheal tube for a few hours sufficed. When I told them that we did this under halothane anaesthesia, with some positive pressure on the airway. I received considerable applause. I think they changed their approach in Toronto after that.

I visited Massachusetts General Hospital in Boston. I never met my supposed host. He was off duty and had obviously forgotten that I was coming. Fortunately Michael Davies, who had been a registrar with us, was working there and organized my visit. I had a good day and met Nick Goudzousian who had a special interest in muscle relaxants, Ian Todres in Intensive Care and Jeff Cooper , their engineer who did the interesting work on human errors in anaesthesia and designed a machine to eliminate them. Unfortunately they sold it to a company who suppressed it and never produced this valuable machine.

I should have gone to Philadelphia but I was tiring of travel so went on to Denver to see someone with a common interest in safety packaging of drugs. I then went on to Vancouver to see my relatives before returning home. I was just in time to see my uncle, three days before he died.

I was invited to join the Association of Paediatric Anaesthetists (APA) which was a British organization, when they first allowed overseas members. These could not exceed the number of home members. I think it had 47 members when I joined. Unfortunately I only managed to attend four of their

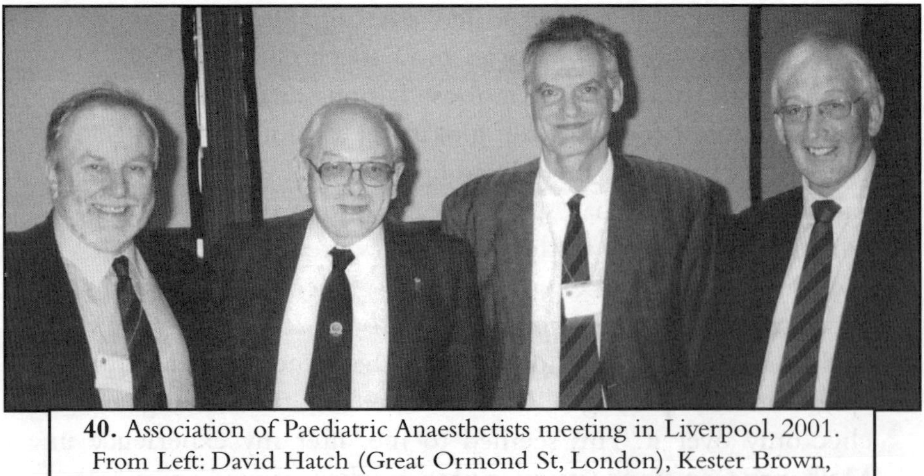

40. Association of Paediatric Anaesthetists meeting in Liverpool, 2001. From Left: David Hatch (Great Ormond St, London), Kester Brown, Ted Sumner (GOS, London — incoming President), Douglas Arthur from Glasgow (President).

regular meetings — in Aberdeen (1984), Dublin (1985), Newcastle (2000) and Liverpool in 2001 when they conferred honorary membership on David Hatch and me (40).

Their meetings are usually in March which is not an attractive time to visit Britain. I tried unsuccessfully to get them to change it. I was more successful in getting them to change the President's term from three to two years, allowing more of their eminent members to hold office. In addition, three years is a long time to hold a senior office.

The Dublin meeting was a rather special being held in May. After it, my wife, Janet (Figures C28) and I we went to Galway with Topi and Pirjo Suutarinren and Olli Meretoja and Eija, all from Finland. Our car was upgraded to one that could carry five people comfortably but six? Anyway ,we all went together because the others could not get another car. "It is the weekend, you know." the lady told them when they asked! Bill Wren, the leading paediatric anaesthetist in Dublin, had arranged fancy accommodation at Casheil House for Topi but not for the rest of us. When we all arrived the lady was rather distressed. No rooms. I said "Not to worry. We would find a B and B." That distressed her more but then, after some careful consideration, she said she had rooms in the cottage, which used to be the staff quarters. They turned out to be fine, even having en suite bathrooms. It was a beautiful place with rhododendrons in full bloom all round the spectacular garden with a stream running through it. I went out to paint and ended up doing a watercolour in the soft Irish rain sitting under an umbrella! Ireland is the only place where one would do that! When we returned to Dublin we visited Bill Wren at his hospital. When I discussed the fast cars taking the middle lane on a dual carriageway, and a tractor appearing out of a field without warning, he said that he meant to warn us that they drive in the middle of the road and that the tractors regard the roads as part of their fields. No wonder there are Irish jokes!

I had many such trips although none as long as the first two, which each lasted ten weeks. Sitting idly in an airport recently, I counted that I had visited at least 80 childrens hospitals around the world. I had met many interesting people and learnt things from many of them. I occasionally saw some awful surgery, but also some very interesting operations. If one is receptive one can absorb much information in a short time. I also had the opportunity to teach. If one can make several visits to a hospital they become more effective. I was invited to Mendoza in Argentina to give a symposium. Once they knew what I could teach them they invited me back. I had an opportunity between meetings in Cordoba and Santiago so went for two days and was able to guide them through eight nerve blocks. I had a further opportunity to return when I had been to the Argentinian Congress in Mendoza. I showed them some more nerve blocks and was just about to leave when a child with burns came for skin grafting. I offered to demonstrate the leg blocks so the surgeon was asked if he minded. He sat and watched. I felt he thought he had been pushed but when I told him that I had been doing burn anaesthesia for twenty years he suddenly became quite animated and interested. He realized that I knew what I was doing. During my visits I had seen a number of burn units — in Montevideo, Buenos Aires, Cost Rica and Bombay. In the latter I learnt that they used sterilised potato skin laid on bandages for dressings for fresh burns. What was interesting was that these could be changed without anaesthetic or sedation suggesting they have some analgesic (pain relieving) property.

One can visit people, go to conferences or bring outstanding people to your hospital for a meeting. Seeing people in their own environment with time to talk and discuss things with them is probably the most useful way to learn and pick up ideas. In Beijing I saw five epidurals inserted during my short visit to the Childrens Hospital. It is no wonder that the Chinese can report a series of 10,000 cases, as one of their anaesthetists did at a World Congress.

On my trips I was always on the look out for good speakers who I could invite to our meetings in Melbourne and potential ASA visitors. John Stocks had organized one for the Hospital Centenary following the Asian Australasian Congress in Canberra in 1970. After I became director I organized one every three or four years. The first was in 1975 when Gordon Bush came as guest speaker.

Our next meeting was in 1979 (26) when I invited John Inkster and Topi Suutarinen. Before the meeting I took them to the ASA meeting in Adelaide via the coast to see the great cliffs, arches and pillars carved by the sea in Port Campbell National Park. We had lunch on the second day at a little place called Robe. After lunch John was sitting in the front with me while the others had a siesta in the back. They found out that Topi and John's wife Eileen both had birthdays while we were to be in Adelaide. On the Sunday morning I met John who approached me in a state of humorous agitation and said " First that fellow Suutarinen slept in the back of your kombi with my wife and now he has appeared with flowers for her birthday before I have even remembered about it!!" John has a wonderful sense of humour.

On the way back we passed through the Grampians which is a range of big hills/mountains in Western Victoria. While on a walk a koala appeared and then its baby came rushing through the bushes and jumped on its back. On our return to Melbourne we launched our book, *Anaesthesia for Children*, which Graham Fisk and I had edited. John Inkster spoke at the launch.

In 1981 Topi Suutarinen (Figure C7) extended my idea of taking paediatric anaesthetists for a trip as well as attending a meeting. The paediatric anaesthetists tours have helped many of us to get to know each other much better. He invited the APA to Finland for a joint meeting with the Finnish Society. This was his retirement meeting. Those who could stay went on a week-long trip to East Finland. It was a simple trip where we travelled by train, bus and then a hired bus. We were met and looked after by the local anaesthetists in Kuopio and Joennsu. We visited the Russian border (the Cold War was still on) and then spent two nights at a biological research station. One day we visited a friend's fishing camp where some of the group fished. His friends put on the most amazing lunch with about a dozen different fish dishes. The other day we went down the rapids of a large river in big boats. We returned to Joennsu so that Topi could march with his regiment in the 40th anniversary parade from the winter war with Russia. During the trip we met a friend of Topi's who had been awarded the Mannerheim Cross for bravery during that war. The Finns lost some land but were not defeated. Topi was a hero amongst them, something like Weary Dunlop in Australia. It was a wonderful trip. I left them to proceed to Oulu for a visit with Arno Hollmen and then on by train, bus and boat to Narvik, Trondheim and Bergen and so to Oslo where I attended the Scandinavian Congress.

In 1982 Peter Morris and Ottheinz Schulte Steinberg (24) came as visitors. This time our meeting followed the ASA in Hobart so I took them over and had them speak at that meeting as well. We flew to Launceston and drove with Stewart Bath round the east coast, so that they could see some of the country. They were lucky to see a wombat while on a walk. It was amazing how most of my visitors saw some wild animal while travelling with me.

Whenever one of the senior paediatric anaesthetists was retiring from around the country I asked them to give a valedictory address, unless they were having their own meeting at home. Thus we honoured Tom Voss, who came to Australia after years as the leading paediatric anaesthetist in Capetown. He had a great range of experience.

Another was Tom Allen (23), Director at Adelaide Childrens Hospital and co-author of one of the first papers on prolonged intubation. He had spent many years in Fiji and I remember him telling me about premature infants surviving there without all the modern care.

Nerida Dilworth (26) was Director at Princess Margaret Childrens Hospital in Perth for 30 years. She was one of the few anaesthetists to become head of the surgical division in the hospital and she was also a prominent member of the Board of the Faculty of Anaesthetists for several years as well as being an examiner.

Each meeting we also had a John Stocks Memorial Lecture which was given usually by some one who had worked in the department, like Geoff Barker who went to Toronto, and Geoff Mullins who also went to Toronto and then became Director in Perth. The others, such as Bill Cole, Ian McDonald, Noel Cass, and Mary Dwyer (20), had been members of the department for many years.

In 1988 we invited the APA from Britain to join our meeting (41). At that time I had access to funds from WFSA, the ASA and our meeting. I therefore arranged for two of our visitors to stopover in Singapore, Bangkok, Kuala Lumpur, Hong Kong and Manila on their way to teach for a couple of days. Peter Morris and Roddy McNicol had an unsuccessful visit because a typhoon hit Manila while they were there. In addition, Fritz Berry from the USA visited Brisbane and Claude St Maurice and Marie Madeline Deleur from Paris visited Perth. They all

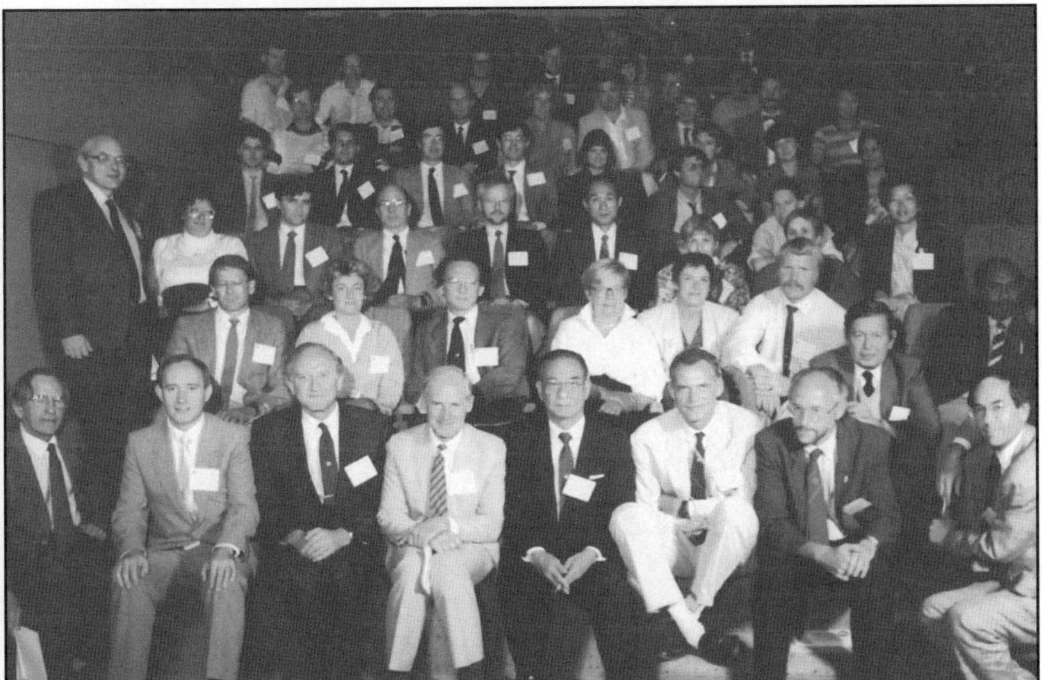

41. Visitors and Speakers at the 1988 Melbourne Paediatric Anaesthetic meeting. *Front row*: Ian MacDonald (RCH. Melbourne), George Meakin (Manchester, UK), Bill Glover (GOS. UK), Noel Cass (RCH), Jake Iwai (Japan), Ted Sumner (GOS, UK), Paulo Busoni (Florence, Italy), Rob Eyres (RCH). *2nd row*: Kester Brown (RCH — standing), Johan van der Walt (Adelaide), Marie Madeline Deleur (Paris), Mario Govaerts (Belgium), Barbro Ecstrom Jodal (Sweden), Angela Mackersie (GOS, UK), Bosie Bosenberg (South Africa), Claude St Maurice (Paris), Jaffat Fa'Arondo (Soloman Islands). *3rd row*: Dolly Hansen (Boston, USA), Peter Booker (Liverpool, UK), Fritz Berry (USA), Olli Meretoja (Finland), Genichi Susuki (Japan), ?, Brian Anderson (RCH and Auckland), Kim Ottaway (Auckland), Teresa Wong (Taiwan).

contributed at the ASA meeting and then to our meeting in Melbourne. In between there were two days during which I arranged for them to do a tour through the Grampians and back by the Great Ocean Road with all the magnificent coastal scenery (Figure C8). This trip was obviously a great success, as people still talked about it years later.

We had further meetings at RCH in 1991, 1995 for the Hospital 125th anniversary (43), 1996 as the Fourth World Paediatric Anaesthesia Conference (40), which has traditionally been associated or followed the World Congress, and in 2000

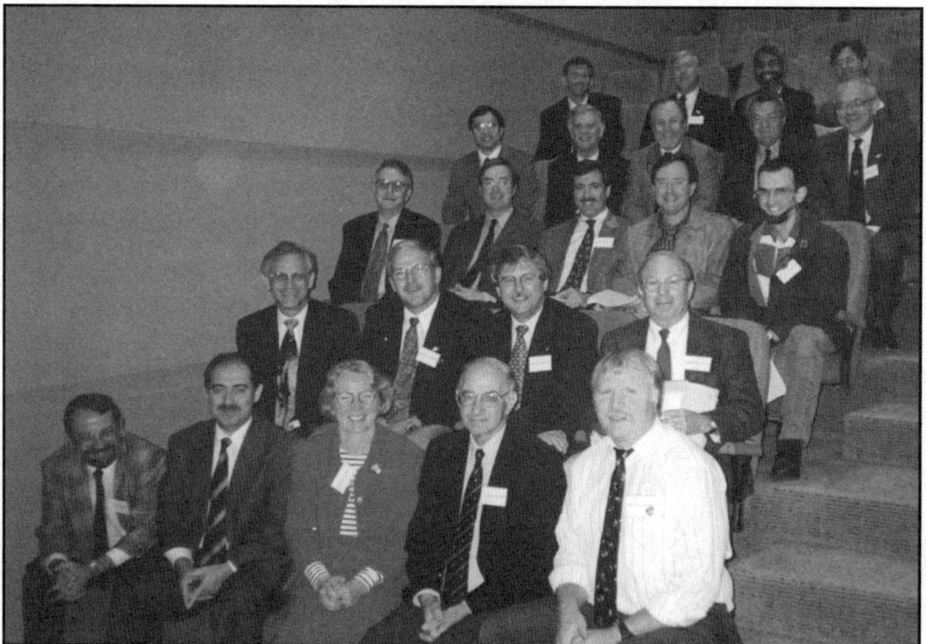

42. Melbourne — 4th World Paediatric Meeting following the 1996 World Congress in Sydney : *Front row*: Marcin Rawicz (Warsaw, Poland), Carlos Riquelme (Chile), Anneke Meursing (Rotterdam, Netherlands), David Steward (Los Angeles, USA), Adrain Bosenberg (South Africa). *2nd row*: Charlie Coté (Chicago, USA), Pierre Limoges (Montreal, Canada), Gerry Goresky (Calgary, Canada), Fritz Berry (USA). *3rd row*: Carlos a Silva (Florianopolis, Brazil), Peter Kempthorne (Christchurch, New Zealand), Jeff Moray (USA), David Baines (Sydney), Francis Veyckemans (Belgium). *4th row*: Masao Yamashita, (Japan), Peter Morris (UK) David Hatch (UK), Martin Marx (Uruguay), Kester Brown (RCH). *5th row*: Sergei Rajev (Moscow), John Overton (Sydney), Dilip Pawar (Delhi, India), Ian McKenzie (RCH).

when I retired. These meetings had significant overseas input.

In 1995 we had invited speakers from five continents — Krister Nilsson from Sweden, Carlos Riquelme from Chile, Kats Miyasaka from Japan, Adrian Bosenberg from South Africa and Estela Melman from Mexico (43). It made for an interesting program and discussion. Estela Melman spoke on foetal surgery and told us how cleft lips heal and do not leave a scar if repaired in utero. After a presentation about conjoined twins I asked the audience if anyone else had experience of this condition. Rob Eyres in our department had three. I was astounded when we found a total experience in the room of 27 cases. Maseo Yamashita from Japan had seen ten himself and Tom Voss had seen five when he was in Capetown.

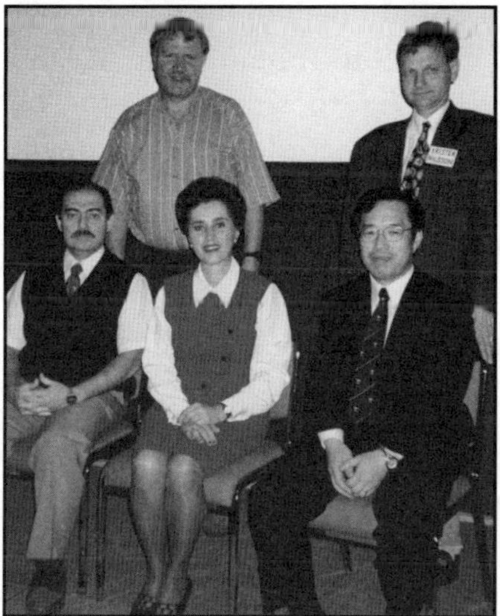

43. International speakers at the 1995 meeting. *Standing* L : Adrian (Bosie) Bosenberg, Krister Nilsson; *Sitting* : Carlos Riquelme, Estela Melman, Kats Miyasaka.

The 1996 meeting was rather special with people coming from many countries following the World Congress in Sydney (42). We had speakers from sixteen countries in a two day meeting.

My retirement meeting in 2000 drew a large crowd from 24 countries. The program was divided to have speakers from the department, from those who had worked with us from overseas and a session from other Australasian departments. It was a great meeting. They all had been scientifically stimulating over the years and were great occasions for Australian paediatric anaesthetists to get together. The photograph of those who had worked in the department with me shows what a wonderful send off I had when I retired as Director. (36)

I attended other paediatric anaesthetist meetings. Anneke

Meursing, after her time in our department arranged the first two European Paediatric Anaesthesia Congresses. I went to one she organised in Rotterdam. At dinner David Hatch and I went to the toilet where I found a most magnificent commode built like a throne. I was going to photograph it and asked David to sit on it.(44) The memorable record of this moment arrived in David's office when he was made professor at Great Ormond Street. "I hoped his new chair was as good as this one!"

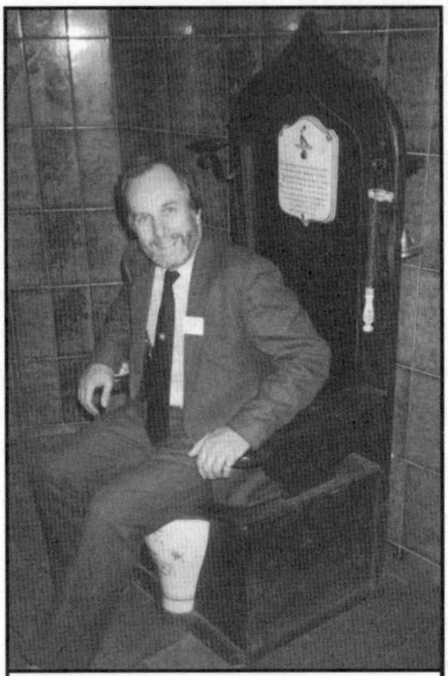
44. David Hatch

Congresses are occasions when we meet friends and colleagues. Some of these appear in the following photographs of well known paediatric anaesthetists. (45,46,47)

We had a delightful time visiting Helsinki again for another European Paediatric Anaesthetic Congress in 2001. Before it, I had a few days to spare, so went to Vilnius, Lithuania to run a workshop for them. Vidunas Daugelavicius had all my talks and slides translated so that the people could get the maximum out of the workshop. It was a wonderful visit to a city which was pulling itself out of the dullness of Soviet occupation and the people were so appreciative of my visit.

After the World Congress in Montreal in 2000 John Muir arranged a now traditional paediatric anaesthetists' tour for participants to be able to go by train and bus to Quebec City, Prince Edward Island and tour through Cape Breton Island in Nova Scotia to Halifax where we held the Fifth World Paediatric Anaesthesia meeting. A highlight was the arrival of an uninvited famous Canadian singer attracted by the lively Nova Scotian music at our dinner. He gave us a free rendition of some of his songs which greatly excited John Muir (who is a Scotsman)

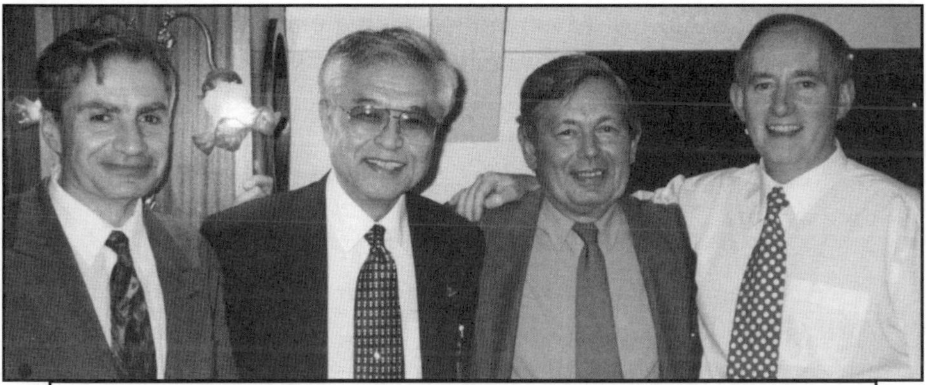

45. 1997 European Paediatric Congress, Paris which was Claude St. Maurice's farewell meeting. *From Left* : Nick Goudsouzian (M.G.H., Boston — an authority on muscle relaxants in children), E.K Motoyama (Pittsburgh, USA — author Smith's textbook), Claude St Maurice (St Vincent de Paul's Hospital, Paris — interested in regional anaesthesia), George Meakin (Manchester, UK — muscle relaxants)

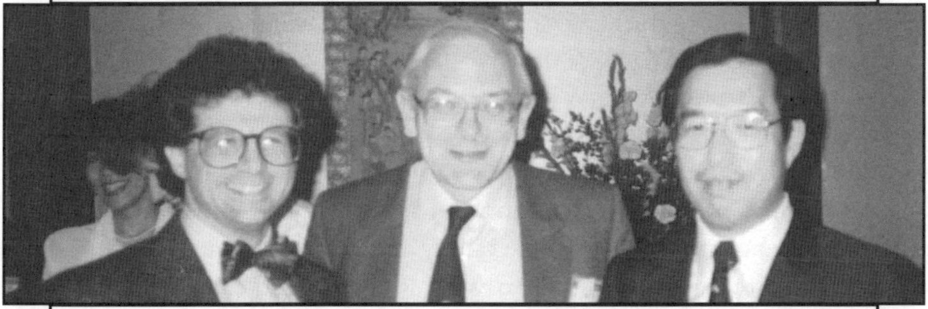

46. Jerry Lerman (Toronto, now Bufffalo), Kester Brown, Kats Miyasaka (Tokyo — responsible for development of paperless Childrens Hospital)

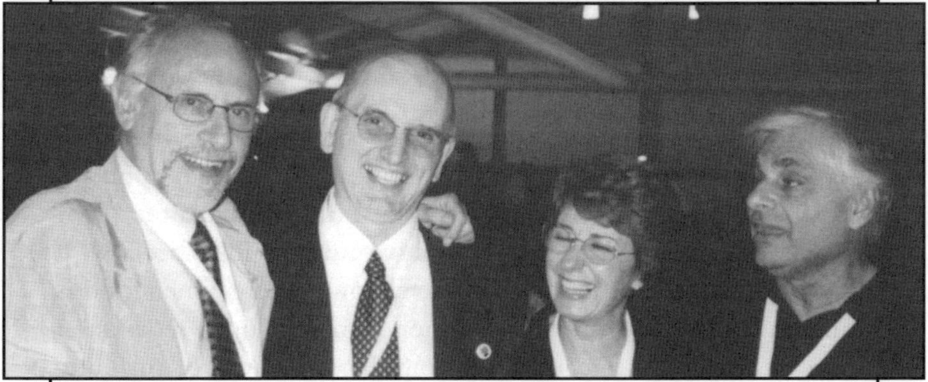

47. Regional anaesthesia experts: *From left:* Paulo Busoni (Florence — who pioneered caudal catheters after O. Schulte Steinberg), Bernard Dalens (France, now Quebec — author on textbook of regional anaesthesia in children), Elizabeth Giaffrey (Marseille, France), Narinder Rawal (Sweden)

because he could not have paid for such a performance.

I was invited to give a valedictory address after which Gerry Goresky presented me with a beautiful silver medal which was inscribed, "For lifetime achievement in paediatric anaesthesia." I was very touched (Figures C18, C29). It is one of my most treasured awards.

Another paediatric anaesthetists' tour took place in South Africa in 2001 when a group travelled from Durban after the All Africa Conference to Bloemfontein for a meeting there. We spent a night at a lovely hotel in the Drakensburg mountains amid magnificent scenery and gardens. We had time to walk in the hills in the morning. That evening we visited a Basuto village where I took portraits of the chief and some of people in the soft evening light which highlights their dark features.

Before the World Congress in Paris I undertook my final visits as President of WFSA — two days teaching paediatric anaesthesia in Slovenia, a lecture in Lucerne and finally one where my interest in anaesthesia began, Inverness in Scotland. After the Congress we had another excellent 6th world meeting in Bordeaux followed the next day by a visit to the fascinating old wine town of St Emillion with its sandstone cave dwellings. At the dinner held at one of the famous vineyards Ted Sumner (38), who is Editor of Paediatric Anaesthesia, and I were presented with medals from the University of Bordeaux, another surprise.

I have been fortunate to be able to combine teaching trips and pleasure. Long service leave is a typically Australian concept. Many people have received four to six months leave after 10 or 15 years continuous service. It is a wonderful idea because it allows one to do something or travel somewhere when one is young and fit enough to do it, rather than wait until retirement when health could already be failing. I used much of my long service leave to travel, usually incorporating teaching visits and conferences. I enjoy teaching and participating in conferences where one can often gain new ideas and have informal discussions on topics of interest. The people one visits usually show one around in a more personal way than a tour. I have lectured and taught in 66 countries.

People from some of these places have subsequently come to train with us, while in others, people had already been to our hospital. On several occasions I have been able to run workshops with former fellows in the department, particularly with Dilip Pawar (34) in India, and on others I have run them on my own for half or one day.

Chapter 17

Other Activities at the RCH

I was involved in many other activities at the hospital apart from anaesthetics. As well as being Director of Anaesthesia for 26 years I was concurrently Director of Theatre Services for 20 and Chairman and then Director of the Division of Specialist Services for 17 years from 1979.

After over 30 years I knew the history of the period of the "new hospital" well. I often found it useful to have this knowledge so that I could give historical perspective to discussions.

I think that one of the most useful roles I played was as an unofficial ombudsman and conciliator. I was often asked to help solve disagreements and disputes. This can often be achieved by hearing both points of view and then helping the parties to understand where the other is coming from. When this is done the other person's reactions may not seem so hostile. It is also useful to demonstrate the positive points on both sides of the argument. I was not always successful. On one occasion when I tried to bring two people together to discuss their differences, one blankly refused saying, "I am not going to talk to him". I believe his response was evoked by a fear of his view not being able to stand up to a logical discussion. He achieved his objectives by imposing them on others and basically he behaved as a bully. It is unfortunate when this happens as it can disrupt an otherwise harmonious working environment. The role of conciliator can be satisfying but can also be quite wearing.

My approach to *administration* was regarded as unorthodox by some who have been brainwashed by modern methods. I believed in delegation to responsible people, to trust those to whom responsibility was given and to deal with them personally. That meant visiting them, preferably in their own office, at least some of the time. This made them feel more at ease and made communication less strained. Unfortunately many administrators today do most of it by email and notices and thus don't gain a real understanding of the people with whom they are dealing. A little time for discussion on more personal matters will often help cheer up someone who is under a lot of stress. Also, telling people in higher positions about your attitudes and how you run things often results in them being more inclined to listen to your ideas in future. If you can gain rapport with them, negotiation becomes easier.

Visiting the department heads when I was Divisional head saved many hours in meetings which are often held because they are scheduled rather than because there is a real need. One can calculate the cost of a meeting by multiplying the hourly pay by the time of all those attending. Is the expenditure justified? Sometimes it is and sometimes it is a waste.

Reducing conflict and recognizing the contribution of everybody in the team helps to make a happier working environment, something we all would like to enjoy. Unfortunately there are people, sometimes in senior positions, who create conflict and disrupt the harmony so that the working environment of others becomes less enjoyable. These people don't care but they seem to fail to realize that happy people work better and more willingly go the extra mile. Low morale results when people are unhappy and discontented.

I taught many groups in the hospital including anatomy and physiology to the student nurses who had just completed their preliminary training school from 1968 -72. I continued teaching nurses in theatre and gave a lecture to them before their finals until the nursing school in the hospital closed on its hundredth anniversary. In many ways that was a sad day because nurses trained in hospitals seemed to be dedicated to their work and towards patients. College trained nurses regard it as a university course. At the end they can continue nursing or use it as a stepping stone to something else.

I was also involved in teaching medical students. I managed to arrange to have a session with them all and then they came individually to theatre for a session with us in their fifth year, during their paediatric surgery term. Students can learn so much from anaesthetists because so much of our work is applied basic science and the technical parts are useful in resuscitation. My simple book, *Anaesthesia and Patient Care*, published in 1983, resulted from these experiences. The cover was designed by one of the nurses who had shown her talent by doing a cartoon of me on a theatre whiteboard.

Pharmacology was a special interest for many years. I used to be consulted on matters relating to drugs because I had a background in research in that area and wrote one of the early papers on drug interactions. John Hurst, who was Director of the Casualty Department, asked me to help with tutorials for the residents on common drugs. These were done with a pharmacist and covered the basic use and side effects of common drugs. One of the most dramatic results of these tutorials was the sudden change over from aspirin to paracetamol for children with temperatures and minor pain after we pointed out the potential dangers of aspirin in small children. From time to time we had children who had been overdosed. Another development from these was a study done by one of the pharmacists, Elizabeth Creber, to determine the effective antipyretic (temperature lowering) dose of paracetamol. Ten mg/kg seem to be appropriate.

At the hospital centenary in 1970 I helped Ian McDonald to put on a display "Evolution and revolution in anaesthesia". My contribution was about new drugs which raised some interest among the *pharmacists*. The end result was that I gave a talk to the Hospital Pharmacists Association. After that I began having a monthly continuing education session with our pharmacists. I was the catalyst. Eventually, they took over and ran it themselves. We also arranged for them to come to the theatre to see us using the drugs they supplied to us, which they never otherwise saw in use. Two of them, Anne Leversha and Elizabeth Creber, later helped me with research projects in the laboratory. They both did very well in their field. For many years I was treated as an honorary pharmacist!

Janet, my wife, is a physiotherapist and so I was always aware of how they could help us in managing patients. I had worked with Anne McCoy in the Burns Unit and when she took over the Physiotherapy Department I also helped her with some continuing education. I arranged for one of my registrars to collaborate on a research project with one of them. I think it was their first research project . It compared various forms of physiotherapy used for clearing secretions from the chest. We found that vibration was very effective and I subsequently used it during bronchoscopy when children had retained secretions. We could see the beneficial effects directly through the bronchoscope.

Another outstanding registrar, Peter Kempthorne (36) from New Zealand, also worked with the physiotherapists. He developed the tibial nerve block to help reduce muscle spasm in the calves of children recovering from head injuries so that they could plaster the feet in a normal standing position. When they regained consciousness this enabled the physiotherapists to stand the children earlier and thus regain their postural reflexes sooner. Peter spent two and a half years with us after he had done his basic anaesthesia training in Dundee. He was elected to the Executive Committee of the WFSA in 2000.

I even helped my surgical colleagues with ideas based on ergonomics or on basic principles used by others which could be applied to their operations. I saved many hours, probably days, of my and their lives by instituting some of these. Unfortunately, on at least two occasions, my suggestions were superceded soon afterwards by new equipment developments.

The simplest suggestions were to use continuous instead of interrupted stitches in an operation for craniostenosis performed by Geoff Klug, a neurosurgeon with whom I reckoned I had worked for about 6,000 hours. My suggestion saved about half an hour each time. The other time-saving tip which I gave to Russell Taylor when he was a young surgeon was to use an appropriately short length of suture for a short incision so one did not waste time pulling an unnecessarily long piece through with each stitch. He has passed this on to all the trainees who have worked with him. It must have freed up several days of his life.

Staphylococcal pneumonia in infants occasionally went on to form pneumatocoeles — large cavities in the lungs due to break down of rotten lung tissue. Occasionally these ruptured into the pleural cavity making it difficult to ventilate the patient due to the air leak. They usually died. One night I suggested to the surgeon, Keith Stokes, that he should remove all the dead tissue and sew it up rather than trying a more conservative closure of the hole in the rotten lung. Although a significant amount of lung was removed the patient recovered and the management of these patients was revolutionized. They lived. The concept was later written up with a few cases by a surgical registrar with no reference to the fact that it had been my idea!

In 1974, when I became Director of Anaesthesia, life changed as it always does when one takes on administrative responsibilities. It was not as busy a job at the start as it became later. I decided that I should always devote at least half of my time to working in the operating theatre giving anaesthetics because I believed that one had to do at least that amount to retain one's expertise and credibility if one is going to teach and lecture.

Shortly after my appointment an independent enquiry on the operating theatres was held which came up with the recommendation that the Director of Anaesthesia should be in charge of the theatres. I then formally took over this responsibility

My appointment as Director of Anaesthesia also conferred a position on the *senior medical staff* which was a fairly influential body in putting forward proposals to the hospital administration at the time. This led to my appointment to the Library Committee. Later I became chairman through some difficult times — $30,000 dollars worth of books disappeared in a year, the cost of journals began to escalate, our librarian changed and we had extensions built. These matters all had to be dealt with.

In 1977 a landmark weekend conference was held at *Lorne*, a coastal resort to the west of Melbourne, when members of the Committee of Management met with a wide selection of hospital staff to consider the future of the hospital. It was a breakthrough in management /staff relations and also recognized the importance of staff other than the doctors who had dominated suggestions regarding policy up till then. The major recommendations were to build an enlarged car park, which has been an ongoing problem for most hospitals, to establish a divisional structure in the administration and to replace the Senior Medical Staff with a Medical Staff Association which included all consultant medical and dental staff.

I was a member of the Conjoint Committee at the time. The medical members were given responsibility for setting up the Divisions. Needless to say there was some opposition to their formation. We had to decide what divisions would exist and which departments would be in them. I almost succeeded in having a division of Anaesthesia and Intensive Care but at the last minute the physicians, led by Tom Madison, objected and the investigative group of pathology and radiology were joined with us. Within a two years Pathology was separated off and neonatology joined us. Although this seems an unusual grouping we were eventually all on one floor in the hospital so for us it worked well. It made it easy for me to visit the departments.

I was elected Chairman of this division and later, when the function became serious administration with budget control and responsibility, I was appointed Director. Colleagues who might have taken over the role of Divisional Director either left or would not take it on, being more than willing to support my continuing in the position. I ended up holding the roles for nearly 17 years. During the last three years I was also the Divisional Director who attended the Board of Management meetings.

Changes to the Board by recent governments has removed the old style Committees of Management and made them government appointees and now the staff are not even represented. How can these boards understand the critical issues without some input from people who are actually working with the patients? It is a new era of management style which replaces patients with clients, continuity with constant change, and which neglects the history and reduces the spirit of belonging which used to permeate the hospital, giving it a great family spirit. People worked effectively for 30, 40 and even, in one instance, 50 years for the hospital. There are still some long stayers around. One day I was working with a surgeon and three nurses in theatre. Our total service to the hospital added up to 150 years.

Later, non medical groups were added to the divisions and Biomedical Engineering and the Central Sterilizing Department joined us. One benefit of this was that Ron Wall, the chief Biomedical engineer, had just completed an MBA. I asked him to review all equipment in the division, to assess when and how often it should be replaced and the cost. It was a big task but it gave us a realistic basis for equipment budgeting. The only problem was that we never had the necessary funding. Later, the next CEO, Ivor Davies, thought a similar review should be done for the whole hospital, probably the first of its kind in the country. Unfortunately, during my time there was never nearly enough money to fulfil the plan but it had one major benefit. The hospital knew what it had and what was most urgently needed. A priority list was made so that when the Health Department decided to give an extra lump sum for equipment we knew what we needed immediately.

We went through several periods of economic hardship. We even built our own ventilators in the early 1990s.(Figure C 15) When pulse oximeters became essential for monitoring in theatre we had to buy on hire purchase and were saved by having them as first big cost item to be paid when we received an extra grant. One year the hospital only had $300,000 for equipment. The real estimate was four million dollars. It was hard to believe we were supposed to be living in the affluent world.

Then the Health Department "kindly" gave us an expensive Magnetic Resonance Imaging (MRI) machine but no money to run it. We had to find that out of our budget. It was not cheap. These were difficult matters to handle.

In 1988 it was decided to expand our operating theatres and build a new front building. The money was to be raised. Unfortunately the economic downturn at the time meant that we did not raise enough and building costs escalated. The Government was not forthcoming with funds as they were to some other hospitals. Ivor Davies arrived as Chief Executive in 1990 to find a $19 million deficit. He and his finance manager, Alan Studley, did well to balance the budget in three years but we went through some severe hardship and had to sell off many good assets.

It was working through such times that made me even more frugal. If you are not responsible for the budget when it is tight it is hard to understand what the problem is. Most people just want the government to give more money. It then raises the question of how much should be spent on health. Wages are the largest item but treatment of some conditions is also very expensive. Should the health budget be restricted and thereby developments in medicine slowed or discouraged? Are they really worth it when one thinks that in the poorest countries as little as $3 per head per year is spent on health. It is a major philosophical point that many people do not really grapple with. They probably could not understand my concerns with cost. I was brought up with the philosophy that if you look after the pennies (cents), the pounds (dollars) will look after themselves. I jokingly tell people that they have kept me on part time after I retired from full time work to teach because the money I save on drugs pays a substantial part of my salary! Actually it does.

The divisional system was most effective under a very capable leadership of Ivor Davies, as he let the divisional directors, which by then included a nursing one in each division, be responsible for their administration supported by their departmental heads. Much of the hospital policy and budget distribution was decided at the meetings of the Divisional Directors and senior management. I was lucky to have Lucy Cuddihy as our Nursing Divisional Director. Once she realized that my style of not having meetings all the time worked, we functioned very well together.

Imagine my relief of not having to attend 8am meetings every Tuesday with all these problems to solve when I finished as Divisional Director after 17 years! I would have finished a year earlier but a major conflict emerged and I was needed as an independent negotiator.

The Medical Staff Association was much more representative of all the medical and dental staff but its influence declined with the advent of divisions where nursing and other paramedical groups were better represented. Geoff Tauro, Director of Haematology Laboratory, and I wrote its initial constitution.

In 1977 I proposed that we should have beds for *day surgical* patients. It was the beginning of the appreciation that children preferred to be at home, that it was economically sensible to have fewer patients staying overnight with the additional nursing costs and that many operations were minor and there was really no need to stay overnight. It began with six beds but gradually evolved to twelve, to a ward and then a separate unit . Unfortunately the advice of nearly everyone involved to build the unit next to the operating theatres when extensions were being built in 1990 was rejected and it was built in the new front building away from theatres and easy supervision. The bridge across to the new unit on the second floor was only built on my insistence because the essential communication with the theatres would have been hopeless otherwise.

Another interesting role was my involvement in *hospital planning*. This interest was inherited from my father who planned and oversaw the building of much of his hospital. Several major extensions were made in my time with which I was involved including the development of a separate Intensive Care Unit, additional operating theatres and a new anaesthetic department. The plans for the original hospital building had not included Intensive Care which only started about the time the hospital moved to its present site in 1963. Eventually another block (North West Building) was built and the plastic surgery unit moved into it creating space for Intensive Care next to the Recovery Room. It had reached the top of the priority list. Then one day several of us were called to a meeting where we were told it was now fifth on the list and there was only money for four projects. There was an uproar. During the next two weeks Jim Breheny, who was acting Medical Director, negotiated it back on to the priority list and another hostile meeting was avoided. This success was the beginning of a long and successful career for Jim Breheny as a medical administrator. It also taught me something about handling hostile meetings — Stop, think and meet again, possibly with a reasonable compromise to offer.

On the theatre, Anaesthetic Department and CSSD extensions we had a wonderful architect, Sergei Holahoff, who consulted frequently with those who worked in the area with good results. Many architects fail to use this valuable consultation process. Rod Westhorpe and I managed brief but vitally important input into planning the new Day Surgical Unit. If we had been allowed more input some basic errors would have been avoided, such as painting the anaesthetic rooms blue. This makes the patients look blue which is a bad sign. From all this I learnt the *importance of the architects consulting and listening to the people who work in an area.*

My involvement in *research* led to being on the Animal Laboratory Committee and later being in charge of it. We oversaw the work in progress and ensured that it was well run. George Cauchi, who had begun as an anaesthetic technician, did an excellent job in looking after the animals and maintaining a high standard of care.

I represented the medical staff on the *Board of Research* for 6 years. This was an interesting time, because during it, David Danks established the Murdoch Birth Defects Research Institute aided by a large contribution from Dame Elizabeth Murdoch, who was a former President of the Hospital. It became a world leader in this field.

The Royal Childrens Hospital has had many outstanding people working in it in all branches of paediatrics. I made many friends among all levels of staff and in many different departments. I collaborated in writing scientific papers with 36 people from other departments. My life there was often very busy but I had great enjoyment in my work, as well as having, at times, the stress of excessive work, the occasional conflict and rare, short periods of depression. All these seemed unavoidable.

On one occasion, when I was down, an astute friend asked me if I was all right. Someone had shown that he cared. It was Neil Campbell, a very caring doctor who was the first full time neonatologist in the hospital. His question was enough to make me snap out of it. Sometimes a few sympathetic, understanding words will be of immeasurable help to someone who is down. On another occasion I lost interest in my clinical work. I suddenly realized this when, at a meeting, people started talking about interesting cases such as I had been doing. My equanimity returned when I realized how fascinating some of my cases were.

When in conflict, I always found it helpful to remember, and even acknowledge, the other person's good points and the useful things he or she had done. This policy helped me greatly during one period of conflict, which caused me much sadness because the individual concerned had been a good friend and colleague. However, remembering all the good things he had done helped me to continue supporting him. Eventually we became friends again.

If I helped to make the hospital and the operating theatre environment a happier place to work then I achieved something useful. I gave a lot of myself for the hospital but I received much in return. It has been a great place to spend most of my working life.

CLINICAL AND RESEARCH INTERESTS

Chapter 18

Intensive Care

When I was a student cardiopulmonary resuscitation as we know it today had not been introduced. Intensive care began with the poliomyelitis pandemic in 1949-51. Patients who could not breath as a result were put in negative pressure tank ventilators. I saw some of these patients still in tanks in 1967 at Fairfield hospital. It was a terrible disease. One of Kenya's leading tennis players came to coach us at school. Three weeks later he was dead. The first intensive care units were established in Scandinavia in response to the polio epidemic. In 1958, when I was a student, we hand ventilated for an hour each an old polio patient who was in respiratory failure.

The first patient to be ventilated at the Royal Childrens Hospital overnight was in 1960 when Ian McDonald hand ventilated a baby. Intensive care for children began about 1962 in Göteborg, Sweden and 1963 in Melbourne, at the time the new Royal Childrens Hospital opened. It started in Toronto about the same time, in part of the Recovery Room in both hospitals. Adelaide also started prolonged intubation that year but their patients were kept in the wards. Controlling the airway with a tube passed through the nose into the trachea and assisting the patients breathing with a ventilator after a major operation was the beginning, although as time went on, patients with other diseases and trauma, including head injuries, benefited as well.

The concept of keeping the airway clear was not new. Tracheostomy (making a hole into the trachea below the larynx — voice box) was performed by Asclepiades in 100 B.C. and by Cornelius Celsus in A.D. 14 to relieve obstruction due to quinsy. Several others used it though the ages — Paul of Aegina in the seventh century, Rhazes, an Arab physician in the ninth century and Avenzoar, a Muslim physician in the twelfth century. Chevalier Jackson, a very famous otolaryngologist, popularised the technique for relieving airway obstruction in his paper in 1909. Later it was used to remove secretions from the airways in unconscious patients and to reduce "dead space" (the part of a breath that does not reach the alveoli in the lungs to oxygenate the blood)

Others recommended passing a tube through the larynx even as far back as Hippocrates. Between 1879 and 1884 Joseph O' Dwyer developed a set of brass tubes (Figure C 11) and a special device to insert them into the larynx of children whose life was threatened by the formation of a diphtheritic membrane over the larynx (airway). This could obstruct the airway leading to suffocation and death. His idea was not widely accepted although in 1927 Dr Scholes in Melbourne reported using them in 1175 patients at Fairfield Hospital. An antitoxin was developed in 1893 which proved effective in treating the disease and later, immunization eliminated the disease in countries where the children were immunized.

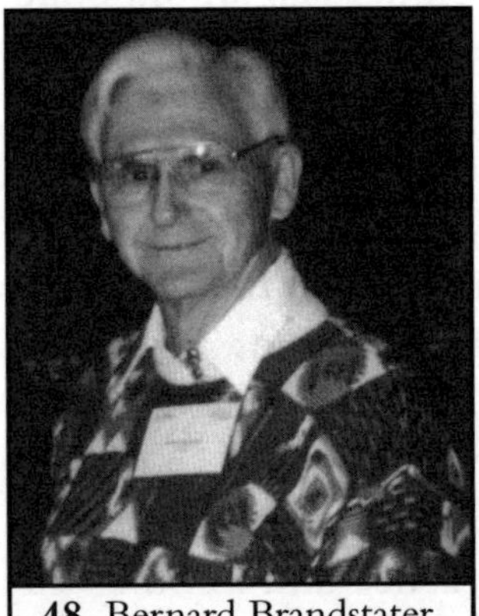
48. Bernard Brandstater.

The modern use of tubes for prolonged intubation was started by Bernard Brandstater (48) an Adelaide graduate who was working at the time in Beirut, Lebanon and subsequently moved to Loma Linda in USA. He reported a small series at the European Congress of Anaesthesiology in Vienna in 1962. This was followed by the reports from Melbourne (McDonald and Stocks), Adelaide (Allen and Steven (23) and Toronto (Markham, Blackwood and Conn) in 1965-6. These methods were not without problems. Secretions could collect and dry in the tubes blocking them with serious consequences if not recognised — the patient could not breathe air into the lungs. A factor in drying the secretions was that the normal mechanism for warming and moistening the air being breathed as it passes through the nose was bypassed. To overcome these problems the gases had to be warmed and moistened. This meant passing the gas over warm water in a tank. Another problem was produced — if the water was too hot the patient could be overheated by the hot gases. Methods for detecting the temperature of the gas were developed. The temperature at the point where the gas entered the patient had to be kept warm but not too hot (34°C). As the temperature dropped during transit from the heater to the patient one could not reliably assess the heating by measuring the tank temperature, although it could warn of overheating. Then some smart engineers in New Zealand thought that they could set the water bath temperature and keep the gas at the correct temperature and fully humidified by having a heating coil in the tube carrying the gas to the patient. Then another problem arose. The previous tanks were heated to about 56 degrees and basically pasteurized the water so that bacteria could not grow. Now the water bath was at a lower temperature ideal for organisms to grow, so that contamination and infection resulted. Life was not meant to be easy. Nowadays circuits carrying the gas to the patients are regularly sterilized, the staff wash hands between patients and suction catheters are frequently changed. Modern intensivists are barely aware of all the problems we had to work through to develop safe methods.

We had to evolve methods to hold the tubes in place so that they would not fall out accidentally with consequent dire results. Probably the most elaborate one was designed by Jackson Rees in Liverpool, UK (Figure C13). It was cumbersome and not easy to insert but Jack was a great thinker and this reflected his attempt to find a solution. There were several problems. Relatively heavy tubing attached to the tube could pull it out if not well positioned. Secretions from the nose could accumulate under the tape used to strap the tube in and loosen it. Much discussion occurred on the best method of securing the tube. Tunstall in Aberdeen developed a clip to hold the tube. Eventually we used a piece of string or thread tied tightly round the tube at the point where it came out of the nose. The tube was positioned so that the tip was in the mid trachea and not down in one bronchus so that only one lung would be ventilated. The ends were fixed on each side of the face with tape attached after the skin had been painted with tincture benzoin co. to protect it and make it more adherent to the tape. Two strips of tape cut down the middle to half way were used. One leg of the tape was placed across the upper lip. The second leg was wound round the tube tightly and then placed up the nose to prevent downward pull on the tube. This was then fixed more securely by passing the upper leg of the second tape across the nose and then winding the lower leg round the tube and across to the other side of the face. All the tape was then covered with a longer piece of Elastoplast with a hole in the middle through which the tube emerged. This had to reach beyond the limits of the under tapes to stick near the ears to provide maximum attachment. If this was done correctly the tube should stay in place and withstand pulling both down and outwards. It is hard to believe that so much thought could be put into achieving an effective method. In my view the strip up the nose is the key to optimum security. Even after all this, secretions collecting under the strapping loosened it so that re-strapping was often necessary every day or two.

How long could these tubes be left in? This was a much debated topic. The longest we had in a baby was for about seven months.

Two newborns who arrived on my first two days at the hospital had oesophageal atresia. This is a congenital abnormality where the oesophagus (the tube between the mouth and stomach) is incomplete and there is often a connection into the trachea, usually from the lower end of the oesophagus, which can cause difficulty to the anaesthetist because air can travel down the trachea, through the fistula into the stomach. If the stomach distends it interferes with the babies breathing because babies depend mostly on their diaphragm to breathe. The difference with adults is that the ribs slope downwards so that when they breathe in the ribs rise, increasing the cross sectional area of the chest, allowing the lungs to expand. The diaphragm (the muscle between the chest and abdomen) moves down at the same time, also increasing the volume in the chest and lowering the pressure so that air is sucked in. In babies the ribs are horizontal and so they cannot increase the cross sectional area much and thus the diaphragm produces most of the expansion that draws air into the lungs. If the diaphragm is pushed up in a baby by, for example, too much air in the stomach, the volume of air taken in is reduced and breathing becomes difficult. Another problem that these babies have is that the blind ended upper oesophagus can fill up with secretions or milk in its first feed and overflow into the lungs.

One of these babies had an unusually large upper pouch so that it pushed the trachea forwards kinking and obstructing it. A nasotracheal tube was needed to relieve the obstruction. In those days these patients had their operation delayed because lung complications were common. Nowadays they are operated on early before the lungs become soiled with food or secretions, joining the two ends of the oesophagus when possible. Occasionally the gap between them is too long and a later operation is done using some stomach or colon to bridge the gap. The diagnosis is easy if a catheter is inserted through the mouth because it will not pass the obstruction.

The second one had a cleft in the larynx which caused the airway to collapse when the patient breathed in, if the tube was removed. It remained in for 7 months, until her larynx grew sufficiently. Nowadays they would probably do an operation before that to solve the problem. These two patients stayed for several weeks

Before prolonged intubation tracheotomy was used to relieve obstruction of the upper airway. Its' use disappeared except when a tube could not be inserted. Later, a tracheostomy was used if a prolonged artificial airway was needed because it was easier to manage and it did not inhibit the development of facial expression caused by prolonged use of strapping on the face.

Epiglottitis is an acute infection and results in swelling of the tissues around the larynx. This is so painful that the children cannot swallow their saliva. Because they find it easier to breathe sitting up they usually adopt that position and the saliva drools out of the mouth.

In 1968, the doctors who usually did the tracheostomies in these patients at our hospital were all away at a conference, so we inserted a nasotracheal tube. Following antibiotics the condition rapidly resolved, the swelling decreased and the tube was removed within 24 hours. Only once after that was a tracheostomy used for epiglottitis, when the swelling was so severe that the airway was not visible, a tube could not be passed and the child's condition was critical.

Epiglottitis used to be the anaesthetist's nightmare, because we had a patient with an increasingly narrow airway through which we had to give oxygen and the anaesthetic. Eventually we used halothane with some positive pressure on the anaesthetic ventilating bag. The latter helped to keep the airway open to its maximum while the anaesthetic was deepened enough to intubate the trachea. This technique overcame the problem. The condition has almost disappeared, because children can now be vaccinated against the disease. This is a relief because it was a life-threatening and occasionally fatal disease.

Ventilators were not built specifically for children so we had to adapt the Bird and Bennett PR2 for use with them. They needed to be pressure cycled so that the inspiratory phase cut out when the required pressure was reached. This enabled the ventilator to be set to compensate for leaks in the circuit as we used tubes without cuffs. The narrowest part of the airway in a child before puberty is at the cricoid cartilage in the larynx which is circular. This allows a reasonable fit to be obtained without a cuff. In adults the airway is irregular at the narrowest part so a cuff is attached to the tube which, when inflated gives an airtight fit.

Loosco in the Netherlands made the first small ventilator for neonatal use.

One complication which was encountered in three of the first sixty cases, but none of the next 300, was subglottic stenosis (a narrowing of the larnyx below the vocal cords.) At first we wondered if there was something toxic in the tube and tests were done to see if tissues reacted to subcutaneously implanted pieces of tube. None developed. It was caused by using too large a tube in sick patients, so that the blood supply to the area became inadequate and ischaemia (lack of blood supply to the mucosa) resulted. This was followed by fibrosis and stricture formation. After we instituted a policy of ensuring that a slight gas leak could be heard when positive pressure was applied to the airway this complication virtually disappeared except in premature babies who have very narrow airways and sometimes a compromised circulation (poor blood supply).

Paying more attention to fluids and nutrition, particularly when administered intravenously, also improved the outcome of very sick children. Access to veins to give the fluids was necessary first. The "Court" needle designed by one of the paediatri-

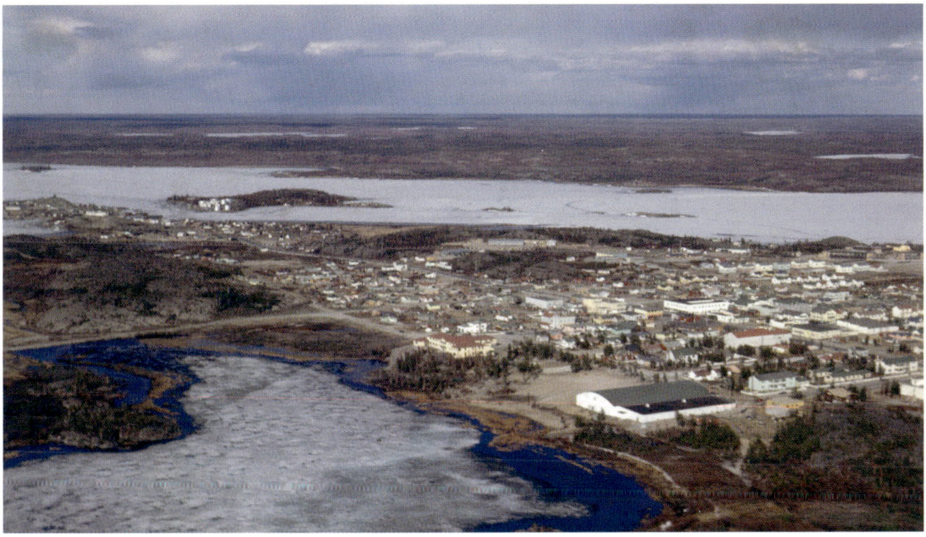

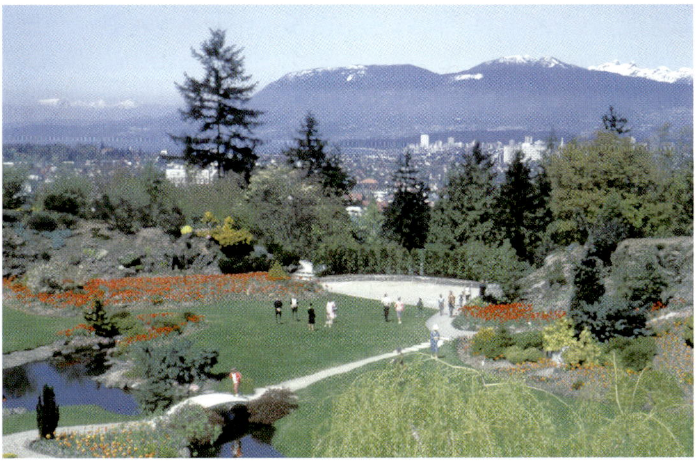

Above: **C1**
Yellowknife, NWT, Canada from the air. The hospital is in the middle overlooking Frame Lake.

Above: **C2**
Vancouver from Queen Elizabeth Park.

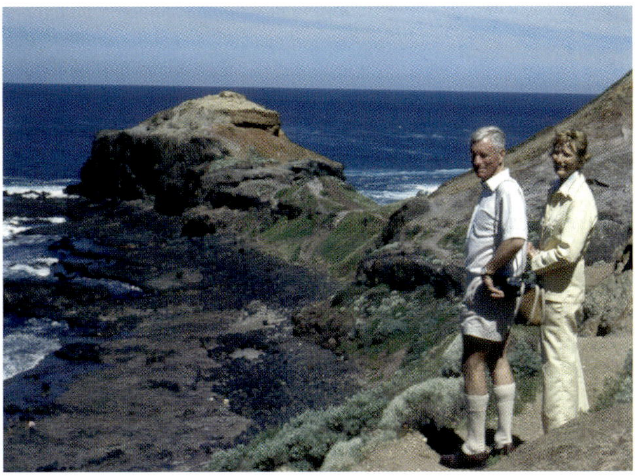

Right: **C3**
Ken Leighton and his wife, Nancy, at Cape Schank, Victoria during their visit in 1980.

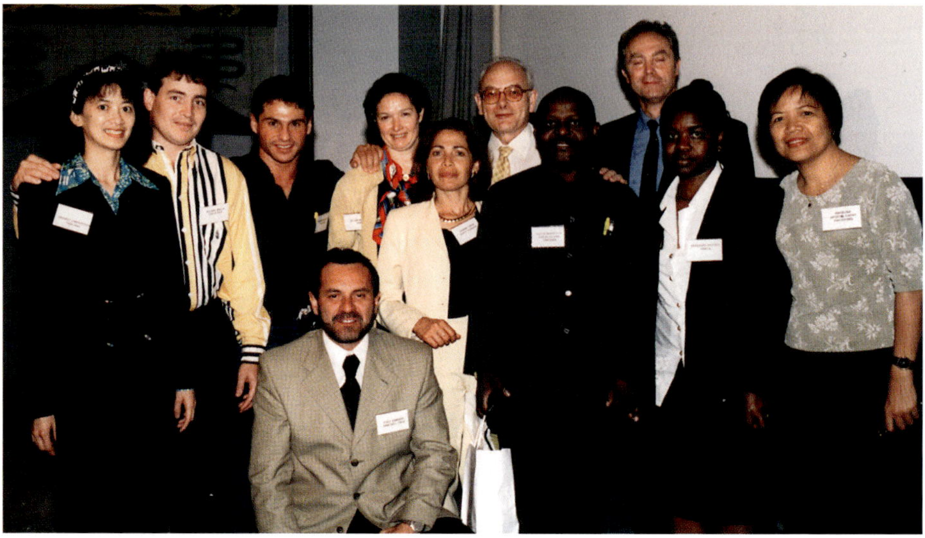

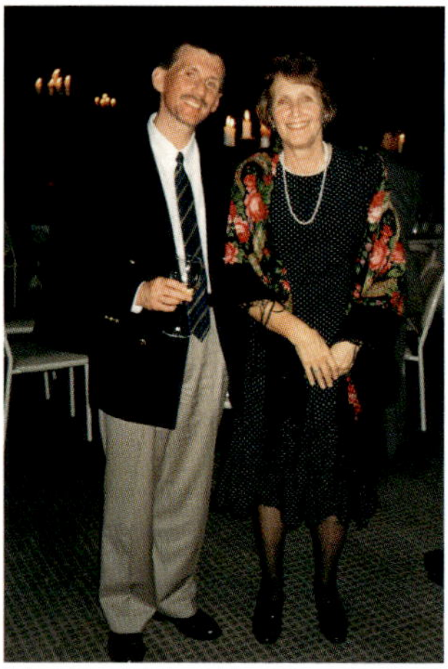

Above: **C4** Former overseas fellows who attended my retirement from full-time anaesthesia meeting in November 2000: *from left* L Jiriwat "Pia" Limprayoon (Thailand), Alvaro Brilla (Costa Rica), Guillermo Galeotti (Argentina), Sylvie Herbeau (Paris), Susana Cueva (Ecuador), KB, Victor Mwafongo (Tanzania), Christian Herbeau (Paris), Praxy Okutoyi (Kenya) and Angie Gapay (Philippines). *Crouching* Italo Zamudio (Chile).

Below: **C6** Bangkok. *From left* Prof. Thara Tritakarn of WFSA Education Committee and founger of the Bangkok Training Centre, Prof. Kameang Chaturachinda (obstetrician, fellow student of St Andrews), KB, Sirilak, Yodying (Chiang Mai), Thitima, Anchalee and Suwanee (Bangkok) – all former RCH fellows.

Above: **C5** Sergei Rajev (Moscow) and Janet.

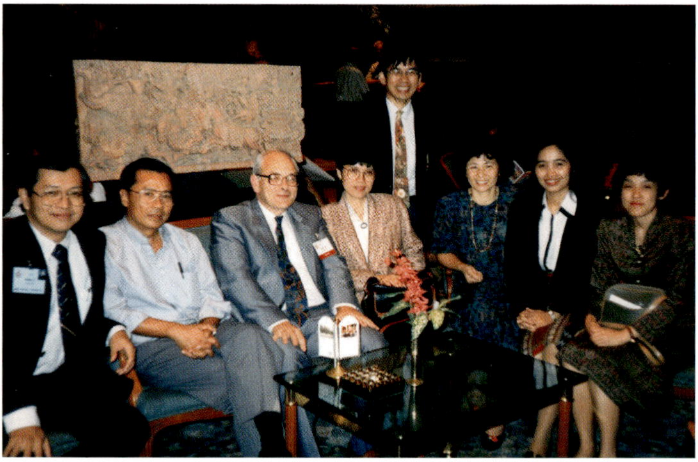

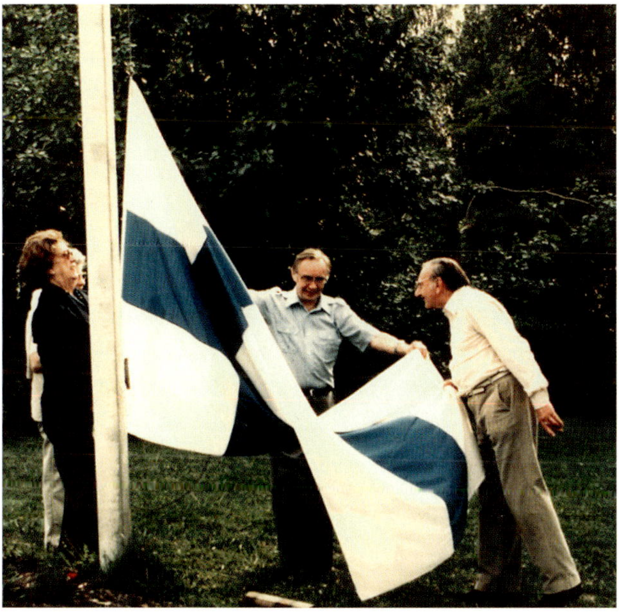

Left: **C7** Toivo Suutarinen taking down the Finnish flag at the end of the APA visit to his country house watched by Jackson Rees and Sheila Anderson (Great Ormond St, London).

Below: **C8** APA tour at the Twelve Apostles, Victoria, in 1988. *From left* ?, Brian Anderson (Auckland), Susan Jones (Birmingham), Adrian Bosenberg (South Africa), Peter Booker (Liverpool, UK), Seizo 'Jake' Iwai (Kobe, Japan).

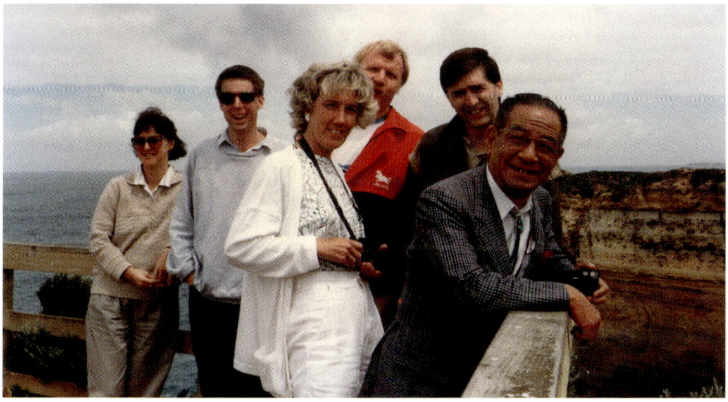

Below left: **C9** Jackson Rees, Liverpool, UK.
Below right: **C10** Kester Brown anaesthetising for a myringotomy with Warner Mooney, who was wearing a cap with his VFL team, South Melbourne, colours.

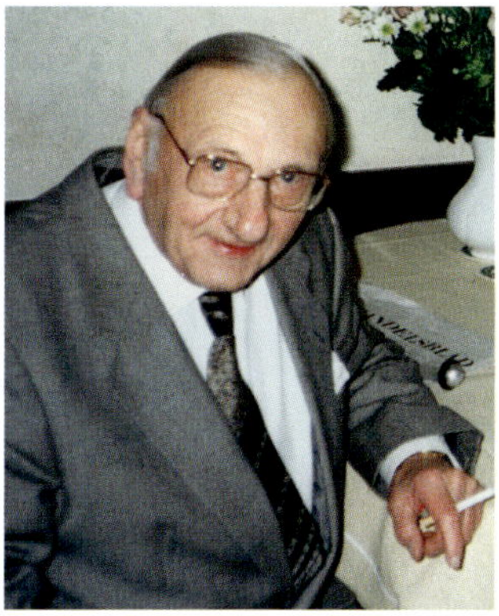

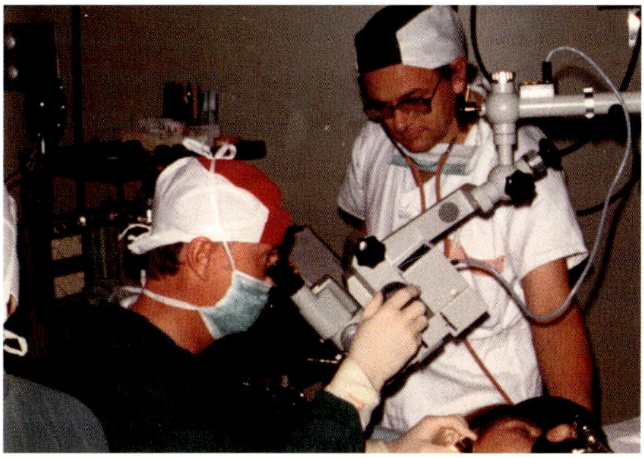

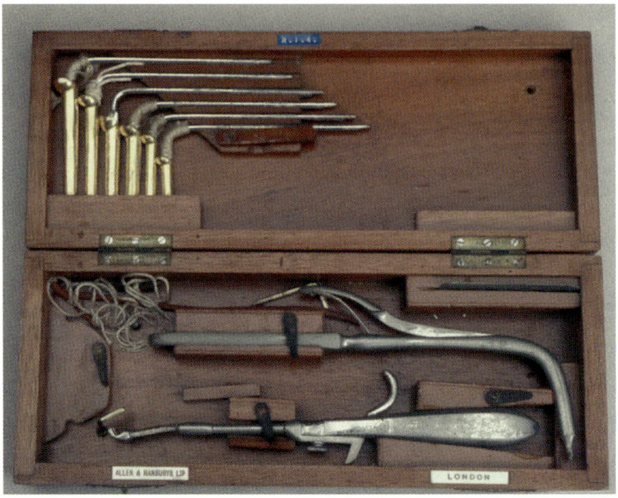

Left: **C11** A set of O'Dwyer tubes and the equipment for inserting and removing them in patients with diphtheria

Below left: **C12** Paediatric anaesthetic equipment of the 1960s – red rubber tube, mask with metal frame, and gas delivery apparatus with T piece and valve designed and made by Dr McClelland and Harry Adams at CIG.

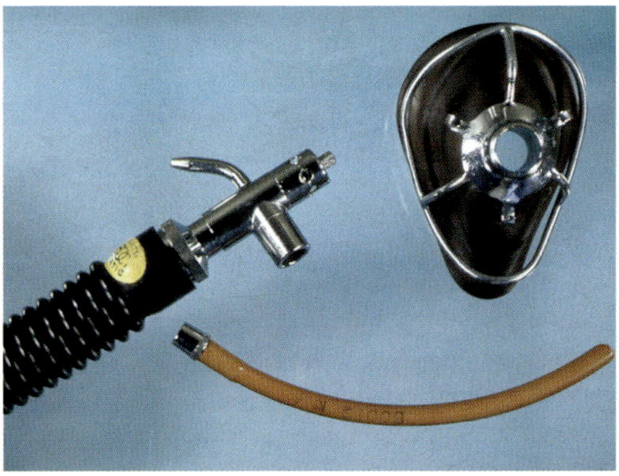

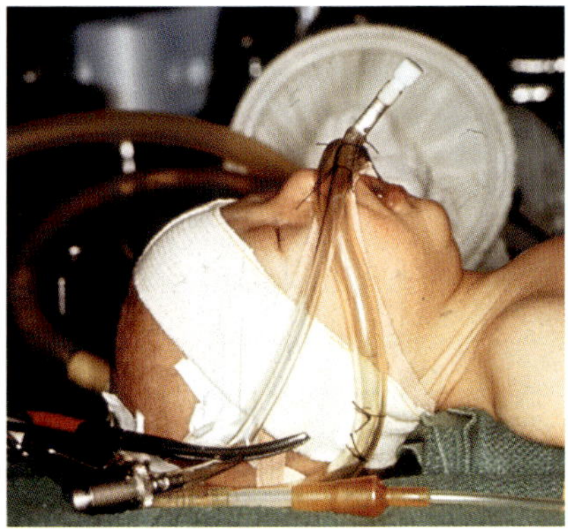

Below: **C14** Denis Clare with the Clare Ventilator at the stand during the ASA meeting in 1995.

Above: **C13** A neonate with tetanus (1965, Toronto) being ventilated via a special Jackson Rees tube for prolonged intubation. The wide bore tube is for gas delivery and fixation, the suction port in front going directly to the endotracheal tube.

Below: **C15** Clare ventilator built at RCH.

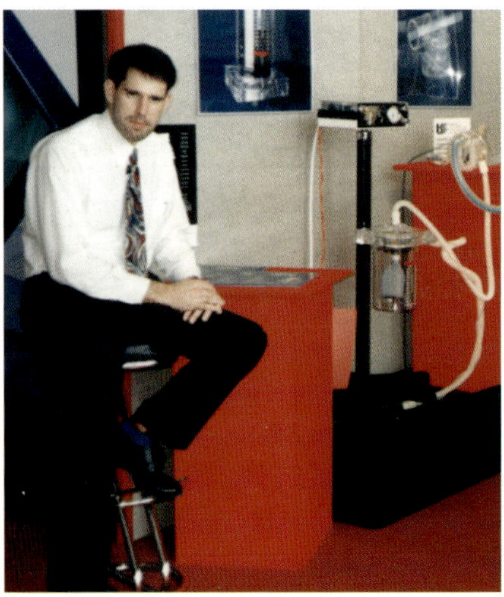

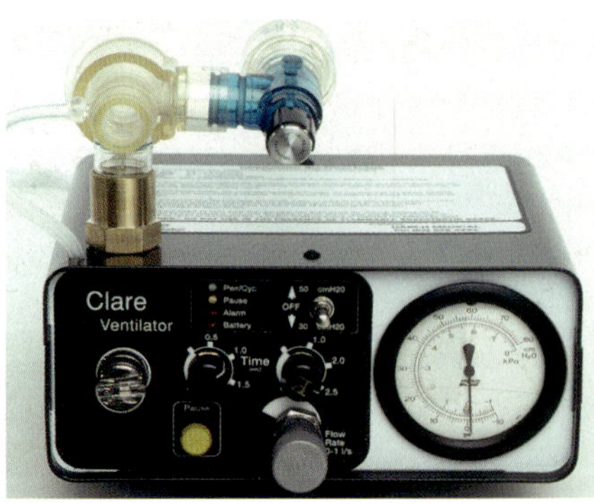

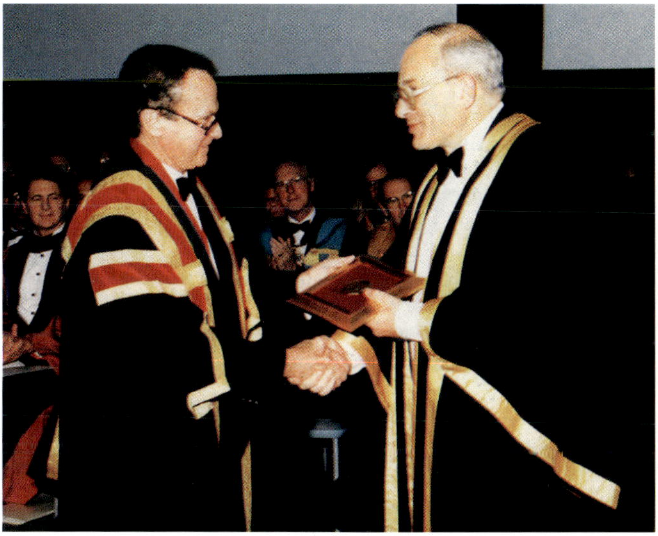

Left: **C16** The author receiving the Orton Medal from the President, Peter Livingstone, at the ANZ College of Anaesthetists annual meeting in Canberra in 1992.

Below: **C17** The author receiving the Fellowship of the Royal College of Anaesthetists in London from the President, Alaistair Spence, in 1992.

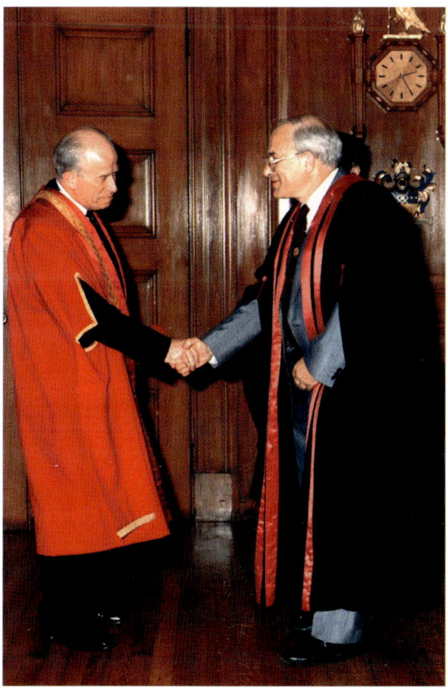

Below: **C18** Medals (clockwise) – Royal Childrens Hospital Gold Medal (1997); Medal presented at world Paediatric Anaesthetic meeting, Halifax, Canada in 2000; Ben Barry medal for distinguished service to the journal *Anaesthesia and Intensive Care* (1996); the two sides of the World Congress Speakers medal; the ASA Gilbert Troup medal (1996).

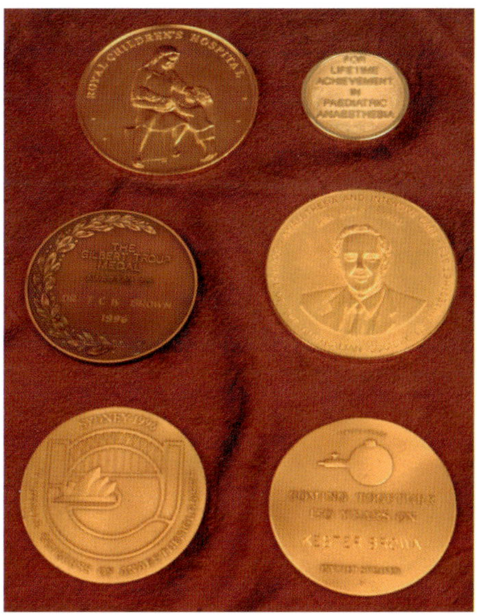

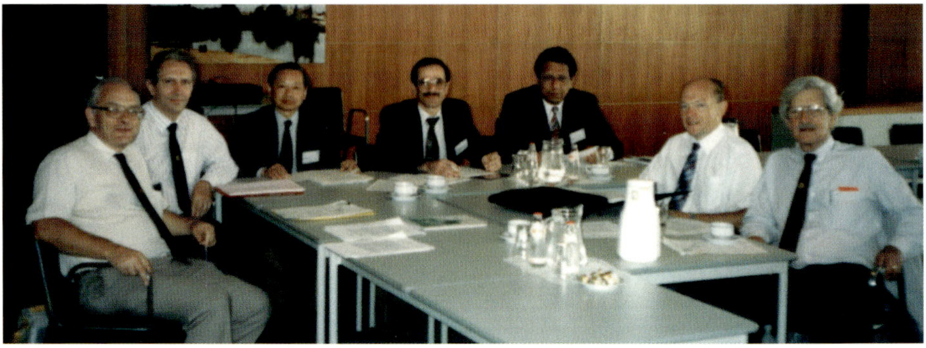

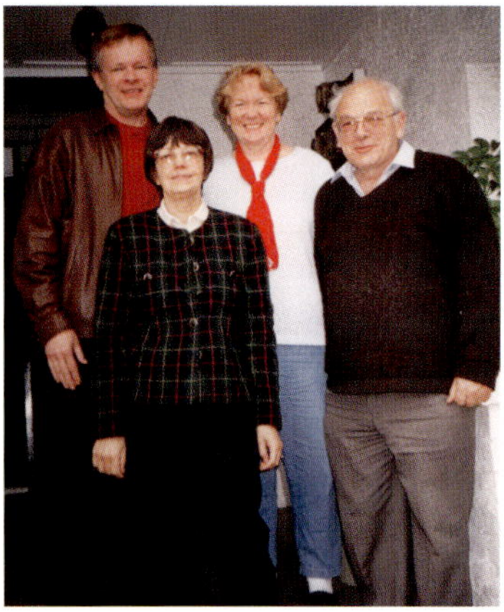

Above: **C19** Education Committee (1988-92) meeting in the Hague 1992. KB (chairman), Philippe Scherpereel (France), M Fujimori (Japan), Jamal Shariff el Shenableh (Jordan), Virgilio Paez (Ecuador), Roger Eltringham (UK) and John Couper (South Africa).

Left: **C20** WFSA Officers meeting at the author's home in Melbourne in October 2003. Richard Walsh (Treasurer, Aust.), Maria Janecsko (Chair, Exec. Committee, Hungary), Anneke Meursing (Secretary, Netherlands), KB (President).

Right: **C21** The author meeting the Icelandic President during the Scandinavian meeting in Rejkjavik in 1995.

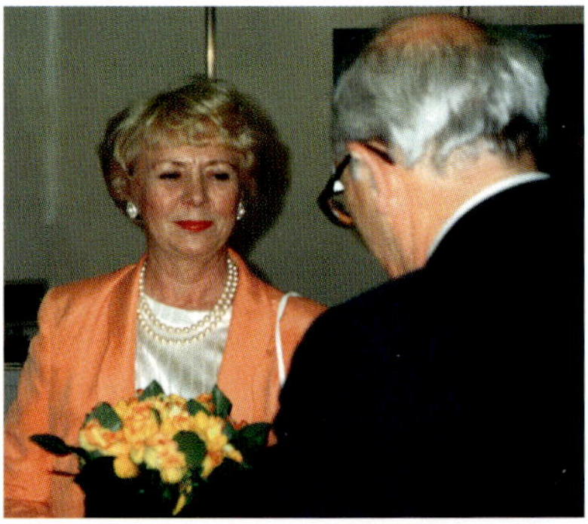

Below: **C22** President's dinner at the conclusion of the Montreal WCA, 2000. Lorna Eltringham, Peter Kempthorne★ (NZ), KB^, Bobby Kempthorne, Karen McMurchy (WFSA office), Janet Brown, Roger Eltringham^ (UK), Elvira and Martin Marx (Uruguay), Victor Mwafongo★ (Tanzania), Dilip Pawar★ (India). [★ Worked at RCH, ^ St Andrews graduate.]

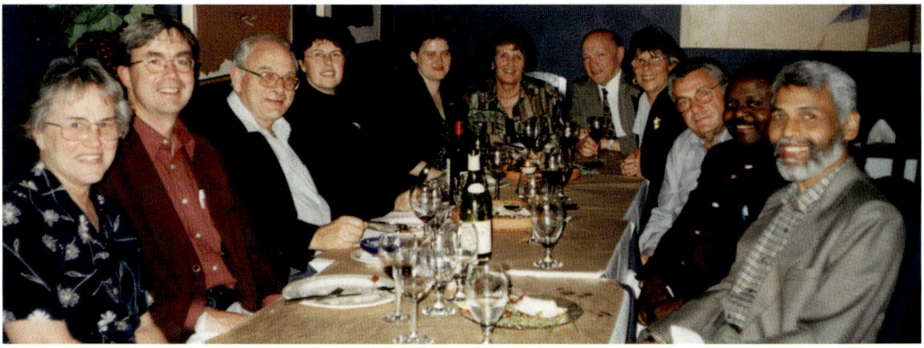

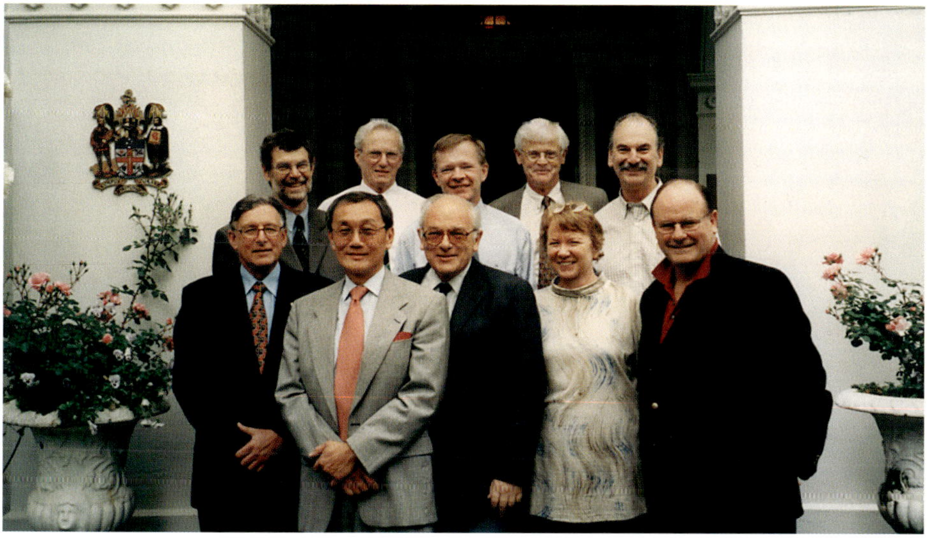

Above: **C23** WFSA officers meeting at the ANZ College of Anaesthetists, Melb. Photograph taken with the College Executive. Back: Richard Willis (President 2002-04), Garry Phillips (President 1996-8), Richard Walsh (President 1998-2000, Treasurer WFSA 2000—), John Gibbs, Rod Westhorpe (President ASA 1998-2000). Front: Michael Cousins (President 2004), Teik Oh (President 2000-02), KB (President WFSA), Anneke Muersing (Secretary WFSA), David Bevan (Chair WFSA Executive Committee).

Below: **C24** Torsten Gordh (Sweden, one of the founders of WFSA), Carlos Parsloe (Brazil, Past President WFSA), and John Severinghaus (USA, CO2 Electrode). Behind: David Bevan (Canada), Patricio Kelly (Argentina), Martin Marx (Uruguay) and Edith Parsloe. At the World Congress in Sydney, 1996.

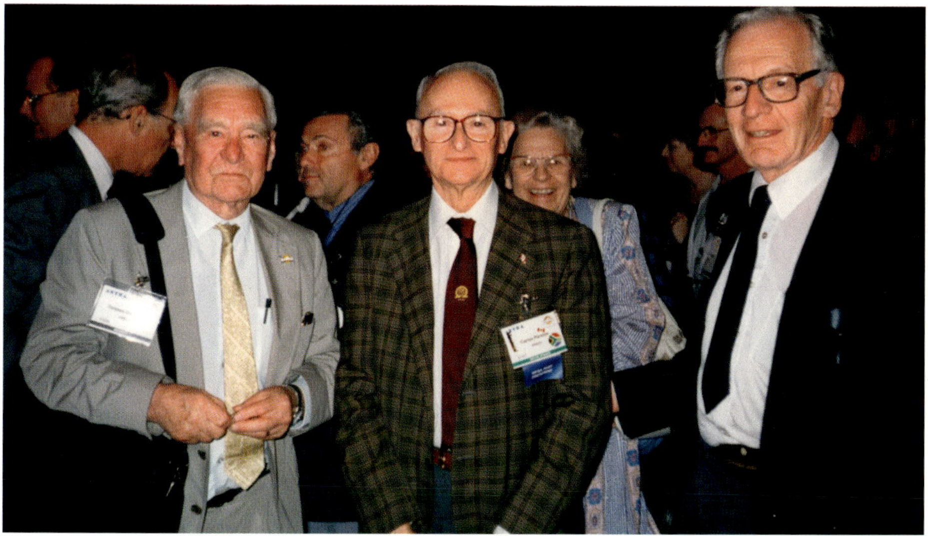

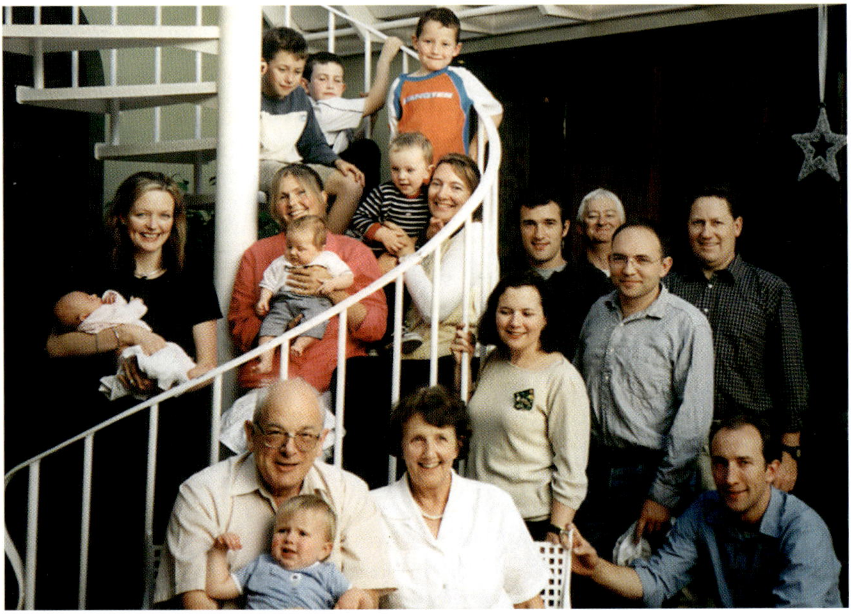

Above: **C25** Kester Brown and Family, 2002.
Below Left: **C26** Painting of the smoke over the blown-up fuel tanks during the coup in Manila in 1989, painted at lunchtime from the Conference Centre.
Below Right: **C27** With Janet, being presented with a medal inscribed "For lifetime achievement in paedriatric anaesthesia" by Gerry Goresky in Halifax, 2000.

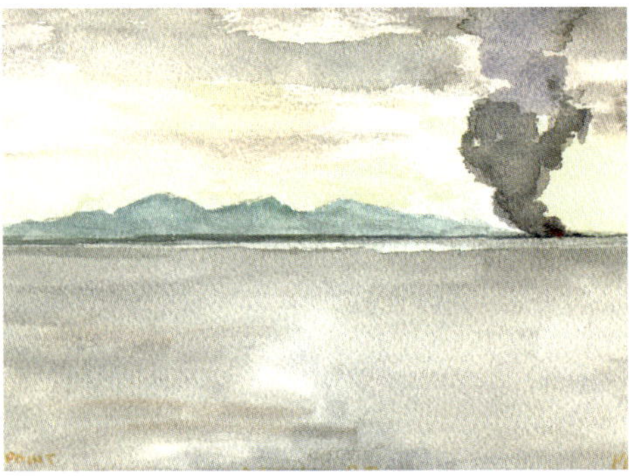

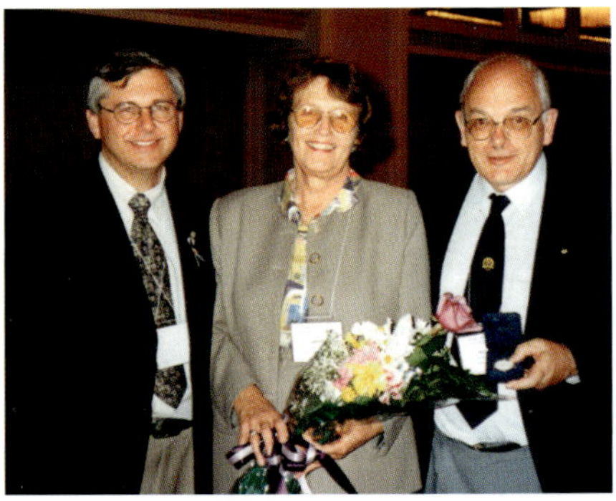

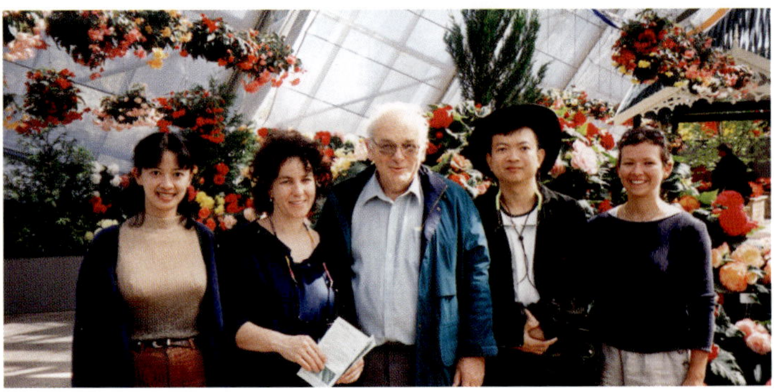

Right: **C28** In the begonia house at Ballarat Gardens; Jiriwat "Pia" Limprayoon (Thai), Guiliana Fognani (Italy), KB, Vorakran (Thai), Inneke van Mol (Belgium.

cians at the hospital, was one of the early developments. Umbilical catheterisation was commonly used in babies as it was easy to access in newborns, but it was not without its complications. Intravenous cannulation was a skill which gradually more and more people developed. Central venous cannulation was also used but less often. The internal jugular route so often used now was developed later. Better cannulae were developed with smoother tips and thinner, more flexible walls. In the first edition of Anaesthesia for Children published in 1979 there is a section written by Noel Cass on the electron microscopic features of cannulae tips — it was a topic of interest at the time. Some had very rough edges.

Parenteral nutrition (giving essential nutrients intravenously) was controversial when it was first introduced because of the cost. It was an example of an expensive treatment which could be justified because the patients ended up being hospitalised for shorter periods. Helen Noblett , a paediatric surgeon who later emigrated to Bristol in England, was at the forefront of the developments in intravenous fluid therapy.

Head injuries were more common at that time due mainly to the lack of restraints in cars. The reduction in the number of deaths and serious injuries from motor vehicle accidents resulted from the outstanding work of Dr. John Birrell, the Police Surgeon, and as a result of a seminar, initiated by Bill Hughes (later Sir Edward, President of the College of Surgeons and then Professor of Surgery at Monash University) and organized by the Royal Australasian College of Surgeons. It was attended by all interested parties — medical, ambulance, police, lawyers, road builders and government representatives. The first result of the workshop was the introduction of seat belts in Victoria, the first place in the world to make them compulsory. Then child seats and baby capsules on the back seat were introduced, followed by helmets for motor cyclists and then cyclists, then alcohol and speeding limits. Gradually the death toll dropped from 1061 a year to about three hundred, despite increasing traffic. The first drop to 900 per year followed the introduction of seat belts and the second drop of about another 200 occurred when random breath tests were introduced.

One of the saddest cases that I remember was an eight year old boy from Mildura who was out walking his beloved dog. It went on to the road and was hit by a car and killed. He went to pick it up and he himself was then hit by another car. He died later in Intensive Care from his injuries.

In 1967 we had 750 patients in the unit for over 24 hours. Intensive Care occupied half of the area planned as a recovery room. Occasionally we had no patients and rarely would we reach our capacity of eight. In the early 1970s the numbers gradually increased so that the excess patients spilled over into the Recovery side of the ward. The situation was becoming critical. The cardiac surgeons then developed a three bed unit across the hall but that was soon not enough. I have mentioned elsewhere the battle to have a new unit built in the adjacent ward. This was finally done in 1974-5 in an enlarged ward area. A later extension was made to make a 24 bed unit, but we cold never afford the cost of the staff and it has remained about sixteen beds. When John Stocks died, Geoffrey Barker (18), one of his proteges who had been in Toronto, took over and developed the new unit. About year or two later he resigned and returned to Toronto where he eventually became Chief of Intensive Care at the Hospital for Sick Children. He went on to have a very distinguished career, becoming Chief of staff at the Hospital for Sick Children and then overall Head of Critical Care in Toronto University. He also organised the second World Congress of Paediatric Intensive Care. He is a man with a good sense of humour who has been a great friend and colleague. He was succeeded by Geoff Mullins and then by two other outstanding doctors — Alan Duncan, who returned to his home city of Perth and later became Dean of the Faculty of Intensive Care and Editor of Anaesthesia and Intensive Care, and Frank Shann, a brilliant paediatrician, who has also acted as a consultant to the World Health Organization and is on the Editorial Board of the Lancet.

Frank Shann's appointment brought an end to having anaesthetist trained Directors of the unit. There are now four consultants, two anaesthetists and two paediatricians. Sadly, after many years, the involvement of anaesthetists in the unit has gradually decreased and economic factors finally led to the end of our consultants being involved. This seems to be the way things are going in this field. In countries where intensive care is less developed anaesthetists still usually play a dominant role but it does draw some of the manpower away from the operating room. As medicine progresses, the particular skills that the anaesthetists have in ventilation, airway management and cardiovascular problems do not cover all the medical problems that present in such units and other specialists become involved.

Intensive care is a fascinating field because so many challenging and complicated problems present but it is physically and emotionally demanding.

Difficult ethical problems arise. Should this patient's treatment be continued? What factors should be considered? Which of these are the most important in making the decision? They include: likelihood of survival; quality of survival — unconscious or uncommunicative, a constant demanding burden on the family; quality of life expected; effect on siblings and the rest of the family; did the parents have difficulty conceiving this child; these are all important considerations. Others come into it too — religion, environment and economics. The parents need rational guidance but they may have overriding beliefs. Even the staff can have divergent views.

About 1980 I was once asked to speak to a group which included people such as chaplains and social workers. Afterwards I asked why they asked me. I was told it was because they thought that I had some controversial views! I suppose I had because I concluded a discussion along the above lines by saying that the day would come when economics would come into the consideration of who is treated.

I am very sensitive to the tragedy of someone losing a much loved child. However, I personally do not believe in saving life at all costs especially when the quality of life afterwards for the patient is not going to be meaningful and where the rest of the family will suffer. I am not in favour of embarking on complex, difficult and expensive medical treatment that may cause the patient and parents much misery particularly if the outcome is likely to be bad. I know that my views are at variance with many colleagues in the advanced world, but there are also many who agree with me, especially in less affluent countries where the money could be expended more effectively for the benefit of many more people. My upbringing in Africa has influenced my views. Sad though it may be to lose a child it may be easier let it go and avoid suffering and to have another hopefully normal child. I once heard a talk in India about neonatal surgery. There were about 20,000 babies born with oesophageal atresia each year. Few were treated because in their environment it is usually easier to have another normal baby than struggle through with one with complications.

It was wonderful to be in at the beginning of paediatric intensive care. While I worked in Intensive Care I enjoyed the challenge, especially if a worthwhile outcome resulted but I came to the point where I did not enjoy struggling to keep a patient alive when I thought the outcome was bad or tragic suffering would follow. I felt my major contribution in preventing accidental drug overdosage was extremely worthwhile. My dilemma was resolved when I became Director of Anaesthesia in 1974 — my duties made it difficult to keep up the Intensive care work and I withdrew. I had done my bit and made my contribution.

Anaesthetists took their technical and scientific expertise from the operating theatre to intensive care and developed the specialty. Now we send trainees to intensive care to acquire some of their skills necessary to optimally look after critically ill children so that they can apply them in the operating theatre to provide optimum care for our patients.

It has been an interesting evolution that has progressed at different rates around the world. In Australia and New Zealand, Intensive Care is now an independent specialty with its own qualification, but in many other countries anaesthetists still play a major role. This leads to confusion, because in these countries the doctors often relegate the importance of anaesthesia and favour intensive care in their work, with the result that other non physicians undertake some of their duties in the operating theatre, to the detriment of the specialty.

Chapter 19

Drug Overdosage and Envenomation

Most drugs used in medicine have an ideal dosage range which lies between that which produces a desired effect and a toxic level. This may vary with age, particularly in infants and small children, because the mechanisms for breaking the drug down or eliminating it from the body may not be fully developed. In addition, the effect may be greater at a given dose because it can be taken up more easily by the organ where it works. This applies to some depressant drugs, such as morphine or the intravenous induction agent thiopentone which enter the brain more easily in babies. Smaller doses are given, otherwise the effects of overdosage occur, such as depressed breathing. It is thus important in a field like anaesthesia, where we give drugs intravenously in our daily work, to know these variations in dose requirement.

Drug overdosage is a problem seen in Intensive Care when the consequences are serious and sometimes require sophisticated management. Sometimes overdosage is lethal and this is the reason some people take large doses of drugs when attempting suicide.

In 1970 the antidepressant drugs of the tricyclic group (based on the chemical structure) were made available in Australia on the Pharmaceutical Benefits Schedule (PBS). Soon afterwards we began to receive increasing numbers of mainly small children who had gained access to these pretty little tablets and eaten several of them. The effects varied, depending on how many were taken, but the serious overdosages presented with irregular heart rhythms, low blood pressure, convulsions (fitting) and even unconsciousness. One third of our 192 patients over the next seven years had one or more of these manifestations. We even had a death, one of two boys whose neighbours were moving house and disposed of the unused tablets into the rubbish bin. These little boys found them and, as they looked attractive, ate them. It was a tragedy which highlights the importance of disposing of drugs by returning them to a chemist.

Whose tablets were being taken? Often they were the mother's, who had been given them because the stress of looking after active little children had become too great. Some were grandparents' and some were even prescribed for the child or a sibling to prevent bed wetting. They increase the bladder sphincter tone. This treatment is inappropriate in children under five years old which is when the drugs are most toxic. Occasionally they belonged to father, other relatives or visitors.

The number of these patients increased from two or three a year to ten to eleven when the drugs were gaining popularity, to 36 and the 45 in the years following their addition to the PBS. The majority were under four years, the age when children experiment and put things in their mouths.

Something had to be done both about prevention and treatment — the arrhythmias were often difficult to control. This led me into a field of research for the next seven years during which time we had one of the biggest reported series of patients.

I undertook a study on children of 2, 3, 4 and 5 years to see how quickly they could access sweets or tablets from different types of containers or drug packaging. It demonstrated that the most effective method was foil wrapping because the children could not see what was inside and the manual dexterity was such that they could not open it easily. Subsequently John Stocks , L.E.G. Sloan, the Medical Director of the hospital and I wrote to the Minister of Health and the Director General of Health explaining the problem and proposing the solution would be to have these tablets foil wrapped. They acted promptly telling the pharmaceutical companies that these drugs should be safety packaged. All the companies except one put them in foil (one company advertised their product as being packaged in the safest manner) and the other put them in a blister package.

Two years later legislation was passed making it compulsory to safety package not only these drugs but also iron, paracetamol and aspirin which all caused problems in children when taken in excess. By then the incidence of overdosage had declined to its previous level despite the fact that the prescription rate had

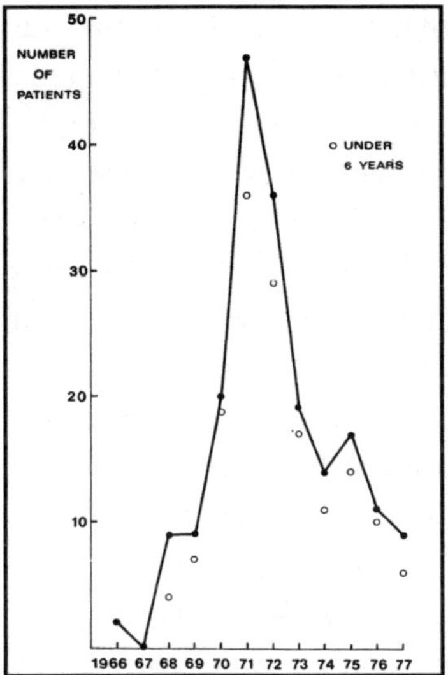

49. Graph showing the dramatic increase in tricyclic antidepressant overdosage after their addition to the Pharmaceutical Benefits list in August 1970, and the decline after the introduction of safety packaging.

increased by fifty per cent. The time taken undertaking this study was probably the most useful two hours work done in my life! The reduction in accidental overdosage in children was accompanied with a reduction in successful drug induced suicide in young adults at the same time. In those days there were no ethics committees which nowadays might not approve such a project. The opportunity to demonstrate a life saving procedure might thereby be lost. It is important that ethics committees are not so conservative that the quest for useful knowledge is inhibited.

The dysrhythmias (irregular heart beats) proved difficult to control at first until we happened to see a short note in a journal referring to some work done in France. It showed that an intravenous bolus of sodium bicarbonate would revert the rhythm and ECG pattern to normal. Many other suggestions for treatment were made by authors all over the world.

My research for several years aimed to determine which was the most effective method. Sodium bicarbonate, surprisingly, proved the most consistently effective. It is normally used as a buffer to correct metabolic acidosis (when free hydrogen ions in the blood increase outside the normal very narrow range the bicarbonate neutralizes the excess). In this situation it did not appear that it worked by correcting metabolic acidosis because arrhythmias could be produced in the same subject with the same dose at different pH levels (hydrogen ion concentrations). It may be that it caused acute shifts of ions so that the balance between the inside and outside of the cells resulted in less irritability.

We found that a bolus of intravenous sodium bicarbonate would stop the dysrhythmias. We had several successfully treated cases and had done some experimental work to back up our observations. We submitted the resulting paper to the Lancet, then the British Medical Journal, both rejected it. It was eventually published in the first volume of Anaesthesia and Intensive Care. Later, someone returning from England suggested that I should write up all our successfully treated dysrhythmia cases because they didn't know how to treat them in Britain. We sent the paper to the Archives of Paediatrics, a British journal, which rejected it. Despondent, I threw it in a drawer. Some months later I found it and sent it to the Medical Journal of Australia where it was published. You can imagine my surprise when a colleague came and told me shortly afterwards that a leader (special comment) had appeared in the Lancet about our work published in the Australian Medical Journal! Never give up!

I had the opportunity to visit the Toxicology Clinic in Paris, where these ideas originated. I found out that they had struck on this treatment accidentally because they gave their overdose patients a solution with sodium lactate which has buffering activity, but not sodium bicarbonate. They thought it had something to do with sodium but my experiments showed conclusively that it was the bicarbonate that was important.

Three years after that, in 1977, there was a World Intensive Care meeting in Paris which I attended. I offered a paper for the toxicology section of the meeting. It had to be unpublished work so the one I offered was comparing the cardiotoxicity of three antidepressant drugs. It was not accepted. When I arrived at the session a few minutes early I was warmly greeted by the co-chairman, Dr C Bismuth from the Toxicology Clinic. She expected that I would be speaking. When I told her that my paper had been suppressed (the expression used in the proceedings where there was a blank quarter page representing rejected papers) she was quite upset as she knew of my work. She spoke to the co-chairman, who was Professor Gaultier from her department. When the presentation of the papers concluded he announced, without warning, that Dr Brown would now speak for six minutes! I was somewhat surprised, but was able to comment on some of the papers and compare their findings with mine. It was an unusual experience.

Following that session there was an informal case discussion session. One doctor from London told a remarkable story from their clinic. They had a patient with a respiratory condition they had been unable to diagnose, but which was becoming progressively worse. The social worker was visiting the ward. As she was leaving she asked the nurse in charge what was wrong with him. When she said that they did not know, the social worker suggested they should think of poisoning, and left. Subsequently they found that the man's wife was bringing him barley water each day which she had laced with a substance which causes pulmonary fibrosis (stiffening of the lungs). He died and she was found guilty of murder!

The same drug was involved in another story. When I went to school at Heriots, in Edinburgh in 1947, I had a friend called Stanley Lewis who invited me home on at least one occasion. When I left to return to Kenya he gave me a book. Years later, sixteen to be exact, I was driving down Captains Road, Liberton in Edinburgh when I remembered that he had lived at No 95. I had had no contact with him for years. I knocked on the door and his mother answered it. She told me that he was working at John Bartholomew's, the well known map and atlas producers, with his father. My father had taken me to visit this publisher in 1956 because my father was a map enthusiast. He transmitted this to me and I, in turn , to two of my sons. It was a very interesting visit and the original John Barhtolomew gave me a little autographed atlas of Edinburgh, which regretably has disappeared. I did not know that Stanley Lewis was there. During subsequent visits to Edinburgh I looked out for Bartholomews in the area where I thought it was situated, around Salisbury Place. Then in 1984 I was driving past and saw John Bartholomew and sons, a grand building with impressive pillars at the front door. I went in and asked the girl at the desk if Stanley Lewis still worked there. She looked extremely blank! As I admired the foyer an older man came down the stairs and asked if he could help me. I told him that I was looking for Stanley Lewis. He then told me that his father had retired and that young Stanley had gone to live at the Borders (southern Scotland) but had later died of poisoning with the same drug. I do not know whether it was an accident or not. It is strange how lives can cross — sometimes something happens to make them connect and other times the chance is missed.

By 1978 I had so much material on tricyclic antidepressant overdosage that I requested permission to submit a thesis for a Doctorate in Medicine at Melbourne University. This was finally accepted and I graduated in person (I missed my original graduation as I had to leave for Canada) MD in 1980. It was a satisfying experience to receive a higher degree and to know that the information in the thesis had been of practical benefit in saving lives.

Another spin off from my work on toxicology was as a member of the Editorial Board of "Anaesthesia and Intensive Care". This is the Australian anaesthetic journal which also includes intensive care because anaesthetists did most of it when the journal was started by Ben Barry in 1972. In the early days they decided one issue per year would be a symposium. The first attempt failed so I took on the task of being sub editor. The first was on paediatric anesthesia, which I thought would be useful as there was a dearth of books on the subject and we had a strong field of potential authors, one of the prerequisites for organising symposia. Only two of nineteen papers sought did not eventuate. Unfortunately one was on fluids.

The next issue was on toxicology, another field which I felt was rather neglected. It was interesting, because as well as having papers on drug toxicity we had two on envenomation. Struan Sutherland worked at the Commonwealth Serum Laboratories on snake and spider envenomation and was involved in developing antitoxins. When approached he told me that he had been thinking of writing a review article for some time and this gave him the impetus to do so. It was a very comprehensive paper. It led on to greater things. Some time later he approached me to collaborate on some laboratory work on his antivenins. I was unable to do so because of lack of time but I organised Jim Tibballs, one of the intensivists to help him. Their collaborative research flourished and eventually they produced a large, authoritative text book on envenomations. Struan Sutherland was awarded an Officer of the Order of Australia (AO) for his work but unfortunately he died just before it was announced although he knew he was to receive it.

The other paper in that issue was by John Williamson AM. (17) from Townsville. His interest was on marine envenomations, of which there are plenty on the Queensland coast. The third symposium that I organised was on education in anaesthesia.

The times in the laboratory were an enjoyable diversion from my other clinical and administrative work. I was helped by George Cauchi and two young and very able pharmacists, Anne Leversha and Elizabeth Creber, who helped with the experiments. I had been involved in helping the Pharmacy Department to set up a continuing education programme and I thought some research involvement would add interest to their work. Liz Creber also helped me conduct a study on the optimal antipyretic dose (temperature lowering dose) of paracetamol. This dose of 10mg/kg was commonly used but was found later to be too low to be effective for paracetamol's other main use — pain relief. Several people contributed to that research which showed that three times the dose at least was needed. One of the leaders in the field was Brian Anderson (Figure C8) from Auckland, who spent a year training with us. He was a very enthusiastic and dynamic registrar.

During my early years at the hospital I was often consulted on pharmacological matters. I was involved in many studies on new drugs, some of which were related to specific areas of clinical interest which I will recount later. Unfortunately, after I stopped working in Intensive Care where we used so many drugs, and having less time, I was not able to keep up with all the advances that have occurred and thus lost this area of expertise.

Chapter 20

Cardiovascular Developments

Imagine walking into an operating theatre to find the surgeon operating on a baby whose heart was not beating. There was no ECG or blood pressure trace on the monitor screen and, if you had looked, you would have found that the pupils in the eyes were dilated; all signs of death. Was the surgeon crazy? Read on!

It is not surprising that by the time I began at the Royal Childrens Hospital (RCH), I had an interest in Cardiac surgery and anaesthesia. I remember seeing a narrowed mitral valve being opened when I was a student. Those were very early days in cardiac surgery. I remember when I was a student looking after a little blue boy, David, who remained blue because surgery for the condition (Fallot's Tetralogy) had not developed at the time. (50)

Then, when I was interning in London Ontario, I worked with the Cardiac surgeon, John Coles — that was exciting but at times sad. I remember looking after a man whose pulmonary artery was huge. He was offered surgery and was told he had a 50:50 chance. Really it was less but he took it as he said he was useless as he was. Watching him with his relatives before the operation was like watching a condemned man wondering if he might just gain a reprieve. He didn't.

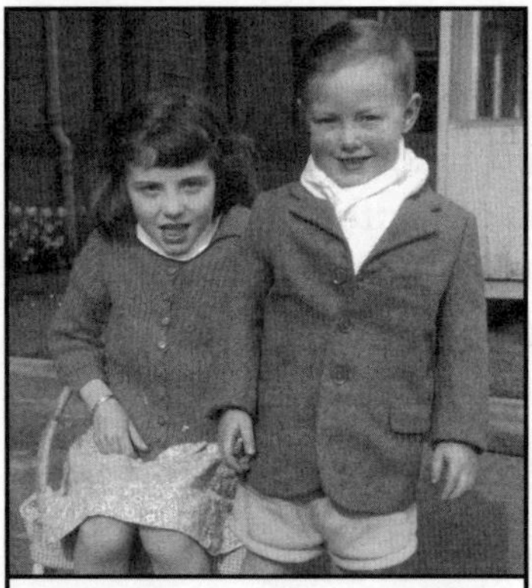

50. My first patients with congenital heart disease when I was doing a locum in Dundee for the resident during 5th year at university.

My time in Vancouver with Al Cox stimulated my interest in heart disease further. At that time diagnosis was dependent initially on recognising the murmurs created by altered flow of blood through the heart, by feeling for different pulses and observing the blood pressure. Cardiac catheters were introduced which could be passed into the heart to measure pressures and allow angiograms showing the blood flow patterns in the heart. Rheumatic heart disease which caused damage to the heart valves was the major problem being corrected. Coronary artery disease was treated symptomatically, with rest and then gradual exercise. If too severe, death ensued.

My introduction to cardiac anaesthesia was in Vancouver with anaesthetists such as Bill Dodds and Jack Nixon, both good teachers.

My real interest in paediatric cardiac anaesthesia developed in Toronto and it was as a result of this experience that I came to work at RCH. It was an exciting time to be involved as several breakthroughs occurred. New operations and techniques were being developed to solve the problems.

Cardiac surgery only became established in the 1950s. Heart lung machines were developed which could add oxygen to the blood and then pump the blood round the body — they performed the functions of the lungs and heart while the surgeons operated on the heart. In Toronto, Dr Bigelow, assisted by Dr Bill Lindsey, who became a plastic surgeon at the Hospital for Sick Children, studied hypothermia (cooling the body) as an adjunct which would provide greater safety in cardiac surgery by reducing the metabolic rate. It was possible to cool the blood to a set temperature when it was being pumped through the heart –lung machine. It could then be rewarmed at the end of the operation to bring the patients temperature back to normal.

In the months following my arrival at RCH we had a run of babies born with *transposition of the great vessels*. Their aorta and pulmonary arteries came off the wrong ventricles (wrong side of the heart). The children were very blue because little blood went through the lungs and therefore it was not oxygenated. At the time techniques to correct this anomaly in newborns had not been developed. An operation (Blalock-Hanlon) was performed to make a hole between the atria (upper chambers of the heart) so that blood could cross to the other side, thus allowing more to reach the lungs and improving oxygenation. It involved putting slings around the pulmonary veins for three to four minutes so that blood coming through the lungs did not spill when the heart was open.

I observed that all the babies developed congestion in the upper lobe of the right lung. Applying principles used in other situations in cardiac surgery, I suggested that if we released the pulmonary vein slings and let a small volume of blood (20-30 mls) off during the procedure, that the rise in pressure in the pulmonary vessels and hence the congestion in the right upper lobe, might be avoided. George Westlake, our cheerful, ambidextrous surgeon agreed to try it. It proved successful in all but one baby. He had a large flow through the bronchial artery (usually the blood supply to the lung tissue).

We had enough cases before and after the introduction of this technique to publish the information. Unfortunately while we were preparing the paper a new development arrived which made the operation unnecessary. A catheter had been developed with a balloon. This could be passed through the atrial septum (the separation between the two atria), the balloon blown up and then pulled back through the septum, tearing a hole in it which allowed the blood to cross over and reach the lungs. And so the first of several of my inventive ideas was just too late and was superceded!

At the end of 1967 I was sent to Adelaide to learn about perfusion (cardio-pulmonary bypass) in Darcy Sutherland's unit. He was the leading cardiac surgeon in Australia at the time. I soon learnt the ropes from his perfusionist, John Waddy, who was a cardiologist. They were brilliant clinicians, doing complex surgery and postoperative care with the minimum of sophisticated monitoring. They used an ECG and blood pressure to monitor the patient and would pull the sheet back and feel the feet to see if they were warm and the veins were adequately filled. I think that the secret of their success was due to Darcy's skill and gentleness as a surgeon and their skill at clinical assessment.I saw a triple valve replacement successfully managed in this way.

It was an enjoyable ten days. I stayed at one of Adelaide's oldest pubs across the road from the hospital, the Botanic, which had been there since the 1850s. It was not luxurious but it was interesting. I also had time to watch some of the South Australian tennis championships, where I saw a rising star, Billie Jean King. She went on to win many grand slam tournaments and was a prime mover in raising the standing of women's tennis

Years later, Darcy Sutherland came to RCH as cardiac surgeon, at a time when we did not have one and were having problems with the unit. It was a convenient time for him as, at the same time, he became the President of the Royal Australasian College of Surgeons which has its headquarters in Melbourne. He was energetic, friendly, firm and reasonable in his demands but I always found him fair in negotiations. Maybe it was that we shared the same birthday and were both Sagittarians! He began to get things into order and then went off around the world to look for someone he could train to take over. Such was his standing that when he found Roger Mee, a New Zealander working in Boston, he was able to persuade the Boston people to let him come on trial for six months and keep his job open for him should either party decide not to continue with the arrangement. As it turned out, Roger stayed and with Bill Braun, they made an outstanding team with the best results in the world. Bill eventually returned to England to become their best paediatric cardiac surgeon. Cardiac surgery depends not only in having a good surgeon but a good team — cardiologist, anaesthetist and technician, perfusionist, who runs the heart-lung machine, nurses and, post-operatively, intensive care staff — who all have an important role in the proceedings.

Deep hypothermia solved the problem of doing corrective cardiac surgery in infants. Years before, in 1970, a Japanese group developed a technique which enabled them to operate on babies' hearts in patients below ten kilograms by cooling the patients down to 18 ° C and then stopping the circulation. The idea was taken up by Brian Barrett Boyes in Auckland, one of the doyens of cardiac surgery at the time. Soon afterwards, Peter Clarke, who had been working with him, became our cardiac surgeon and brought the idea with him.

We immediately started in the laboratory, using the same technique in dogs. We cooled them with ice packs until the temperature was 25°C (normal is 37°C), then put them on bypass (heart lung machine) and cooled further to 18°C to minimise oxygen requirements. The blood was then drained off the dog into the oxygenator. The heart had stopped. It was left motionless for an hour. It was the situation I described at the beginning of the chapter. The pump was turned on again, the heart and blood vessels were filled and the blood was gradually rewarmed. It was one of the most amazing and exciting experiences to watch the heart muscle start to flicker, then gradually to beat irregularly and, as the temperature rose, it became more regular and stronger. Eventually when normal temperature was reached the pump was stopped and the subject disconnected. The dog made a complete and uneventful recovery. After we had done this successfully a few times we were able to do the same with small babies. It was an incredible advance at the time but now it is taken for granted that one can operate on a baby's heart. Modern surgeons have improved their skills so that they can operate with the heart lung machine still going.

An understanding of the physiology of hypothermia helps to explain how it protects the brain and also some of the research which I undertook at the time.

The following paragraphs explain this for those who are interested. Lowering body temperature slows chemical reactions and therefore all bodily functions. Lower animals , like the reptiles, snakes and lizards which do not maintain a constant body temperature, become sluggish when cold. In fact putting a snake in the refrigerator for a while makes it very inactive and therefore easier to anaesthetise! In mammals, including humans, metabolism decreases and oxygen consumption is reduced. This means that the oxygen present in the tissues lasts longer before the damage caused by oxygen deprivation occurs. The lower the temperature the longer the safe period.

Other changes occur. The solubility of gases increases as temperature falls. As the solubility of carbon dioxide, one of the products of metabolism, increases its tension in the blood decreases. This contributes to the acid-base status of the patient which is usually measured as pH. This term is a chemist's way of condensing the figures describing the free hydrogen ion concentration in the blood. It is the negative logarithm of the hydrogen ion concentration which does not give most people any concept of the amount.

This topic proved to be one of the greatest teaching challenges when I taught nurses, many of whom had done little chemistry. If we use the measure of nanomols, which is a quantity that can be compared easily with other chemicals in the body, pH 7.4 is 40 while pH 7.0 is 100 nanomols. Free hydrogen ion levels in the blood over 100 (pH below 7.0) and below 10 nanomols (pH8) usually results in death. The tolerable range is very narrow. It is maintained by buffers in the blood of which bicarbonate is the most prolific. It can react to take up hydrogen, forming carbonic acid, or the latter can release carbon dioxide when necessary to form more bicarbonate.

It is normally a very efficient system and only when someone is extremely ill does it become deranged, except when body temperature changes. Then, in hypothermia (lowering temperature) the free hydrogen ion decreases and the pH rises. One of the consequences is that haemoglobin, which carries oxygen in the red cells around in the blood, releases less oxygen into the tissues. To compensate for these changes we added carbon dioxide to the gases being delivered to the patient and the heart lung machine so that the pH was kept constant. The result was that more oxygen was delivered to the tissues before the heart stopped allowing a much longer time without circulation before the oxygen supply ran out. This is technically known as the *pH stat* system as opposed to the alpha stat system where carbon dioxide is not added and the pH is allowed to change with temperature in the same way as it does with water. The latter is now used in bypass procedures but the circulation is rarely stopped completely so it is less critical. Fashions change and the pH stat system is gaining popularity again.

The longest period of arrest that we had was 84 minutes, and the patient made a good recovery. Maybe the fact that some of these patients with complex abnormalities had been living with low oxygen tensions all their lives provided them with a greater safe range. In addition, I believe adding carbon dioxide to the oxygenator so that maximum oxygen was released in the tissues before we stopped the heart was vital to our success. The body is incredibly clever at adjusting to adverse conditions.

Another example of physiological adjustment is where the patient has an abnormality which prevents adequate volumes of blood from reaching the lungs for oxygenation and so they become blue (cyanosed), as in Fallot's tetralogy. They increase oxygen transport by increasing the haemoglobin that carries oxygen in the red blood cells. This makes the blood more viscous and results in increased resistance to flow. Clotting of the blood might seem to be more likely as a result but the body compensates by increasing the anti-clotting factors (fibrinolytic factors) present in the blood. The consequence is that these patients bleed more when operated upon. However, it has been shown that if some red cells are removed, lowering the haemoglobin and thus viscosity, the clotting mechanism returns to normal in a day or two. The patients will then bleed less. It is fascinating how these fine adjustments are made in the body to aid human survival.

In 1971, I heard Professor Douglas Lampard from the Electrical Engineering Department at Monash University speak on his computer controller for physiological variables which could also be used to give computer-controlled anaesthesia. This was a really exciting development. He was looking for clinical people to undertake collaborative research with him so I expressed my interest. That was the beginning of eight fruitful years as a Research Associate in his department. Doug was a brilliant man who had been a visiting professor of physiology as well as being an academic electrical engineer. He was also a very competent chemist, making perfume as a hobby. He enjoyed Jazz and played a ukulele in a band with my friend and colleague Noel Cass. His research student, John Coles, had built this enormous computer as a PhD project. It consisted of two modules about 150 by 50 cms., which is huge by today's standards but that was in the early days of computers.(51)

Our research with him related to brain blood flow during cooling. We demonstrated, using temperature probes in various parts of the brain, that if carbon dioxide was given during cooling, the blood flow in the brain was more even and the temperature gradients decreased. At lower carbon dioxide levels there were wider variations in temperature and flow in different parts of the brain. The great advantage of the computer controller was that we could keep the end expired carbon dioxide constant. It was able to compensate for changes in CO2 production due to decreased metabolism and also the changes in CO2 due to increasing solubility at lower temperatures.

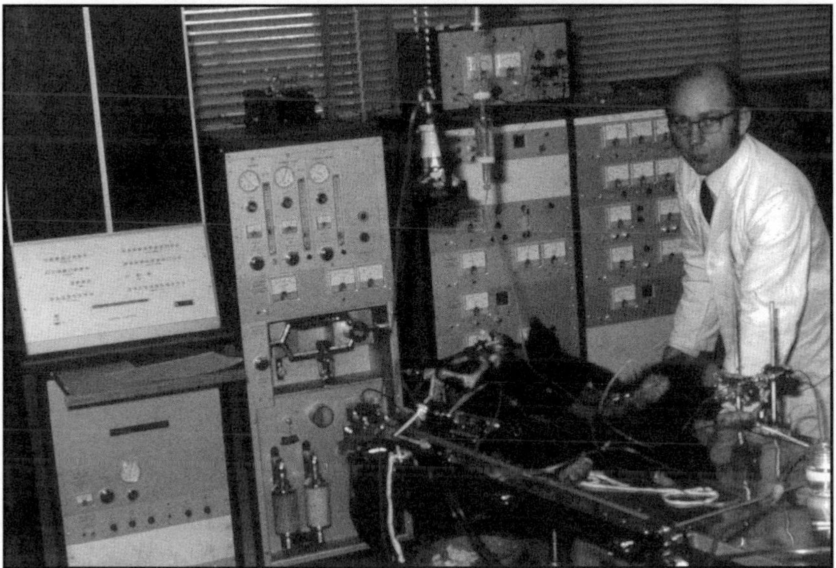

51. Bill Brown, one of our co-researchers with the large computer set up behind which was used for physiological studies and may have been used for the first computer controlled anaesthetic about 1970-1.

At the end of the day's experiments I often had to take blood samples 20 kms back to the hospital to do biochemical measurements which we could not do in their laboratory.

Their department also developed a computer controlled electromyograph which could be used to measure the degree of paralysis in muscle when muscle relaxant drugs were given and control their administration. We showed in a series of experiments which I did with a post doctoral fellow, Stephen Lam, that the dose of relaxants needed was reduced during hypothermia.

I was very privileged to be able to work with this group, Doug Lampard, Bill Brown, John Coles, and Stephen Lam, and to be allowed time to pursue this interesting research for several years.

When the Japanese group developed the deep hypothermia technique they included free fatty acid infusions in their protocol. I could not understand the purpose of this and so decided that if I could find someone who could measure free fatty acids I might find some useful information. I found Marjory Dunlop, who worked as a research biochemist with John Court, who was on sabbatical leave. She agreed, provided she could also measure insulin as she wanted to keep her technique up while John was away. The fatty acid work provided no useful information but the insulin work proved fascinating. Insulin decreased with cooling, rising on occasions when we gave potassium to correct dysrhythmias (irregularity of the heart beat) which sometimes occurred below 27 °C. It appeared that this was new information and we were excited at having made an original observation. Then I found a book with a chapter on the physiology of hypothermia. To my dismay I found that the effect of hypothermia on insulin had been described in 1928, only six years after the discovery of insulin. It must have been a remarkable piece of work as analytical methods were not as advanced. But why was the study done then? It showed that *if you look far enough back many things have been done before*. Many young scientists only go back about five years, so they miss much relevant data. Sometimes it is worth asking older colleagues if they are aware of any earlier work.

I read in the New England Journal of Medicine (1970) that hibernating animals show an increase in plasma magnesium during hibernation. Magnesium is an ion found mostly inside cells and only a small amount is extracellular. It is important in a number of ways. It acts at the neuromuscular junction to decrease the release of acetyl choline, the transmitter substance which carries nerve impulses across to the muscle to cause the muscle to contract. Increased serum magnesium (in the blood) thus causes weakness and decrease muscle activity, something that seems entirely logical in hibernation when activity is reduced.

I wondered what happened when animals were cooled and whether increasing magnesium by infusion might be useful in our work. So we measured electrolytes during cooling. Magnesium did not show any consistant change but potassium did. It regularly declined by 2 mmol/l while the patients cooled from 37 to 27°C. Thus, *when patients developed dysrhythmias (irregular heart beats) we gave some intravenous potassium and they disappeared, and the heart beat became regular again.* This was a very useful discovery as the problem of dysrhythmias during cooling when not using the heart lung machine was a worry. Sometimes serious ones could be life threatening. Now we know that a little intravenous potassium will fix the problem and stop the dysrhythmias.

The other fascinating aspect of this finding was that the insulin level paralleled the potassium level, rising when potassium was given supporting some other research that potassium plays a part in insulin release. We also found that the plasma glucose rose during cooling and decreased when the insulin rose in response to the potassium. Insulin normally lowers plasma glucose by facilitating its entry into cells.

My curiosity about magnesium led to all sorts of other findings. Magnesium has antiarrhythmic effects. One day we were going to use electrical cardioversion to stop a troublesome dysrhythmia in a child. I suggested that we try a bolus of magnesium first. I drew it up in the syringe and was approaching the patient when the rhythm spontaneously reverted to normal. If I had been twenty seconds earlier I would have taken the credit and would have been even more convinced of the benefits of magnesium. It was an interesting example of not drawing conclusions on inadequate evidence!

Magnesium has now been found to be useful in the treatment of *tetanus*. This terrible disease causes spasms of muscles and dangerous rises in blood pressure. The patients have to be kept in a quiet , darkened room for fear of setting off these spasms. The advent of diazepam was a major advance but it did not solve all the problems, especially the hypertensive crises. Magnesium, as I have mentioned, has an effect on the neuromuscular junction by reducing release of the chemical transmitter, acetyl choline. This reduces contractility and weakens the muscles so that in these patients it reduces spasms. It also has a beneficial effect on the adverse cardiovascular effects, mainly hypertension. One possible mechanism could probably be by reducing acetyl choline release at ganglia and reducing activity of the sympathetic nervous system. Tetanus can stimulate the cardiovascular system. So, although an old drug, magnesium sulphate has recently been found to be the most effective treatment for a terrible condition which has perplexed doctors for generations. Of course, immunization is available, and toxoid can be given if the possibility of infection is thought to be high. It is also being used in a number of other situations where cardiovascular stability is required. I sometimes wonder what discoveries I might have made if I had had pursued my initial idea of using it in deep hypothermia.

Hypothermia has many clinical applications but it is not widely used apart from cardiac surgery. It has had vogues in attempted brain preservation after head injury. We used it for many of our patients having liver tumours resected. In the early cases two had cardiac arrests during the operation because they had lost too much blood. One of these had been cooled and made an uneventful recovery after resuscitation while the other, who had not, was brain damaged. I believe that in some cases the extra time taken to cool the patient is worth spending for extra safety.

My involvement in hypothermia caused one amusing diversion. I received a phone call from one of the radio stations suggesting that I was an expert on *cryogenics*. Could I come and participate on their talk back program! I started by saying that as I was not certain of the definition of cryogenics it did not seem appropriate to ask me. "Oh! But you freeze babies, don't you?" was the response. I admitted that I did cool children for heart surgery. "That will do! Will you come?" So I participated in my only talk back show. It was about the development in California of deep freezing someone as they are dying so that they could be preserved until a cure was found for their terminal disease. I was not convinced, particularly after they read out the instructions clients carried with them — " If found dead pack head in ice and call this number". It would be impossible to cool the brain fast enough to save irreparable damage if that was done unless they were thrown into liquid nitrogen as they were dying. I told them that I thought the whole thing was nonsense. Someone was making a lot of money. I wonder how these cryogenically cooled people will be kept? I also wonder if anyone would bother to revive them.

Vasodilators and the use of hypotension to reduce blood loss became a valuable adjunct to our work. It is not often that one can define an occasion as a turning point. In 1971 Ron Katz from New York was the guest speaker at the Australian Society of Anaesthetists Annual meeting in Perth. One of his talks was about the use of a drug called sodium nitroprusside. Surprisingly, it is a very old drug, having first been made in 1888. It is very short acting and works by relaxing smooth muscle in blood vessel walls, causing them to dilate. Its cardiovascular effects were well described in a paper by Johnston in 1927 but yet it had been in oblivion for the next forty years. Its potential was exciting but it was not available commercially in Australia. Some enthusiasts had their hospital pharmacies make it up for them until the commercial potential was realized and it became available on the market.

Before describing why it was so useful, consideration of the application of *Ohms Law* in Physics to Physiology and medicine is worthwhile.

It is volts (potential difference) = current x resistance. (V=IR)

In physiology this can be translated into Pressure = Flow x Resistance. In cardiac physiology this is Blood Pressure = Cardiac Output (amount of blood pumped out of the heart per minute) x Peripheral Resistance.

In respiratory physiology it is Pressure = air flow x airways resistance. Thus, in an asthmatic when the airway resistance increases due to bronchospasm it takes a greater pressure difference to maintain the normal flow or, if this cannot be achieved, the amount of air entering the lungs will fall and eventually oxygenation and carbon dioxide elimination will become inadequate and respiratory failure ensues.

When the blood vessels dilate the blood pressure will fall if the cardiac output remains the same. This is the basis of induced hypotension (lowering blood pressure) which was introduced in the 1960s with the advent of ganglion blocking drugs to lower blood pressure during anaesthesia. These drugs were not as controllable and some disasters occurred so that the technique fell into disrepute. Sodium nitroprusside, on the other hand, was short acting (a few minutes) and easy to control when given by an infusion.

So much interest developed that two years later a group of interested people met in Sydney to discuss their experiences. Major scoliosis surgery (correction of twisted spines) was relatively new. Blood loss was significant with three or four units of blood commonly being needed. The operation current at the time was insertion of Harrington rods — two rods laid along the spine with hooks to hold the back straight. It took about three hours. Janice Peeler (20) provided anaesthesia at RCH for these operations. She introduced hypotensive anesthesia for them. The blood loss was reduced, so that rarely was more than one unit, if that, was needed and the operating time was shortened to 1 — 1 1/2 hours, presumably because the surgeons gained more experience but also because they could see what they were doing better without blood in their field. She did over a thousand cases, possibly the largest individual experience in the world. She became expert at assessing blood pressure by the feel of the pulse when it was measured as the blood pressure was being lowered.

My use of the technique was more varied but having acquired the skill it has proved very useful on many occasions.

I did a small study on cooling anaesthetised puppies. We infused saline in one, 10% alcohol, which we used with hypothermia, in another and sodium nitroprusside in the third. Alcohol decreased cooling time by a quarter, while nitroprusside halved it, demonstrating the relative degrees of vasodilatation with each drug and the benefit in aiding cooling

I introduced nitroprusside and later, phenoxybenzamine, into cardiac anaesthesia, initially to treat vasoconstriction post-operatively where a reduced cardiac output resulted. Dilating the patient and giving extra blood and fluids reduced the load on the heart, improved its output and hence kidney blood flow and urine output. Its effect could be dramatic. We then started putting some in the heart lung machine so that the patient was fully dilated when perfusion from the pump concluded. This resulted in more rapid and even rewarming and the circulation was well filled, because all tissues were dilated.

Previously rewarming the patient was uneven, so that the parts, which were still cool and constricted at the end of the operation, dilated later. The blood volume became inadequate and the blood pressure declined. More fluids were required. In addition the heart had to pump against a higher resistance and thus the energy required was increased.

Later, we added sodium nitroprusside and then the longer acting drug, phenoxybenzamine (which blocked the sympathetic vasoconstrictor effect), to facilitate cooling and rewarming , as well as to avoid the above problems.

I remember meeting Eve Seelye for afternoon tea at the very grand old Melbourne institution, the Windsor Hotel in Spring Street. She was an anaesthetist who worked with Brian Barrett Boyes at Greenlane Hospital in Auckland. She wanted to know about our experience with vasodilators. At that time his opinions and those of Kirklin in Alabama were heeded by cardiac surgeons all over the world, so that our ideas were probably popularised by them.

My first paper on the use of vasodilators in cardiac surgery, written with Rob Burton, a brilliant young surgeon who eventually became Director of the Anti-Cancer Council, was rejected because of the lack of sophisticated monitoring which we did not have at the time. However, it may have been ahead of its time because there were no other reports of the use of vasodilators in cardiac surgery.

My second paper, on the use of short term hypotension in critical situations met with same fate — rejection. How conservative some people are! This paper described several situations when bleeding during the operations was out of control, and by using vasodilators the situation was quickly brought under control. An example was a child with a brain tumour who started bleeding profusely. The surgeon could not locate the bleeding point because the blood welled up in the wound as soon as pressure was taken off the site. I happened to wander in to see how they were progressing to find a stressed anesthetist pumping blood into the patient while the surgeon repeatedly and unsuccessfully tried to locate the bleeding vessel. A massive transfusion situation with no solution in sight was approaching. I told the surgeon to keep pressure on the bleeding vessel while we replaced the lost blood, gave some extra fluids because the volume the circulation would hold would increase when we dilated the patient. We mixed up a dilute solution of sodium nitroprusside (0.1mg/ml) and administered a very small dose. This was enough to lower the blood pressure and reduce the bleeding for two or three minutes. The surgeon then removed the pack and could easily locate the bleeder as the flow was much reduced and in a couple of minutes had the situation under control. The patient avoided a massive transfusion which causes many complicating factors, the surgeon's and the anaesthetist's stress were relieved and the operation ended much sooner. Everyone was better off and yet my paper was rejected.

Occasionally people have what seem like minor head injuries. The blood pressure rises and the heart fails. Then the blood pressure falls and the lungs become congested. The patient needs to be ventilated to keep him alive. The condition is called neurogenic pulmonary oedema. We had such a case, which improved with the ventilator treatment but became worse as soon as it was stopped. Isoprenaline, a drug that stimulates the heart by stimulating the sympathetic nervous system (ß1 stimulant) was given by infusion. The patient improved. It was decided to put a catheter into the left ventricle of the heart and to measure the pressures during these manoeuvres. In addition it was decided to give a small dose of sodium nitroprusside to see what effect vasodilating him would have. He improved with the latter, so phenoxybenzamine , a long acting vasodilator (alpha blocker which relaxes all vessels except those in the brain) was given and by the next morning he had recovered. This was an interesting case as there was much debate at the time on the mechanism of neurogenic pulmonary oedema. Our studies supported the concept that it is due to an acute sympathetic discharge causing severe vasoconstriction (hence the rise in blood pressure) followed by an inability of the heart to pump against the suddenly increased resistance so it fails and pulmonary oedema (fluid in the lungs) develops. Physiologists refer to this as an increase in afterload which has to be relieved or the heart will fail. The vasodilators decrease the afterload. It took the four authors six years to complete this case report and have it published — my second slowest publication!

I had an interesting experience in Italy which confirmed that not everybody believed me. I was invited to give a lecture in Padua, one of the oldest universities in Europe. During part of it I discussed our experience with hypotensive anaesthesia. I had overheads prepared in Italian so they could follow my lecture more easily. At the end the gist of the questions was " isn't this a dangerous technique?" I assured them it was not, particularly in children, if one knew what one was doing. My daughter, who speaks Italian, was in the audience and told me after that there was much discussion around her casting doubt on the veracity of my comments!

The technique is safe if used correctly in appropriate situations. It is generally safe in children. In some older people one has to be careful as it is not always appropriate, especially when they have cardiovascular disease and the blood pressure falls below that critical for perfusion of the brain and heart. Toxic effects were described if certain administration rates were exceeded. We had one small baby whose blood pressure remained low after cardiac surgery. We assumed that the problem related to the surgery, and were not very hopeful of the outcome until six hours later the pressure suddenly increased to normal and the patient made a good recovery. In retrospect, it may be that with slower drug metabolism the small dose given was too much and it took a long time to metabolise. It did not show any of the usual signs of distinctive of nitroprusside toxicity. The only problem was a small pressure sore on the back of the head because the baby's position was not changed. The weight of the head prevented adequate blood flow in the compressed area.

Cyanide is a potential product of nitroprusside breakdown if it happens too rapidly. It was a matter of concern when we first used it but I never saw it occur and am unaware of any cases where it happened. We always restricted the dose and would discontinue if the hypotensive effect was not easily produced. In children I put 1mg/kg in 100 ml in a burette. This was a safe dose. Only once did I stop because the rate of infusion needed was too rapid.

I have used hypotension many times to stem the flow with troublesome bleeding and also preemptively to avoid significant blood loss, so that the surgeon can see what he or she is doing. The technique can be used in conjunction with hypothermia to provide maximum safety in very hazardous operations, by reducing bleeding and decreasing metabolism, in the event blood of blood flow being reduced to critical or lower levels. I did one very complex neurosurgical case where the surgeon told me that 50% of patients had died having it done. I used this combined technique and after ten hours the operation was successfully completed.

In another six month old child, who had a rare condition with a very large tongue (Beckwith-Wiedemann syndrome) which required two operations to reduce its size to normal , we then had to operate to resect a liver tumour. This is a hazardous procedure in small children but the difficulty was compounded by this baby's parents being *Jehovah's Witnesses*. They believe that the Bible says that transfusion is not allowed and if one of their members receives a transfusion he or she will be ostracized. It creates a very difficult situation for the attending doctors, especially when significant blood loss can be expected and the patient is already anaemic from previous operations, as in this case. We succeeded using hypothermia, hypotension and haemodilution where the patients blood is diluted so that any lost will contain less of its valuable haemoglobin. With very careful surgery the operation was successfully completed without transfusing anyone else's blood.

We had a period when the Jehovah's Witnesses were trying to persuade doctors to sign up to look after their patients and guarantee not to give blood. This approach caused some irritation as we tried to go along with their requests anyway. I suggested we should have a meeting with their representatives and this was duly organised. Representatives of the departments most involved with blood transfusion attended. The Jehovah's Witness representatives explained their situation and the doctors made comments from their points of view, which varied. Interestingly, and coincidentally, members of one religion seemed much more hostile towards them than the others. The discussion was informative, courteous and ended by concluding that the hospital staff tried to adhere to their principles, that there would be times when it might be difficult but we had opened a channel for discussion to occur if necessary. I also pointed out that while we respected their religious belief, some of our members held equally strong, but different beliefs and that we hoped that they would respect them. It proved to be a very worthwhile meeting. So often when there is apparent conflict sitting down and listening to the other point of view allows mutual understanding to be reached and a more reasonable attitude to develop.

I stopped doing cardiac anaesthesia in 1974 and used the experience that I had gained with the various techniques to deal with difficult cases in other fields. It had been an interesting period of my career and I had the good fortune to participate in some of the most exciting new developments. One can glean from my comments that anaesthetists can do a great deal to help surgeons in difficult situations. Collaboration, teamwork and mutual respect leads to success and a good outcome for the patients.

Chapter 21
Airway Problems

We are all addicted to breathing oxygen for survival! Because this is so important, overcoming airway problems in patients is a topic paediatric anaesthetists discuss frequently. This has been one of my main clinical interests. It can be very challenging. Most of this work has been with Ear, Nose and Throat surgeons and respiratory physicians.

Routine ear, nose and throat (ENT) operations are regarded as bread and butter work. I often think that the cost benefit of removing enlarged tonsils and adenoids, which obstruct breathing, or doing a myringotomy (draining fluid from the ear), which allows a child to hear and thus learn better, must rank as some of the most worthwhile operations.

In Melbourne I have worked with four very able ENT surgeons. Clive Pyman was a gentle, caring man who had no idea of time. He was always late and often came at 10pm to remove a foreign body from some child's airway — and then he took a long time to do it. He was not aware that the toxicity of local anaesthetics increased at that time. (Science 153:100.) John Floyd succeeded him for a short time as he decided to retire when he reached fifty. He was a delightful, quiet man with whom to work. His father was an exceptional man who ran a regular weekly classical music programme on the radio until he was well over 90 years old. Warner Mooney then took over until he had a coronary at the races. He made a good recovery and we worked together on many interesting and challenging problems for over 25 years. Rob Berkowitz is a thoughtful, meticulous man who took on the challenge of repairing narrowed airways successfully. He made a vertical incision in the trachea and inserted an oval piece of rib (costal) cartilage into the opening thereby opening the airway. In severe cases a cartilage graft could also be placed in the posterior wall of the trachea. He is more active in research than most ENT surgeons doing some interesting work on laryngeal reflexes.

Some fascinating research carried out in the Otorhinolarygology Department in Toronto when my friend David Mitchell was head, demonstrated electron microscopically, that the hair cells in the cochlea, which we are dependent on for hearing, are structurally destroyed by exposure to excessive noise. It worries me to think how young people listening to loud music risk damaging their hearing for ever. I think that this is why bands increase the volume as the evening progresses- they cannot hear the music well enough themselves because they are already deaf. What a tragedy for them. I believe noise pollution is a major public health problem which needs attention. Imagine a world full of humans who cannot hear — I suppose they would just communicate by some sort of sophisticated email or hand signs.

A relatively common childhood accident is the inhalation of a foreign body into the airway. They usually settle in the bronchus (airway leading into the lung). Seventy per cent of these children are in the exploring age — 1 to 3 year olds. They usually have a coughing episode when the inhalation occurs and thereafter may have a wheeze. About a quarter of these are not recognized as inhalation for over a week afterwards. They then present as asthma or with a respiratory infection. In many countries the commonest object to be inhaled is a peanut. These should not be available in the house if there are children under three years of age, if this potential hazard is to be avoided. Once, a child's grandfather had given the toddler peanuts. She chewed them into little pieces and then accidentally inhaled them into both lungs. There were so many pieces that unfortunately we were not able to clear them before she died. It was long before the days of ECMO (Extra corporeal membrane oxygenators) which might have saved her today.

The trachea and bronchi expand when we breathe in and contract when we breathe out. This allows the interesting phenomenon of air trapping to occur because air can pass the object during inspiration when the bronchus is dilated but does not let it escape when the airway narrows in expiration. The lung on the affected side then distends. If the foreign body swells and the tissues around it become swollen air will not enter and eventually the air in the lung will be absorbed into the circulation and the lung beyond the obstruction will collapse. When one side is blocked, one cannot hear air entering. This is one clinical sign that enables the doctor to diagnose the problem and determine on which side it is situated. From the anaesthetist's point of view no anaesthetic gas can be absorbed on that side and so an inhalation anaesthetic takes longer to establish.

Removing these requires good cooperation between the anaesthetist and the surgeon. They have to share the airway to let the patient breathe oxygen and the anaesthetic gases while the surgeon passes a bronchoscope (a metal tube with a light at the end) to look for and remove the object.

The great advances during my career were:- (1) the development of endoscopes which can be used to look into different parts of the body; (2) fibreoptic illumination for them which gave a much more intense light and allowed the light to go round corners, and (3) the operating microscope and the laser which can be directed down the airway to destroy abnormal tissue, like papilloma (warts) which can grow in the larynx and lower airways. I designed a device to use with the microlarygoscope which is used for microlaryngeal surgery (using the microcsope to operate on the larynx). It was an extension with a short tube which slid through the laryngoscope into the larynx so that the laser did not damage the vocal cords when it was being directed on to tissues beyond the cords, in the trachea. I had just had a set made (52) when they produced a microlaryngoscope with a long, narrow extension incorporated — once again I was just too late!

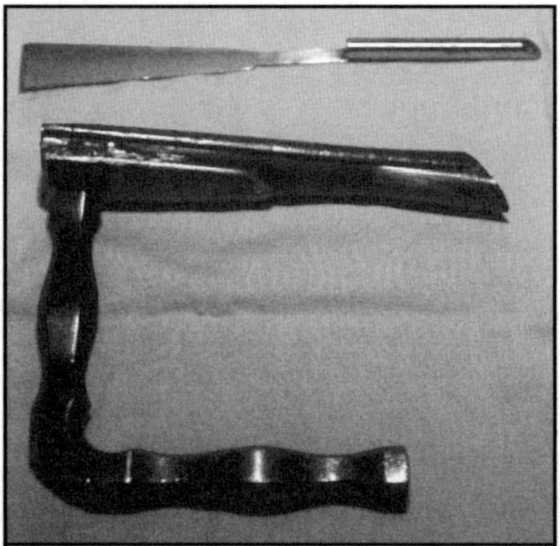

52. Inner tube for the microlarygoscope to protect the vocal cords during laser treatment. It was designed by the author and made in the hospital.

Laryngoscopes and bronchoscopes can be used to study the airways looking for abnormalities. These may include cysts or nodules pressing from outside, something narrowing the airway or some narrowing within the trachea. Among the most difficult conditions are wart-like growths that invade the larnyx, called papilloma. They can behave like warts and be troublesome for a year or two and then disappear. Some don't and just keep regrowing.

Justin became a special friend. He presented first as a baby and continued until he was eighteen having the papillomata removed every four to six weeks. They caused so much obstruction to his airway that he had a tracheotomy (opening into the trachea below the larynx. He eventually had 230 anaesthetics, of which I probably gave over two thirds of them. They were not easy anaesthetics as he often displayed various side effects seen with the anaesthetic agent, halothane, like spasm of his muscles or irregular heart beat. In his younger years he also went through a brief stage of excitement, which is sometimes seen as an inhaled anaesthetic is deepened during induction of anaesthesia. In the last couple of years when I gave his anaesthetic this response was replaced by one I have never seen in anybody else — he put on a broad grin as he lost consciousness. I understand that latterly he became quite agitated when I was not there to anaesthetise him. Eventually the growth spread through the tissues including his oesophagus so that he could not swallow. Despite this he retained a positive attitude to life and continued doing things that boys do. As he grew older we organized for him to come down to the department to help with some electronic work. The last time he came to see me I was busy and so he said that he would not stop and bother me. Unknown to us he was referred to an adult hospital where they decided to do a radical operation to try to remove all the growth which by now had invaded and obstructed his oesophagus. Sadly, he died during the operation but it was a peaceful way to go rather than suffocating, which might eventually have happened. It is rare to have such a close relationship with a patient for so long but it was disappointing to us that the adult surgeons did not even consult us before they operated. I lost a friend, but I was privileged to be able to tell his friends, at his funeral, what a brave and wonderful lad he had been. He tried to live life to the full. I have continued to keep in touch with his mother who helps children with disabilities in school.

Babies sometimes have noisy breathing (stridor) which is caused by narrowing of the airway making the airflow through the larynx turbulent. This can be due to an anatomical abnomality or it can result from unusual function of the larynx. One condition, known as laryngomalacia or infantile larnyx, is caused by the epiglottis, which in these children is curled into an omega shape, becoming even more tightly constricted when they breath in. At the same time two little arytenoid cartilages adjacent to the epiglottis tend to fall inwards. All this makes the entrance to the airway narrower, which causes stridor (noisy breathing). Usually the condition resolves as they grow and reassurance is all that is necessary. Diagnostic examination under anaesthesia requires the patient to be breathing on their own so that the movements can be observed. We had one infant who was deemed to need a tracheotomy because the obstruction was so severe. This was unusual and when we checked the child after a year to determine if the tracheotomy could be removed a nodule was found. Looking over his body, light brown "café au lait" spots were found in scattered patches. These two features, nodules and café au lait spots, are characteristic of von Recklinghausen's neurofibromatosis. I have seen two of these very rare cases with nodules pressing on the larynx.

The part of the airway just below the vocal cords can become narrowed, usually as a result of damage. In small infants, particularly premature babies, this can result from pressure when an endotracheal tube has been inserted as part of life supporting treatment. The airway is so small that even a narrow tube might exert pressure on the mucosa reducing the blood flow to it. If this happens it can fibrose and constrict when the tube is removed. It may also result from other forms of trauma such a transection of the trachea. One boy fell across a wire and hit his neck, resulting in the trachea being divided. Fortunately someone was able to insert an endotracheal tube into the trachea so that it could be repaired. The problem was that scarring narrowed the hole which we then had to try to keep open by repeatedly dividing the scar tissue with the laser. He had a tracheotomy which we were not able to remove permanently. He was a wonderful boy but attempts to remove the narrowing failed. He continued to play sport with a tracheotomy.

A few babies are born with narrow segments of the airway which can be very difficult to manage, especially if they are long segments in the chest. The surgical solution to these difficult problems vary. They require close collaboration with an experienced and very specialised anaesthetist to cope with the varying situations that arise during these operations. Tubes may have to be removed and replaced and the patients kept oxygenated while it is progressing.

One child, with a narrowed lower end of the trachea, had the stricture resected under hypothermia. This gave the surgeon more time to do the resection and place the posterior sutures without the child suffering from a lack of oxygen. Sometimes they are even done with cardiopulmonary bypass (using a heart lung machine).

Some babies lack the cartilages which hold the trachea and bronchi open. We devised a simple but novel method to assess the degree of the tendency to collapse called a tracheobronchogram. We could instill some radio-opaque dye and then apply varying degrees of positive pressure to determine what pressure was needed to keep the airway open. One such baby had collapsing main bronchi after the airway divides at the

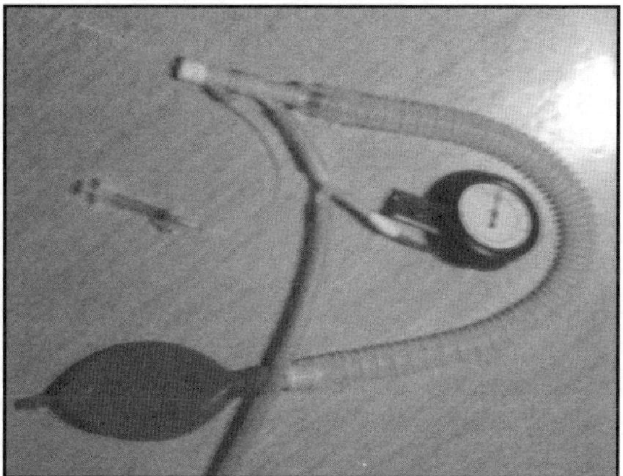

53. Circuit arrangement for tracheobronchogram. Note double Portex Y connector — one for anaesthetic with a pressure guage in the inflow side arm and the other to pass a catheter to instill the radio-opaque dye.

trachea. We had to make a special double lumen tube which had to be placed with one tube going into each side. This was extremely difficult and I was asked many times to insert it, usually at 4 or 5 pm when I was getting tired. By the time it was in place one or two hours later I was exhausted by the stress — probably that was why they asked me to do it! The hope was that when he grew it might be possible to take the tube out. After a year in intensive care it was removed and the baby went home. His mother was fantastic with him and in helping the staff. Everyone realized that he was still at risk but the family were pleased to get him home. Unfortunately he died a few days later.

This is one of those terrible dilemmas faced by doctors treating complex problems. Is it really worth all the effort, costly resources and mother's time sitting in Intensive Care with the child. She was grateful for all our efforts but eventually realized that they were futile and maybe that we should not have continued so long. It is difficult to stop treating such patients once started and it is difficult to know at the beginning what the outcome will be. Her grief was partly consoled by the birth of a normal healthy child not long afterwards.

We had a six-month-old boy who had been fed by a tube passed through his nose into his stomach. His problem was that his jaws were fused shut so an operation was proposed to separate them so he could open his mouth. Our first attempt to pass a tube through the nose into his trachea blind was unsuccessful. After several attempts we decided to abandon the procedure that day and do some x-rays to see if they could help to delineate the reason why we could not pass the tube. We found that the opening to the larynx was one vertebral level higher in the neck than usual, which made it more difficult to negotiate the tube around the tighter bend to reach the trachea. The technique of blind nasal intubation involves getting the patient to a deep plane of anaesthesia breathing an inhalational anaesthetic. The tube is then inserted into the nose and advanced. As it approaches the larynx the breathe sounds become louder and louder. It requires skillful manipulation of the tube towards the larynx which is pressed backwards. The tube is guided towards the position where the breath sounds are loudest. Then, with luck, the tube will enter the larynx. In this case it kept slipping past it.

On the second occasion we decided to cover the larynx with local anaesthetic. This was done by injecting local anaesthetic through a catheter passed through the nose into the oropharynx where it pooled and then pushing the larynx back into it. The excess local anaesthetic was then sucked out. This made the larynx less reactive and then, with more pressure on the larynx we were able to align and pass the tube. We learnt from this incident the value of a lateral neck x ray and how to anaesthetise the larynx even when one cannot see it. Flexion of the neck also helps the passage of the tube.

It is challenging situations such as this that demand the ultimate skills of the anaesthetist and gives great satisfaction when one succeeds. Nowadays, in more affluent countries, a fibreoptic bronchoscope can be inserted through an endotracheal tube and passed with vision into the trachea. The tube is passed over the bronchoscope which is then removed. The problem arises when one is not available. Younger anaesthetists tend do not acquire the skills to perform difficult intubation without the fibreoptic bronchoscope because they never have the opportunity to learn the alternative techniques.

I developed a special interest in a group of patients with series of syndromes (congenital abnormalities) grouped as the mucopolysaccharidoses, because they have abnormal deposits of these substances and abnormal metabolism. The patterns of disease differs with each syndrome but some of them have very difficult airways to manage during anaesthesia. My interest in these patients was aroused by one two year old boy with Hurlers syndrome who was to have two small operations. He did not look particularly well and I warned the mother that if we had difficulty we might stop after the first one. We did. After that we reviewed all our cases and found that a tube passed through the nose provided the best airway. The basic problem turned out to be that children with Hurler's and Hunter's syndromes have abnormal upper cervical vertebrae which makes the neck shorter and the larynx lie relatively higher. This makes it more difficult to see the larynx with the laryngoscope. After that, we tried to ensure that all their anaesthetics were given by a few anaesthetists who developed special expertise in their care. If possible, these patients should be referred to centres with people expert in handling them. Some of the syndromes also have associated heart disease. Hurler's can have coronary artery disease and Hunter's can have abnormal heart valves. Another variety, Morquio's syndrome, can have subluxation (sliding forward of a vertebrae) in the neck resulting in spinal cord compression. These require the utmost care so that the cord is not compressed further during anaesthesia. This could lead to quadriplegia.

Anaesthetists have a great advantage in working with surgeons in different specialties. A solution to a problem used by one specialist may not be known to someone in another field where it could be useful. The anaesthetist can be the conduit for such ideas from one to another.

Various anaesthetic methods and drugs are used in this airway work. Not long after I arrived at the Childrens Hospital a new French drug called gammahydroxybutyrate became available for trial in the hospital. I was fortunate to do these trials, one of two people in Australia to do so. The other was Bill Cole, a sessional anesthetist at the hospital who tested all the new anaesthetic drugs. This drug is a simple compound closely related to ß hydroxybutyrate which is part of the Krebs metabolic cycle, well known in biochemistry. One of its most useful properties was that it provided good conditions to observe the larynx without paralysing the patient. The patient takes big slow breaths which made observation of the airway easier. It was useful for microlaryngoscopy and bronchoscopy. Its major disadvantage was that the patients remained unconscious for longer than required, sometimes two to three hours. It had been observed that ß hydroxybutyrate, given before it, counteracted its effect. I decided to try giving it afterwards to see if it would reverse its effect. Because we only had a limited supply I decided to study it in a small animal, so I chose a rabbit. I gave a dose over ten times that which I had been giving children and all that happened was that the rabbit's ears drooped. Obviously we had an example of species variation to the response to a drug and so abandoned the experiment. (Shortly afterwards the rabbit was offered some lettuce and, immediately, its ears pricked up!)

People working in Dunedin in New Zealand later found that the anti-cholinesterase drug, physostigmine, reversed its action.

Unfortunately this drug has now appeared as one of the drugs young people take as a recreation drug, not realizing how dangerous this is.

My first venture into film making, in 1972, was *Gammahydroxybutyrate Anaesthesia for microlaryngoscopy for removal of laryngeal papilloma in children*. It was wonderful to be able to show the vocal cords moving as the patient breathed. It was technically much more difficult to show this before the days of fibre-optic light sources and flexible endoscopes which were developed later.

It was also before the convenience of video was introduced for recording such events. It is now so easy to record things that young people do not realise that it was not always so. The 16mm film gave very clear images when projected, much better than video, but it was a much more complex and slower process editing 16mm films than video. In addition the commentary had to be read word perfect straight through, a very difficult task.

I undertook some other research related to the airway work. I spent some sabbatical leave at the Veterinary School at Queensland University with Professor Michael Rex. He was a wonderful and very talented man. He had a rugby blue from Cambridge, was musical as well as having his veterinary interests of which anaesthesia for animals was a major one. He also played an active role in the Australian Anaesthetic Research Group which provided a forum for researchers to meet for about 15 years from 1977. It was very sad that he died while waiting for cardiac surgery.

We used a model of his where we implanted electrodes into the cricothyroid muscle in the larynx in anaesthetised cats. Elaine Robinson, one of his research students, helped with these experiments where we sprayed the vocal cords with the local anaesthetic, lignocaine, and stimulated the muscle periodically until activity returned when the cords were stimulated, indicating that the local anaesthetic effect had worn off. It was an exhausting but worthwhile week as we showed that the duration of action of the local anaesthetic was related to concentration, being longer with higher concentrations.

An interesting aside while I was there was a "paraplegic" snake which was brought in for x rays of its spine! It had a tumour compressing its spinal cord and it was decided to put it down. The x rays were taken under injected ketamine anaesthesia. Snakes can be given a general anaesthetic. It is advisable first to sedate them, which is most easily accomplished by putting them in a refrigerator to slow them down, and then a fine catheter can be inserted into a small hole under the tongue and the inhalation anaesthetic administered through it.

Even the common upper respiratory infection in a child can be a challenge to the anaesthetist. Should one proceed with the anaesthetic or postpone it. Usually if the child has a temperature, has a bad cough and looks sick it will be postponed. The difficult decision is to which children can one give the anaesthetic and what problems might occur by doing so. Risks have to be balanced with other factors — how urgent is it; has the family traveled a long way for a minor operation; has the parent had to take a day off work; has it been difficult to arrange baby sitters? All this has to be assessed against a risk which is often small, but occasionally the anaesthetist may have difficulty with an irritable airway. Fortunately we are trained to deal with the problems. Sometimes the decision is easy, at other times it is not.

Postoperative hypoxaemia was a subject which was widely discussed when I was training. This is a subtle reduction in the oxygen saturation of the haemoglobin which occurred after anaesthesia. A paper in the Canadian Anaesthetists Society Journal (1965) by Dery, Pelletier and others explained the importance of maintaining nitrogen in the lungs to prevent a reduction in functional residual capacity — really the prevention of areas of collapse following anaesthesia. (This is one of a few key papers, which have significantly influenced my practice.) Nitrogen diffuses into the blood much more slowly than oxygen and nitrous oxide and so splints the alveoli so they do not collapse. In 1976 I came to the conclusion that the elimination of nitrogen from the lungs was one of the reasons that premature babies went back to having apnoea (not breathing) spells after anaesthesia. These could be avoided by ensuring that the lungs were inflated with air (which contains 80% nitrogen) at the end of the anaesthetic. Later, when we had air available on the anaesthetic machines, it could be used to carry the anaesthetic vapours. The apnoea problem virtually disappeared, except in those babies who were having frequent attacks before anaesthesia when respiratory centre immaturity played a greater part.

Many years later we decided not to re-use disposable face masks in the recovery room for administering oxygen. We then decided, as an economy measure, not to use them anyway when the oximeter reading was 94% or higher because that indicated that there was plenty of oxygen reaching the tissues. Ventilating with 50% air at the end of the anaesthetic seemed to lessen the need for oxygen administration. The nitrogen was keeping the alveoli open.

Another application of this knowledge relates to blowing up the cuff on a endotracheal tube to create an airtight seal. Wally Thompson (61) in Perth demonstrated that if air is used nitrous oxide will diffuse into the cuff, causing an increase in volume and hence pressure in the cuff. This leads to greater ciliary dysfunction and an increase in likelihood of secretions being retained in the airways. If the cuff is filled with the gas that is being used for the anaesthetic diffusion does not take place and then only the warming which occurs in the body will raise the pressure, but by a much smaller amount.

These may seem like fine details but I have always thought they are important. Attention to detail is an essential requirement of a good anaesthetist.

Respiratory and airway problems constitute some of the anaesthetist's greatest challenges, particularly in children, and it is important for patients that the anaesthetist knows how to handle them. Collaboration and discussion with the surgeon is vitally important.

Chapter 22
Neurosurgery

Enormous advances have been made since I began neurosurgical anaesthesia. At that time none of the complex scanning techniques were available. The common neuroradiological investigations were *pneumoencephalography* and *cerebral angiography*. The former depended on doing a lumbar puncture at the lower end of the spine with the patient sitting up in a special seat. Some cerebrospinal fluid (CSF) was removed and replaced with air. This, being less dense than CSF, rises until it reaches the ventricular system in the brain. X-rays show where it is. Because the ventricles have a complicated shape the patient had to be somersaulted, turned face down and then face up again to allow the air to move into each part of the ventricles. In each position x rays were taken. In children all this was done under anaesthesia which makes them relaxed and floppy so that they have to be carefully supported during each manoeuvre. When completed one could tell if the size of the ventricles was abnormal or if their position or shape were altered. Cerebral angiograms, which outlined the arteries in the head, could also be done to show whether they were in the normal position or were being pushed aside by a tumour, clot or other mass in the brain, The angiogram, which is achieved by injecting radio-opaque contrast into the arteries, could also outline aneurysms, narrowing or other abnormalities in the vessels. The neurosurgeons were much more dependent

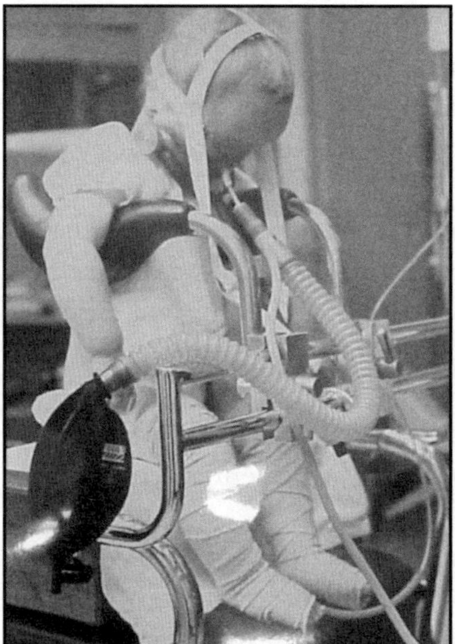

54. Patient in special apparatus for doing pneumoencephalography.

on the history and examination of the patient. If there was the suggestion of some abnormality in the head and some mass seemed to displace the structures from the usual position the surgeon opened the head and looked for the lesion.

How primitive this all seems today when CAT, MRI and other forms of scanning can be performed to show all the tissues. Tumours can be seen easily. Now the surgeon, with the aid of a few placer dots, can put a probe in the brain and move it toward the lesion, suck it out with a special sucker and then check with the probe to see that it has all been removed. The precision is remarkable compared to the old way. These techniques have been used to remove hypothalamic hamartomas, a relatively inaccessible tumour that causes fitting throughout life. The pioneering work in this field done by Jeff Rosenfeld attracted patients from all over the world to our hospital for the operation.

Children with localised epileptic foci in the brain can now have these located accurately by implanting recording electrodes on the brain. The recordings locate where there are abnormal areas which can then be removed.

Nowadays, if the abnormality is very vascular with many abnormal blood vessels these can be embolised, under radiological imaging, with small particles which occlude them, so that they bleed much less during surgical removal. It makes the operation, if one is needed, easier and less hazardous.

In very challenging cases where much bleeding is anticipated or occurs additional techniques such as hypotension (lowering blood pressure so that less bleeding occurs) or even cooling the patient (hypothermia) can be used to add safety and make the surgery easier. These have been described in a previous chapter.

I worked with some interesting and very able neurosurgeons, two of them women, Elizabeth Lewis and Wirginia Maixner, who were both outstanding in their own ways. But my longest association was with Geoffrey Klug who was the registrar in neurosurgery when I began working at the Childrens Hospital in 1967. When he retired in 2000 I calculated that we had worked together for over 6000 hours, a remarkable collaboration, made easy by his wonderful, equable temperament. I

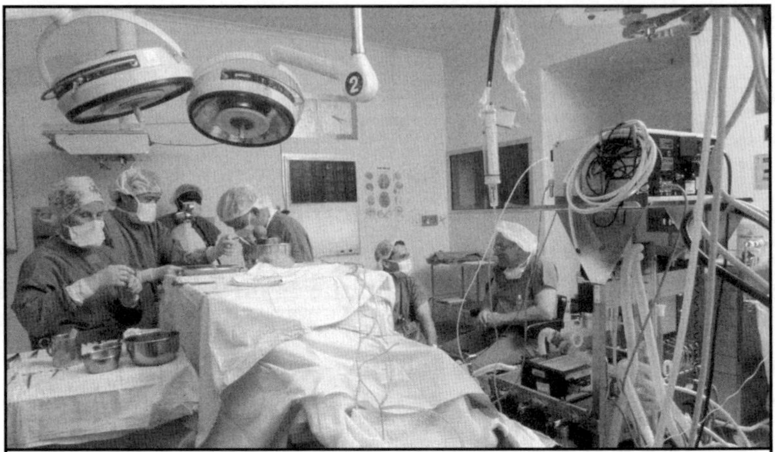

55. Neurosurgical operating theatre with Mr. Geoff Klug operating, with Hilda Jegermanis, who worked at the hospital for over 30 years, scrubbed with him.

never saw him outwardly angry with anyone although I knew he had been occasionally irritated by someone. If our afternoon list went on into the evening he tended to start singing around six o'clock. At other times he entertained us by reciting the whole of "the Man from Snowy River" or telling us how he carried the Olympic torch, when he was a student, on its way to Melbourne for the 1956 Games.

We did some challenging work together. Removing a very vascular choroid plexus papilloma, which took three operations because of bleeding, was one of the most difficult cases. The choroid plexus is the tissue that forms the cerebro-spinal fluid in the ventricles in the brain. We used hypotension using the long acting vasodilator drug, phenoxybenzamine, combined with hypothermia. The drug was chosen because it was long acting allowing smooth control of blood pressure, and because it dilates all vessels except those in the head. If they dilate in neurosurgery the brain becomes more distended with blood which is undesirable. Eventually we removed all of the papilloma. The boy made a good recovery after each of the three operations.

Reg Hooper became a neurosurgeon during World War II. I met him at the Royal Melbourne Hospital where I gave the anaesthetic for his last operation before he retired after 20 years, the mandatory retirement time at that hospital. He was a great photographer and made some excellent teaching films on subdural and extradural haemorrhage. He was a thoughtful and inventive man, who devised a special wheel for patients who had to sit up during their procedure. When he retired at 65 he trained in radiology, a field in which he continued to practice for some years.

One remarkable operation we did together was a three month old baby with a subdural haemorrage. Bleeding was extremely difficult to control. Eventually, after losing half its blood volume, I had the patient's blood cross matched against my own, something that one might have done in Kenya in those days! This was a long time before AIDS and all the restrictions that now exist. The blood was compatible so I had someone take 50 mls off me and gave it directly to the baby. It was fresh and so contained all the clotting factors. Such transfusion would be impossible now, in more advanced countries at least.

Things improved and we were able to conclude the operation. Reg Hooper left a swab in to fill some of the space that had been created by the haemorrhage. Three days later we returned, when all bleeding had ceased, and removed it. This was a particularly interesting patient because he had a twin brother with whom he could be compared. Seven years later Mr Hooper told me that he could detect a minimal difference in their development but most people would not notice any.

Sometimes the surgeon was unlucky as in the following case when he was operating on a tumour. The brain was swollen by its presence. To reduce intracranial contents and make it easier to operate he passed a needle into the fluid filled ventricle to draw off cerebrospinal fluid. Unfortunately he hit a blood vessel and the bleeding worsened the swelling. He removed the needle. The situation continued to worsen and the brain swelled to a worrying degree. He made an opening in the dura, the layer of tissue which covers the brain, and the brain began to bulge out through it. It was a frightening and potentially disasterous situation. I did something probably nobody else would have thought of doing. I quickly mixed up some sodium nitroprusside and gave a very small dose which lowered the blood pressure. By good luck and to everyones great relief the bleeding stopped and the swelling subsided. The operation went on to a successful conclusion.

I also anaesthetised the only child I ever saw with a cerebral hydatid cyst with the same surgeon who, before he realized what it was, punctured it.

One of the most remarkable boys that I had to anaesthetise was Quentin who developed a brain tumour when he was twelve. This was operated on. Unfortunately he lost the fine motor control of his right hand. He learnt to use his left hand and became a proficient painter with it. He later required further surgery and lost the use of his right arm. When he was 15 he won an award as the most promising young artist at the Heidelberg art show in Melbourne. His mother then took him for a trip overseas to see some of the great galleries. While they were away she realised that he was losing his sight. At sixteen he lost his sight so he took up sculpture and playing the harmonica.

I met him when he was about eighteen. We had to do a cosmetic operation to remove the mass of growing tumour. During my visit after the operation I asked whether his sense of hearing became more acute when he went blind. "Yes," he said "but his sense of touch was enhanced even more." It was then that I found out about his sculpture and that he was preparing for an exhibition at school. Unfortunately, I was going to be away when it was on, so he invited me to come and see his work at home when I returned. I took my son, Ken, with me as he was about the same age and also interested in music. They got on well together. The sculptures were impressive — some figures built on wire frames, some musicians similar to ones he had painted and a variety of other subjects such as fish. To ensure the musicians were all the same height he had a bottle that he used as a reference for height. It was amazing that he did all this with his non dominant hand and without sight. A few of the sculptures were painted — his mother had done them for him following very detailed instructions. His painting was bold and some of the more recent ones represented his thoughts about his condition and on his tenuous hold on life. We visited from time to time.

I suggested organizing to take him to the National Gallery

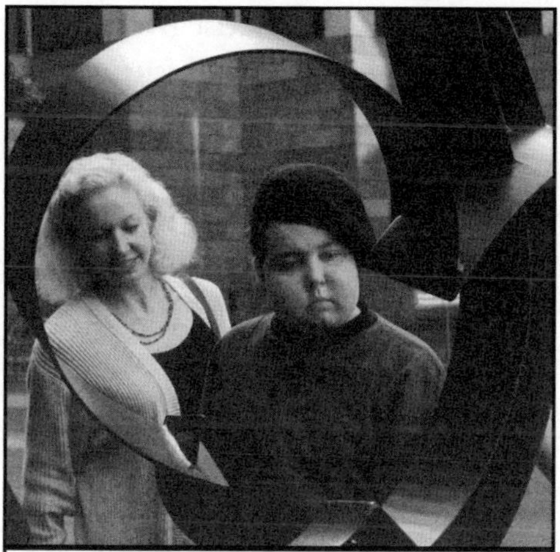

56. Quentin and his mother with one of the sculptures at the National Gallery of Victoria.

of Victoria to feel the sculptures there. At the time he was too busy but some time later we arranged the visit and that he could wear cotton gloves to feel the sculptures. I had had this experience at a show of Henry Moore's work and was astounded at how much I could feel that I had not observed while looking carefully at them. It gives an extra sensory dimension. Unfortunately, when we went the European Gallery with its collection of small Rodin sculptures was closed, so we had to be content with the few in the Australian Gallery and the very large ones in the courtyard. One amazing coincidence occurred when he sat down on the plinth beside a very large Henry Moore figure in the courtyard. He sat in the same pose although he could not see it. He was disappointed that he couldn't feel more, especially the Rodin sculptures.

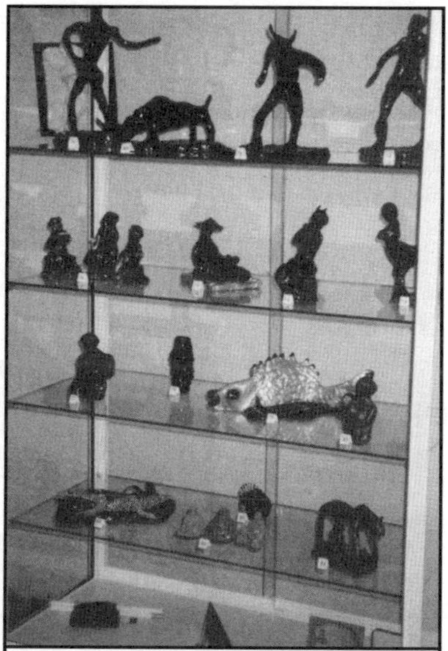

57. Sculptures made by Quentin when he was blind and could only use his left hand.

A week later Quentin died. He had a remarkable personality and a wonderful spirit. He made full use of his short life and said that it was fortunate that he had become blind otherwise he would not have developed his talent as a sculptor. What a wonderful outlook. He seemed to have a spiritual aura about him.

A year later a retrospective exhibition was held in aid of the

Anti Cancer Council. I took a Brazilian anaesthetist friend, Jose Carvalho, to see it. The following year, when I was visiting him in Brazil and we discussed the problem of busy doctors having time to relax and do something different. I persuaded him to try painting and gave him a lesson on the spot. He took it up as a hobby. It is a great outlet, taking ones mind right away from all the problems of life. Quentin's example led me to make a little plaster of Paris sculpture for a surgeon when he retired. He was an orthopaedic surgeon and it represented him in the operating theatre standing with plaster scattered over the floor — he was not a tidy plasterer!

Another challenging anaesthetic was in a 10-week-old achondroplastic baby who had a very small foramen magnum. This is the hole through which the spinal cord emerges from the skull. It was only 3mm in diameter and was causing compression of the spinal cord, a very dangerous situation. If the baby's neck was flexed or extended he would stop breathing. Wirginia Maixner planned to enlarge the opening. I administered the anaesthetic by face mask until it was deep enough to intubate him without paralysing him, which we often do. I inserted the tube. Then we had to place him face down on the operating table with the head in the optimal position to keep him breathing. This we determined using the capnograph which showed us when the expired CO2 was at its lowest level. The operation was successful but it took a couple of days for the swelling to recede before the problem was cured.

Another uncommon problem in neurosurgery is when air enters the circulation through an open vein. This is more likely to happen when the operation is performed in a patient sitting up and when the blood volume is reduced. The air goes to the heart where it may collect in the right ventricle or in the arteries going to the lungs. In both situations the amount of blood reaching the lungs is reduced and so the amount of carbon dioxide released will be less. The capnograph reading of expired CO2 will decline by an amount related to the degree of obstruction to blood flow through the lungs. For many years it was advocated that a catheter should be placed into the vena cava near the entrance to the heart so that if air enters it can be sucked out. I have only seen it used successfully once. The problem is that most of the air has already passed the tip of the catheter. To be useful the catheter tip needs to be in the pulmonary artery where it is technically difficult to place it in children. I did some studies which showed that an isoprenaline infusion had a beneficial effect. It stimulates the heart to contract more vigorously and it dilates the pulmonary arteries.

Neurosurgical anaesthesia often takes many hours. It requires meticulous attention to detail if problems are to be avoided. It is a field in which I have enjoyed the challenges of the anaesthetic and the surgeons with whom I have worked.

Chapter 23
Burns

Burns can be devastating to the patient and family. A child who has large areas of skin burnt changes suddenly from normal to one who will be disfigured for life. My interest in the problems of these patients began with curiosity about the abnormal response some patients with large burns had to the muscle relaxant drug, suxamethonium. It sometimes caused cardiac arrest.

The Lara fires in January 1968 were my first involvement in a mass burn disaster. Lara is on the Melbourne to Geelong road which was a dual carriageway. That day the fire leapt across this road and people in several cars were trapped. Unfortunately they did not know that it was safer to stay in their car. They feared the petrol exploding. They emerged dressed for the beach with only minimal clothing. This was inadequate protection from the heat and they were scorched and badly burnt. Some died before reaching hospital and several died later, in one case four months afterwards. We received four children — a brother and sister of eight and eleven years old and seven year old twin boys. One of the latter was already dead, the other arrived singing *Jingle Bells* but sadly he succumbed shortly afterwards, before he could be adequately resuscitated.

Later in the day, four children from one family caught in another fire in the Western District arrived, but fortunately, they had less severe burns. Even so, one of them had a problem with acute sensitivity of the soles of her feet years afterwards. She could not wear or walk on nylon as it pricked her sensitive feet. She had to wear woolen socks. We learnt this some years later when, as a nurse, she came to a meeting on burns and told us some of the problems from the patient's point of view.

A new drug which was still on trial had just become available — CI 581. Later it was named *ketamine*, or locally nicknamed "Kestamine", because I did much of the early work in Melbourne with it! It was a new concept drug called a dissociative anaesthetic. It acted in the brain mainly by preventing impulses from the thalamus and lower part of the brain from reaching the cortex where the information could be recognized. It did not act like other anaesthetics depressing activity at lower brain levels, like the medulla which contains the vital centres controlling cardiovascular and respiratory functions. Because ketamine maintained the activity of the medulla it had certain advantages — blood pressure did not decrease and the airway did not become obstructed when the patient became unconscious. It was later found to have pain relieving (analgesic) actions as well, in low concentrations. We used it extensively in these children, particularly when we had to give them baths. One adverse effect that was described was an incidence of bizarre dreams, which in some adults proved to be unpleasant. One of these children complained of bad dreams so we changed to giving her a general anaesthetic. She then dreamt that we were pouring water down the tubing from the machine so it seems her condition may have contributed to her bad dreams.

In those days big burns became infected and the skin virtually sloughed off after two or three weeks. It was a most unpleasant situation for everyone. New treatments, including bacteriostatic creams (sulphamylon and silver nitrate), had just been introduced to reduce the infection These helped but we had no effective way of killing a bacteria called pseudomonas which occasionally caused septicaemia and sometimes death. Our girl, after weeks of progress, finally succumbed in that way after four months. It was heartbreaking to all, particularly as we had thought that she had a better chance of surviving than her brother.

Burns caused terrible scarring in some children. This was an especially difficult problem when it affected the neck, as the chin would be drawn down towards the chest. This made anaesthesia more difficult, because it took longer to reach an adequate depth of anaesthesia with inhalation agents and they could be extremely difficult to intubate. The solution was to give them a dose of intravenous ketamine which allowed the surgeon to divide the contracted tissue enabling neck extension and then intubation could be relatively easily performed.

One of the great advances in burn care has been the development of close fitting Job suits which compress the grafts and tend to inhibit contracture and keloid formation.

There are several problems with burn anaesthesia — blood loss, finding suitable veins to cannulate, maintaining the patient's body temperature especially when large areas of the body are exposed, ensuring that the patients do not have pain, sometimes having to change position during the operation if the back and front are both burned, and altered sensitivity to drugs such as muscle relaxants.

The most gratifying aspect of working with burns was the wonderful team that looked after these children. It included the surgeons, nurses, anaesthetists, physiotherapists, occupational therapists, dietitians, social workers, psychologists and psychiatrists, orthotists — more groups than are involved than in the care of any other patients. There were many good and caring nurses — two who stood out were the charge nurses when burns were more common and the unit was busier. They were Win Menadue who was a rather boisterous but very efficient and effective leader, and Wendy Swift, who was recognised for her outstanding work in the field. She visited India several times to teach about burn nursing.

The surgical arrangements were rather unusual. John Barnett was the only plastic surgeon who was involved with acute care for any length of time. Murray Clarke, one of the wonderful older surgeons really established the unit and initiated the prevention work that was eventually recognized by the naming of the Murray Clarke Child Safety Centre. He, with Julian Keogh (58) and John Soloman were all general surgeons with a special interest in burns. They ran the unit for many years and contributed to the reduction in burns through public education. They fostered the ideas of keeping the thermostat setting lower on the hot water services in houses with children, the use of non flammable clothing, safety features in kitchens so that hot items could not be pulled over and many other ideas which more than halved the incidence of burns. They were practical and very caring men. Julian was also responsible for airlines having a little tray on which to place your cup while hot tea or coffee is being poured. Before their introduction spills occurred and people were scalded.

Later, Russell Taylor joined Julian Keogh when John

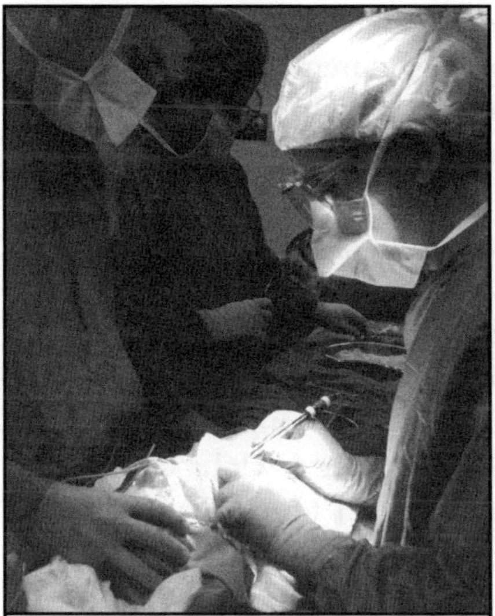

58. Julian Keogh operating.

Soloman retired. He was a friend from an early age, as I first knew him as a theatre orderly in the theatres during his holidays. I taught him about anaesthetics and drugs as a student and later he became a resident, registrar and finally a surgeon.

The patient with the greatest area burnt who survived only had a small area around the groin and his scalp unburned from which we had to gradually graft over 90% of his body. Such patients do not usually survive but this boy had tremendous spirit. A month after the accident when these patients are at the worst stage he was still telling us jokes — quite amazing. Then the boys in his cricket team sent him a bat which they had all signed . This was followed by a visit from Dean Jones with a bat signed by his team mates in the Australian team. I think these helped him to keep going and survive. He did well and went on eventually to have training in some electronic related field. He was selected to present a book, compiled by patients about their accidents, to Princess Diana when she and Prince Charles opened Childhood Accident Prevention Week at the Hospital.

Another boy whose mother died in the same fire had 70% burns. He was in Intensive Care on drugs to keep his blood pressure up. His father had long since left and his only relative was an aunt who lived interstate. We began grafting him and I remember being amazed how well the grafts took, considering the treatment he was on for low blood pressure. However after a couple of weeks he seemed to give up. He had no support. He passed away.

It was sad working with these patients. Another family had several children severely burnt. One, whom I had anaesthetised, died after a couple of weeks. The remarkable comment from his mother was that she felt his spirit left two days before he died.

One of the most entertaining children that I looked after was Jade who came from Tasmania. Her nightdress caught fire on an open bar heater — very dangerous items in the presence of children. She had 50% burns. One day as she was gradually recovering from ketamine following her bath she said to me "Dr. Brown, what are you doing?" I was holding her hand to ensure that the intravenous cannula did not become dislodged. Then she said to the physiotherapist "Jane, what are you doing?" To our surprise, a few minutes later, she became more familiar and asked, "Kester, what are you doing?" After a while she became disenchanted with repeated anaesthetics. I found that if I talked about flowers in my garden she settled down. Then I had to bring her a rose each time she had an anaesthetic. One day she arrived with a plate of cheese and biscuits for her "starving" anaesthetist ! There was a period when her recovery seemed to slow down. We found that she needed more zinc which is an essential ingredient for healthy skin. Soon afterwards her recovery continued and after five months with us she went home. She insisted on having her photograph taken with me and presented me with a copy in a frame which she had made, surrounded by sea shells and painted silver. One day I phoned her to find out how she was progressing. Her twin brother was making a noise in the background. She said "Do you hear that noise?" "Yes", I said. "That is Josh. Just a minute,"she says and then called to Josh to keep quiet. "Don't you realize that I am on the phone?" She says to him. Very grown up for a child of just six. I saw her three years later when she demonstrated how she could do the splits.

A year later we had another girl with the same name and same extent of burn who was with us for nearly as long. That was a hard year for us as we had five children whose faces were burnt. This can be the worst disfigurement, especially if the burn is full thickness, because the face is always exposed. Fortunately, the Job fitted masks help to reduce the scarring and have made a difference to the end result, but it is never perfect. They often need plastic surgery later.

Making the face masks requires a mould to be made under anaesthesia. This provides the anaesthetist with a challenge because the orthotist has to make a resin and then plaster of Paris mould so that a firm fit is achieved with the final garment. This means keeping the child still without using a mask or tubes. Ketamine has often proved helpful for this procedure as there is no need for anaesthetic equipment around the face.

Usually there are two or three surgeons working together. On at least one occasion, when the surgeon did not have any help, while I had a registrar, I scrubbed in to help with the surgery and let my assistant watch the anaesthetic.

Working with patients with burns can be emotionally draining. One has to develop a certain detachment and yet maintain the sympathetic and supportive approach to the patient. Only once did I succumb when we had a significantly intellectually impaired child with large burns who was not doing well. I felt that discussions on his management lacked sensitivity and consideration of the overall situation, which upset me.

Decisions on how vigorously to pursue treatment in major burns create terrible dilemmas. How important is survival if the resulting quality of life is poor or unbearable. It can have awful repercussions not only on the patients but also on the families. The psychologists play an important role in helping families through these problems. From the stories I have told it seems some fight to survive and others just give up. Some will survive and cope well while others will be miserable. Often it is impossible early on to know who is in which group.

My personal contributions to the care of burns, apart from promoting the idea that the same person should give these patients all their anaesthetics if possible, has been in delineating the problems with muscle relaxants and developing techniques for nerve blocks to the thigh, from where many grafts are taken.

My interest in the problem of cardiac arrest in large burns following the muscle relaxant, suxamethonium, began when I was working in Vancouver before I was even working with burns. My early work showed that normally this drug caused only a very small increase in serum potassium. Later it was shown by Americans in the Vietnam War that there was a huge increase in potassium when suxamethonium was given to burned patients. This was the cause of the problem. Later, my studies showed that the degree of the rise in potassium was related to the area of the burn and the dose of suxamethonium given. I confirmed studies done by Jorgen Viby Mogensen and colleagues in Copenhagen that the rise did not occur until a week to ten days after the burn. When the electromyograph (60), developed by the electrical engineers at Monash University with whom I worked, became available, I showed that following very small doses (0.1 mg/kg) the degree of paralysis produced was greater in burn patients compared to normal children of the same age and weight.

My paper on this study was rejected for publication because there were not enough controls! This was another example of how rejection can lead on to other studies and discoveries. One was the first big study to work out accurately what the dose of suxamethonium was for different age groups. The commonly used doses were found to be 2 ½ to 4 times the dose that will usually produce 95% paralysis measured in the hand. Because this drug is short acting this did not matter and probably has the advantages of faster onset and more profound paralysis which makes it easier to intubate the patient's trachea.

The second study found that patients with burns have a period between 5 and 9 days after the burn injury when they are extra sensitive to very small doses of suxamethonium and may become completely paralysed with as little as 0.1 mg/kg or one tenth of the usual dose given. This had not been demonstrated before. My work on muscle relaxants in burns went on over a long period — over 20 years.

My other contribution related to using local anaesthetic nerve blocks to manage pain. It is very painful cutting skin for grafting. There are nerve endings throughout the skin and when donor skin is taken a thin layer is removed which must cut many of these causing pain. An important part of the anaesthetic is therefore to minimize this and to keep the patient comfortable into the post operative period. When possible we took grafts from the thigh or leg. We developed or improved on techniques to block the nerves supplying this area and successfully applied them to provide pain relief (analgesia). In addition, intravenous morphine infusions were introduced in the late 1970s and provide a stable level of pain relief superior to the intermittent injections that patients used to receive.

My work on nerve blocks began with anatomical dissections to show the layers that the needle passes through until it reaches the nerve. These were done by making windows over the site which became smaller as each layer was reached. In this way one can visualize the tissues that are being traversed. I was helped in this work by several people who trained with me including Alex Babarczy, Khoo Siew Tuan from Singapore (36), Corinne de Moerloose from Geneva (31), Peter Kempthorne from New Zealand (36), Bob Dickens, an Orthopaedic surgeon friend, and Patrick Hughes, who both helped to develop new techniques for lateral cutaneous and posterior cutaneous nerves of the thigh respectively. These are described in the British Journal of Anaesthesia in July 1999. When we worked out the latter technique we decided to try it on each other to ensure it worked. It did. The interesting thing that I learnt from that experience was that when the local anaesthetic is injected into a space or potential space no discomfort is felt except the needle entering the skin. In children we usually do the blocks under anaesthesia to avoid the psychological trauma associated with needles.

Subsequently I have made a video of these dissections and techniques, which won the best video presentation at the Canadian Society of Anaesthetists meeting in 1985. They have been translated into other languages (Spanish, Japanese, Arabic and Romanian) and have been shown in many countries when I have been lecturing on this subject.

Recently, there have been new developments in burn management which reduce the amount and frequency of grafting and allow good healing. This is encouraging and is leading to less work for the burn team. In addition, the preventive measures have reduced the incidence in the community significantly but, unfortunately, some accidents will continue to occur.

Not many people willingly take on regular burn anaesthesia for many years. It is very demanding work but it can also be very rewarding. It has been a privilege to work with such dedicated people.

Chapter 24

Pain Management

Pain is a sensation which indicates that there is something wrong in the body or that trauma has occurred. Surgical incisions are one form of trauma which cause acute pain. This used to be treated with intermittent injections of analgesics (pain relievers) such as morphine. The problem was that the blood level, and therefore effect, varied with time. It would rise to a maximum and may reach the level at which undesirable effects such as vomiting occur. It would then decline through the effective therapeutic range to a point where pain returned. Another injection might then be given but there would often be a period when pain was felt. Fortunately, the body can produce some of its own endorphins which have some pain relieving ability and gradually, as the pain declined these might become sufficient so that further analgesics are not needed.

Local anaesthetics can also be used to block pain from the affected part of the body.

In the last twenty five years the management of pain following surgery has received considerable attention. This has been due to a better understanding of drug action, routes of administration and responses related to blood levels. Infusion pumps have been developed which can administer drugs at a rate which will provide a constant pain relieving effect with, ideally, minimum side effects. This management is more labour intensive and its evolution has been slowed in many places, or has not yet developed, because there are not enough experienced nurses and doctors to provide it or money is not available to provide the staff and infusion pumps.

Chronic pain is long lasting and may be more difficult to treat. Again staff and funds influence whether adequate facilities are available in the community to provide for its satisfactory management. Chronic pain is a major factor in loss of working time. Potentially, millions of dollars could be saved if government or some other source provided funds to treat many of these people so that they could return to work. It is less of a problem in children but some do suffer from chronic pain.

Palliative care in cancer patients and some people with chronic painful conditions aims to keep them comfortable in the later days.

An enormous amount of research has been conducted in the latter part of my working life on the mechanisms of pain and its management. I was involved in the management of children with some of these pain problems, which I will describe, at a time when interest in the field was just beginning. I was also involved in helping others in the department to develop an acute pain management team and publish a manual with our colleagues in Adelaide.

My first specific involvement in pain management was when we were asked to do an intercostal block in a teenager with a painful spot in the back to ensure that the proposed sectioning of a nerve would be helpful. The surgeon did not tell us that the child had undergone a Harrington rod operation to straighten her back or that two ribs in the painful area were fused together. I did the intercostal nerve block with local anaesthetic and the patient's pain was relieved, not for a few hours but for six months. I repeated it with a similar result. Pain is a curious symptom to treat. I must have broken some self- perpetuating cycle that caused the pain.

It was several years later that I saw my first patient with what was known as Reflex Sympathetic Dystrophy, now called chronic regional pain syndrome. This nine year old girl presented with a painful foot. The response to my enquiries to friends who were more expert in this area suggested that I inject a vasodilator drug, guanethidine, intravenously into the leg while a tourniquet was on. This seemed to help and she went home to Tasmania. A year later she returned on crutches not having borne weight on her foot for three months. After further consultation we did a series of lumbar sympathetic blocks. A needle is inserted through the back until the tip lies on the front of the vertebrae where the sympathetic nerves and ganglia lie. We located the point with x-ray. Injection and blocking the transmission of nerve impulses reduces the sympathetic vasoconstriction and improves blood flow to the leg. Three blocks were done over two weeks with dramatic success. We used phenol, which has a long action for the last one, and the child was cured. The fascinating feature that this patient showed was a line on her leg x ray, above the epiphyseal line, indicating illness. She also had 1.3cm shortening of that leg. Six months later re x ray showed a third line and a gap of 1cm to the next one described above, indicating catch up growth.(59) The first line was the epiphyseal growth plate. This is the only patient that I know of where this feature was recorded. She made a good recovery.

Another girl had seven episodes affecting different limbs which was very unusual. She had three sympathetic blocks including a stellate ganglion block because her hand was so swollen and painful that she could not hold a pen. I phoned to ask if she could come in to act her limp for a video I was making when her mother told me she was having another attack. I had a genuine limp to film. I had arranged to do another block after filming but she improved so much while repeatedly demonstrating her limp in front of the camera that we decided that physiotherapy would be sufficient. Sometimes these patients improved with physiotherapy, particularly if they appeared to have a significant psychological component. This could be dif-

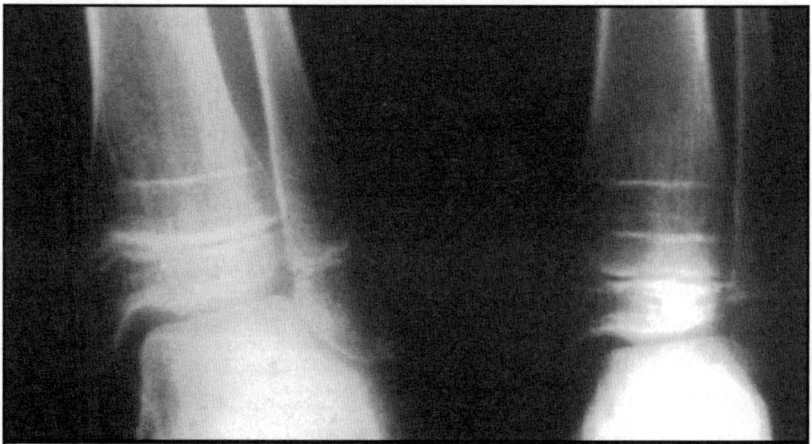

59. X-ray of tibia before and after treatment with lumbar sympathetic blocks for Chronic Regional Pain Syndrome in a 9 year-old girl, showing the epiphyseal plate (bottom line), a line caused by the illness and, on the right, the catch up growth after treatment.

ferentiated by their response to an alpha sympathetic blocking drug, phentolamine, and to skin potential testing which demonstrated a difference in sweating following a sympathetic stimulus, such as a loud noise or asking some mental arithmetic. If these showed a difference sometimes they needed sympathetic blocks to relieve their pain.

I had another 12 year old boy who had a painful knee with a granular feeling like sand under his skin. He was not a typical case but I decided to do a lumbar sympathetic block as a therapeutic trial. Amazingly it worked and on follow up three months later he was pain free and had no granular feeling.

Eventually, I had to pass this work on to others because I became too busy but I was able to encourage the others (Ian McKenzie and Phil Ragg) to set up a Pain Management team which was later taken over by George Chalkiadis. Gradually we built up this service in the department and even changed the name to the Department of Anaesthesia and Pain Management. This service requires people to see and review the patients daily and to respond to calls at any time. We employed nurses to help and then had a registrar predominantly involved for a week. Eventually, after several years we received enough funding to support a team which could cover the service adequately. As well as seeing the patients there is a continual need to train the staff looking after them. Now patients are regularly assessed for pain after their operations and the level is recorded on the chart with the pulse, temperature etc.

Constant infusions, or, in older children, patient controlled analgesia (PCA) infusions, where they could administer an extra dose if required, became commonly used. The wider use of local anaesthetic methods such as caudal and epidurals, especially when maintained for longer periods by infusion through catheters, became an additional useful tool.

Our team produced a *Manual of acute pain management in children* for which Ian McKenzie did most of the editorial work assisted by Phil Gaukroger, Phil Ragg and myself. My contribution was a chapter on local anaesthetic blocks and to arrange the publishers who were Churchill Livingstone. Unfortunately it was during a period of takeovers in the publishing industry and our publisher was taken over by Harcourt Brace and then soon after they were absorbed. There was another similar book produced after ours, published originally by one of the other companies in the group. Their promotion seemed to be lost in the takeovers. It was a sad outcome particularly as the new owners ignored my correspondence about it. So much for big business and takeovers.

One of the most interesting pain clinics that I visited was in Callicut in South India. Professor Rajagopal set this up with practically no support initially, not long before I visited. His concept was to provide pain management for cancer patients. The difference was that once the patient had gone home from hospital the relatives would come each month and report on progress. The doctors would then arrange with the relatives the treatment for the next month. The patient was not brought in each time in order to avoid the uncomfortable trip on the bad roads with poor transport for a sick person. Rajagopal was an exceptional man. I found some funds to enable him to come to Australia for a short visit to pain clinics. He declined and asked me to allow one of his young colleagues to come instead because she would be around longer to utilize the knowledge gained.

He gained financial support from the community and outside. His clinic went on to become a model arrangement for the third world recognised by the World Health Organization and is now a practical training centre for chronic pain management. All this has been accomplished in only a few years. It is a wonderful example of what a dedicated person can achieve.

Chapter 25

Dental Anaesthesia in Children

When I was a medical student in Labrador Dr Paddon taught me how to do dental blocks and pull teeth. This was useful when I was in General Practice in Yellowknife because we were sometimes called upon to do dental work when the dentist was away. The experience also gave me a special rapport with our dentists because they knew of my experience. In fact, because of it I was even invited to sit as a non-dentist member of staff on a selection panel in the Dental department.

In my early years at the hospital I sometimes did anaesthetics for extractions in the dental chair. This required some skills with which many anaesthetists have not been trained. We have to administer the gas while the dentist isolates the mouth from the pharynx, usually with a swab, and extracts the teeth. For some years our registrars went to the Dental Hospital to gain this experience but that stopped when workloads increased.

Although I have done dental cases from time to time throughout my career it was only after stopping full time work that I was asked to do a dental list on which they do the patients with complex medical problems. This was an interesting challenge and has provided me with some of the most difficult patients I have had to anaesthetise.

The reasons for giving anaesthetics to children for dental procedures are to give the dentist unrestricted and easy access to the teeth in children who are frightened, difficult to control or who have some serious medical condition where these factors are important or it makes the patient easier to manage. In contrast, surgical anaesthesia has a much greater emphasis on avoidance of pain from the surgery, and the control of physiological changes consequent on the surgery such as haemorrhage and fluid loss. Both these can occur to a much lesser extent in dental work, particularly when teeth are extracted or have to be surgically removed.

Dental anaesthesia, like other forms of anaesthesia around the head and mouth, requires good collaboration between the anaesthetist and the dental practitioner. The dentists preference is to have a field unobstructed by the endotracheal tube so we often use a nasotracheal tube. Sometimes a compromise has to be reached when there are difficulties or contraindications to nasal intubation. The dentist likes a relaxed jaw where wide mouth opening is easily achieved. There are some conditions where this is not always possible such as when there is some temporomandibular ankylosis (stiffness of the joint).

If an oral tube is used the dentist has to able to move it from side to side. This usually means that it is not secured with tape or that the tape is changed when the sides are changed. I developed an alternative idea which is to attach the tube to a tape which functions like a mesentery so that it can be flipped from side to side without detaching the tape. The tape is fastened round the tube and then the two layers are stuck together for 1 $^{1}/_{2}$–2 cm before being attached to the chin in the midline. The tube can then be swung this distance to one or other side and the tape prevents it being pulled out.

Some children, often older ones, who have cerebral palsy, intellectual impairment or autism may need special handling. I found that if a parent or guardian offered advice on how to handle a particular child it was wise to listen to them because they are with them all the time. They can be of great assistance at induction. Often these patients will not take premedication. Sometimes, kindness and gentle cajoling works. Blowing the weak anaesthetic nitrous oxide over the face until they become dizzy works and gentle stroking of the cheek often helps to calm them. At other times, unfortunately, more severe restraint is occasionally necessary until anaesthesia is induced.

Some contraindications to nasal intubation include previous surgery for choanal atresia, cleft palate repair or pharyngoplasty. There are congenital anomalies where difficulties may be encountered. I have had children with osteogenesis imperfecta who have bones that break easily. Very gentle oral intubation is then preferred.

Intubation may be difficult in the presence of a receding jaw (micrognathia in Pierre Robin and Treacher Collins syndromes), where the larynx is situated higher than usual such as some of the syndromes (conditions such as mucopolysaccharidoses — Hurler, Hunter, Maroteaux Lamy syndromes) or where there is laryngeal involvement with swelling in the surrounding tissues such as cystic hygroma. In such cases it may be helpful to give IV ketamine (1mg/kg) at the beginning to provide analgesia (pain relief) and reduce the amount of other anaesthetics needed. Another small dose (1 mg/kg) can be given near the end of the procedure to provide anaesthesia and analgesia while the inhalation anaesthetic is eliminated. The advantage of this is that the patient regains good muscle tone earlier and airway control recovers before the child regains consciousness.

I used the above method in a child with Ondine's curse where the child stops breathing when he goes to sleep. They have to have home ventilation to support them at night. This child responded well with the small dose of ketamine and started breathing before he was fully conscious.

I have had several patients with epidermolysis bullosa which is a hereditary disease with a deficiency of collagen in the dermis of the skin. Physical contact, especially of a shearing nature, to the skin and mucous membranes in the mouth can result in large blisters or bullae forming. The condition varies in severity but extreme gentleness and avoidance of shearing is essential. In severe cases the blisters break down and may leave open oozing lesions which go on to fibrosis. The face mask should be covered with vaseline to make it less adherent to the facial skin, the laryngoscope blade may need to be treated likewise to prevent sheering on the surface of the tongue and the endotracheal tube should be passed very gently to avoid mucosal trauma. It must not be a tight fit otherwise trauma may occur leading to stenosis of the airway. Fortunately this is very rare but it has occurred. Adhesive tape should be avoided, especially in more severe cases although tegaderm has been used in some mild cases to hold an intravenous drip in place.

Some children have other other medical problems such as congenital heart disease, bleeding conditions, diabetes or Down's Syndrome which can add to the challenges. I had one child who sometimes developed a prolonged Q-T interval on his ECG. These patients may develop serious arrhythmias if they become excited or have stimulation of their sympathetic nervous system. One of my colleagues made me nervous by telling me that these patients sometimes collapse with venticular fibrillation watching very frightening programs on TV or exciting sporting events. I made sure my patient was well sedated so that he was tranquil when he arrived!

The most difficult patients that I have had to handle on this list were 14 year old twins with fibrosis ossificans progressiva. This is an extremely rare condition where trauma, even an injection, can lead to fibrosis followed by ossification (bone formation in the tissues). I had never come across it before. These girls both had rigid cervical spines, some scoliosis, severe limitation of jaw opening (28mm) and one clinically looked as if she could have limited respiratory reserve. Direct oral intubation would have been impossible. As the naso-pharyngeal angle was acute (about 80 degrees), it would be difficult to manipulate the nasal tube around the corner into her mouth without trauma and if this occurred fibrosis, ossification and stenosis might result. We decided to use ketamine and insufflate oxygen in the nose. Careful use of a rubber dam would isolate the mouth and airway from the operative field. Ketamine was administered, but we could not open the mouth. Ketamine tends to maintain muscle tone. Propofol, another intravenous anaesthetic, was then given and satisfactory conditions were obtained although access for the dentist was limited. I had to support the jaw throughout to ensure a clear airway.

The second twin was less scoliotic and we thought would be easier, but she developed laryngeal spasm. This is a situation where the vocal cords close tightly, preventing air reaching the lungs. If the spasm does not break spontaneously the patient may need to be paralysed to relax the cords. When the spasm was overcome the dentist found that when he opened the mouth by the amount she had been able to while awake, the jaw compressed the fibrous tissue over the trachea obstructing the airway. He had to work with less mouth opening and reduced access. It was a strenuous morning but the procedures were accomplished successfully. The dentists were obviously serious when they wanted to utilize my years of experience on this list. They have certainly provided me with many interesting challenges.

Chapter 26

Tumours and Muscle Relaxants

This and the previous chapters give you some idea of the interesting clinical work with which I have been involved for 40 years. Interest depends on being receptive to things going on around one, and observing and dealing with the unusual and sometimes difficult problems that occur. The challenge is to learn to understand their significance and handle the problems safely.

Patients with tumours pose many problems, some affecting anaesthesia. They often need multiple anaesthetics for investigations, chemotherapy and surgery. It is better for the child if one or two anaesthetists look after them as they come to know each child's individual needs.

My special interest in hypothermia (cooling) and hypotension (lowering blood pressure to reduce blood loss) proved very useful in a number of these patients when major blood loss could occur and the dissection was likely to be difficult. These adjuncts were most commonly used in children with liver tumours where major blood loss sometimes occurs. On one occasion the vena cava was inadvertently opened as the liver was dissected away. In a few minutes the hole was safely repaired because the patient had been cooled and we were able to stop the blood flow in the vena cava temporarily. In the early days two patients had cardiac arrest from blood loss. One, who was cooled, recovered normally while the other at normal temperature was brain damaged. It is often worth the extra time taken to cool the patient to 32 — 34°C. to ensure safety. Fortunately tumours of this type are rare.

Patients with large masses in the chest (mediastinal tumours) need special care to avoid potentially catastrophic problems. Sometime just lying down will cause the tumour to compress the airway or the inflow of blood to the heart. Anaesthesia can aggravate these problems because the tissues may become more relaxed. I had one girl who I had to anaesthetise with her positioned half sitting and rolled to one side to prevent these problems. Fortunately she did well. I had to anaesthetise her a second time for another biopsy after the tumour had shrunk to ascertain if she was cured. I received a card from her after that in which she thanked me for keeping her alive during her two big operations. It went on "You are my hero. With love from your greatest nightmare!" It is nice to receive such appreciation.

I made an interesting observation on children with tumours. I noticed that some of them did not relax as readily or as quickly following the usual doses of non depolarizing muscle relaxants. These drugs usually prevent the transmitter substance from the nerve (acetyl choline) from reaching the receptor on the muscle so that paralysis occurs. I studied over two hundred patients with tumours using electromyography with the now old drugs, tubocurarine and alcuronium. Tubocurarine, which has now been discontinued, gave the most definite results. It was subtley different to the other non depolarizing relaxants. When a child with a *malignant* liver, kidney or bone tumour received these drugs the onset to a standard dose was slow indicating that a larger dose was needed.

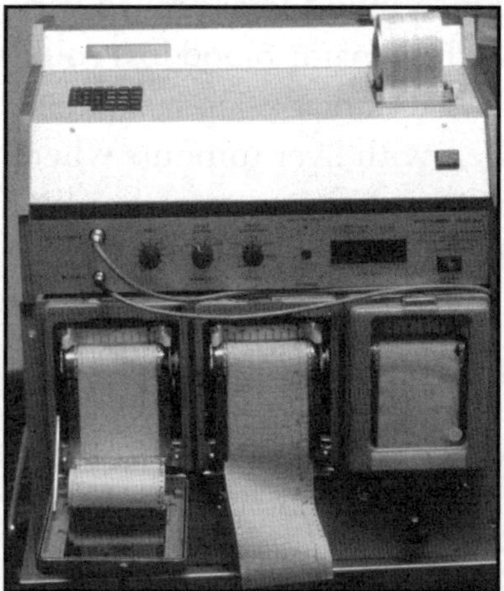

60. The electromyograph (EMG) with its original computer controller built at Monash University Department of Electrical Engineering (Prof. D. Lampard and colleagues) about 1979. It drove a syringe pump to deliver every minute if the set activity level was exceeded.

Unfortunately I was not able to undertake the research to determine why this happened. I even went to the manufacturers in Basle to obtain radio-active tagged relaxants to determine if they were taken up in the tumour. They had none available and it was not worth their while making some for me. One of the most likely possibilities was that the tumour contained chemicals to which the drug became attached in large amounts (acceptor sites). If this had been the case, there was an exciting possibility that if the chemotherapeutic drug attached to the muscle relaxant it would be delivered to the tumour where the chemotherapy could produce its maximum effect. Regretably, no-one has followed the idea up.

The next fascinating finding in this research was that when the muscle relaxant was given to patients with benign tumours they had a normal response. When the patients had been treated with chemotherapy, and in one case amputation, the slow response reverted to normal if the treatment was successful. When we studied the tissue from some bone tumours under the microscope we found that the treatment was only partially successful. In these cases the electromyographic response only partly recovered towards normal indicating a correlation between the response to chemotherapy and the patient's response to the muscle relaxant. So we had a test which we could do during the course of our anaesthetic which could give an indication whether the tumour was malignant or not. We had one child with a large mass in the upper abdomen which felt like a liver tumour. No one knew what it was so it was decided to operate. Our EMG study suggested it was benign. It turned out to be benign nodular hyperplasia of the liver. I found this all very fascinating but the information made very little impact on the anaesthetic community.

Another interesting pharmacogenetic study which we did with suxamethonium showed that patients with abnormal pseudocholinesterase, the enzyme which breaks down the drug, required reduced doses, the amount depending on whether they were homozygous or heterozygous for the abnormal enzyme. Failure to reduce the dose resulted in prolonged paralysis. Heterozygous patients (one abnormal gene) were paralysed for about 20 minutes instead of 4-5 minutes while homozygous patients (abnormal genes from both sides) could be paralysed for three hours. These patients often carry warning cards to avoid the drug when really the correct modification of dose would enable them to have it without problems. A homozygote needs about one seventh of the usual dose.

We were very fortunate to have the collaboration with the Electrical Engineers at Monash University who built and provided us with, maybe the first, the electromyograph and its computer controller to enable us to do all this interesting research.

Involvement in Anaesthesia Organizations

Chapter 27

Organizations in Anaesthesia

Our society is built around organizations, often useful but sometimes there are too many of them. Anaesthesia is no different.

Anaesthesia is a relatively young medical specialty and while there were some famous anaesthetists many years ago like Snow, Clover, Magill, Waters, Lundy, Guedel and many others the specialty only really emerged after World War II. The first chair of Anaesthesia was established by Lord Nuffied in Oxford in 1948, in appreciation of a successful anaesthetic he received from Robert Macintosh, a New Zealander, who was appointed the first Professor. I had the good fortune to meet him in Oxford after he retired. We attended a departmental dinner with Keith Sykes who took over as professor, Robert Macintosh, and John Severinghaus. Janet sat next to each of them during the evening while I sat next to their wives! I also met Dicky Salt there. He was an old man by then but still full of enthusiasm, who had been the departmental technician and helped in the development of the Oxford tube and some of the anaesthetic equipment and vaporisers that emanated from that department.

A handful of societies formed in the 1920s and 30s. The first, started by Frank McMechan in the USA. was the National Anaesthesia Research Society, later I (International)ARS which produced the first journal, Current Researches in Anesthesia and Analgesia, in 1922. His organizational drive evolved from the fact that he developed arthritis and had to give up practicing anaesthesia so he turned to organizing it instead. His enthusiasm and that of Ralph Waters in Madison, Wisconsin influenced young Geoffrey Kaye (born 1903) in Melbourne.

Kaye was an enthusiast, particularly in the development of anaesthetic equipment. After meeting McMechan he eventually contacted other more senior colleagues devoted to anaesthesia in Australia encouraging them to meet and present papers. The Australian Society of Anaesthetists evolved from a meeting in January 1934 at Hadley's Hotel in Hobart, when a group of seven met to discuss the formation of the Society, its aims and constitution. These were Gilbert Brown from Adelaide who became the first president. He had been appointed honorary anaesthetist to Adelaide Childrens hospital in 1920 and Royal Adelaide Hospital in 1921. He is commemorated through the Society's highest honour, the Gilbert Brown Award, which I received in 1986. The others present were Geoffrey Kaye, the first secretary, Gilbert Troup from Perth, Harry Daly and Ivor Hotten from Sydney, Leonard Lillies from the Alfred Hospital, Melbourne and Cedric Duncombe from Hobart.

I had the good fortune to meet Geoffrey Kaye when I was organizing the Societies Jubilee Congress in 1984. He opened it 50 years after being involved in founding the Society. He was very excited about the occasion. He had only intended to come to the opening ceremony but stayed for the full two days. He had a speech written out but couldn't see to read it so spoke ad lib for twenty minutes. He had memorised it. I also met Harry Daly when I was a young. It is interesting that all this occurred during the latter part of the Great Depression. The Australian Society was one of the earliest along with the American, British and French Societies. How thrilling it must have been to have been part of this important development. I have experienced the same satisfaction when I look back on the introduction of some of my own innovations such as the dedicated time during the week for tutorials in the hospital in 1968 and the starting of the Anaesthetic Registrars meetings in 1971.

It is interesting that several of the scientific papers presented in Hobart in 1934 were about basal sedation with rectal Avertin (tribromethanol) which had just been introduced. A fascinating aspect of anaesthesia history is that the period of the great depression (1929-1935) was one of the most fruitful. Nupercaine, a long acting local anaesthetic used for spinal anaesthesia, was introduced in 1929; the barbiturates, hexobarbitone (1932) and then thiopentone (1934); cyclopropane (1933); the first trial of trichlorethylene (Trilene) was published in 1934; and Avertin (1933-4) were all introduced during this era. Endobronchial intubation and thoracic anaesthesia developed soon after, probably facilitated by being able to reach a deep level of anaesthesia quickly with cyclopropane.

The society grew gradually and now plays an important role. It is the organization which deals with the government on the business side of anaesthesia — conditions of employment, fee scales as well as dealing with national and international standards organizations and being involved in continuing education and overseas aid programs.

In 1952 the Society moved to have a Faculty of Anaesthetists set up in the Royal Australasian College of Surgeons in a similar way to the British Faculty, to organize the training programs and examination system and to issue a specialist qualification. Before that the only specialist qualifications were the Diploma of Anaesthetics at Melbourne and Sydney Universities. This move effectively took the higher qualification from the tertiary level at the Universities to a quaternary level in the College. Seventeen years later the last Melbourne DA was awarded. The Faculty became an independent College of Anaesthetists in 1992. It also plays important roles in setting standards of practice and in continuing education.

Many countries have more than one organization such as a Society and a College or Boards, the latter looking after training and examinations. In some countries there is only a Society which may also oversee training or the training may be in the hands of universities so that an national standard may not exist, or the qualification may be under government control. One factor which I have observed is that the relationship between two organizations is not always harmonious because of conflicts at the top, which is regrettable, because most of the membership is common to both groups. These groups should be working together for the welfare of their members, the anaesthetists.

About the same time as the Faculty was established the Society sent representatives to meetings in Paris in 1951 and Brussells in 1953 which led to the formation of the World Federation of Societies of Anaesthesiologists (WFSA).

In my time I have also had the privilege of helping to set up two regional organizations — the South Asian Confederation and the African Region of the World Federation which I will discuss elsewhere.

There are now an ever-increasing number of regional and specialty organizations. They tend to be established to bring people with common interests together and to provide continuing education congresses. That is what many of them do but some go further and deal with more grass roots needs, particularly in education and training at a more local level and may produce some scientific or information journal.

Congresses certainly bring people together and if friendships are made across boundaries of nationality, race and religion there should be a benefit to mankind as well as the educational and intellectual benefits to the individuals.

All these organizations have committees, some of them numerous. Much time is spent in deliberation but their ultimate value can only be assessed by the useful outcomes that are achieved. Often this is the work of a few hard working individuals.

I have worked with all these organizations for many years, mainly through my interest in teaching and education. My involvement will be discussed in following chapters.

Chapter 28
The ANZ College of Anaesthetists

My first involvement with the Faculty of Anaesthetists, later to become the College, was attending courses in preparation for my fellowship examinations. I had not sat any in Canada because they had a terminal examination and I had not completed the required time there. By the time I reached Melbourne I had more training than most registrars but I decided to wait for a year so that I was thoroughly prepared for the examinations. I sat and passed the primary in February and the final in October 1967. I believe I was the last person to sit both parts in one year.

After I had passed my Faculty of Anaesthetists Fellowship examinations in 1967, I became involved in teaching in the hospital and on courses run by the Faculty. I decided that I should try to develop one new topic to teach each year on Faculty courses. Drug interactions was one of the first. People were just beginning to realize the importance of this problem after it was noticed that patients on monoamine oxidase inhibitor antidepressant drugs developed high blood pressure when they ate cheese, which contains tyramine. The enzyme monoamine oxidase normally prevents the absorption of excess amounts of this substance. It is absorbed more freely when MAO is inhibited and, as tryramine causes the release of noradrenaline, blood pressure rises. It was then realized that many patients were on multiple drugs which may be interacting causing deleterious side effects. I published a paper on the principles involved in the Royal Australasian College of Surgeons Journal. Noel Cass had just negotiated a specific section for anaesthesia articles in this journal as we did not have an anaesthetic journal then. The need was short lived as *Anaesthesia and Intensive Care* came into existence soon afterwards.

This lecture on drug interactions was useful for a tour of New Zealand for their Post-graduate Medical Federation which Noel Cass asked me to do in 1969. This tour was an interesting challenge as it was my first one overseas. In many places there were only one or two anaesthetists and other doctors and even dentists attended my talks. The trip coincided with the first landing on the Moon. I visited several smaller centres. As I missed Dunedin, three of their anaesthetists came to Invercargill in the far south for my lectures — I imagine it was a rare event! I had a weekend in the beautiful resort of Queenstown and took a flight over the snow clad mountains to Milford Sound in a Cessna. I was a perfect day. The trip cost $20. In Wanganui the surgeon conveniently arranged a case so that the anaesthetist could not attend my lecture! In Rotarua I saw children walking to school in bare feet on a frosty morning. I took the bus from there to Gisborne on the East coast. As I was the only passenger the driver obligingly stopped at scenic spots for me to take photographs. In the tearoom at the hospital a teaspoon was chained to the wall. Obviously they kept disappearing. I was surprised some years later to find that a New Zealander, Noel Hosking, who came to work with me had chained it there.

In 1970 an opportunity arose which I has hesitant to accept at first because I thought I was rather junior. I was invited to become the first Education Officer for the Faculty of Anaesthetists in the state . I held the position for five years. It was an exciting task for me as I had to organize all the courses. I established a new introductory one for people just beginning anaesthesia who were working in smaller hospitals which did not have any formal teaching. I believed that they should be taught some basic principles at the beginning of their training. It served its purpose but as training became better organized in hospitals over the next few years it became unnecessary.

I was aware that many people who were teaching on our courses had never had any instruction on how to teach. My next idea was to provide some training for them. The first year Professor Kwong Lee Dow, from the Centre for Higher Education at Melbourne University, taught us about the basic educational principles — aims, objectives and assessment. The following year we used two teaching films made by the British Navy — *A class of your own* and *Visual aids* — which showed some useful points, good and bad, in teaching and highlighted the value of good visual aids. Forty eight anaesthetists, who were teaching, attended in three groups.

These activities led on to other things. I was asked to go to Malaysia to teach pharmacology to trainees preparing for their primary specialist anaesthetic examinations. There was to be a physiology teacher as well but in the end I was the sole teacher for two weeks and had to teach both physiology and pharmacology. My *summary answer tutorial technique* made this easier for me. The students wrote a summary of questions which then formed the basis of the discussion. They had to work and they produced much of the information themselves. As the sole teacher for two weeks I became well acquainted with the students. I still meet some of them at meetings.

After five years as Education Officer I became Chairman of the Victorian Regional Committee for two years. During this time the government began to raise the matter of peer review in medicine and Brian Howe, the Minister of Health, told the medical profession to introduce it. I was then asked to chair a joint Faculty / ASA Peer Review Committee. How this could be achieved was not an easy question to answer. Would re-certification be necessary and if so how would this be done. There was definite resistance to re-examination because the work in anaesthetists' practices varied so widely. During one committee meeting on this subject I learnt something important. There was much discussion, mainly by three of the members. At the end I decided that this was an important topic and everybody's comments should be heard. We went around the table. Two people who had said nothing now came out with the most pertinent comments. It taught me to seek the views of all members on a committee when important topics were discussed.

It was the beginning of demonstrating continuing competence and maintenance of professional standards, something that is now widely accepted. It was a logical and important development at a time when knowledge and the complexity of our work was increasing. Our first step was to gauge anaesthetists activity with a questionaire which asked about reading journals and books, attendance at meetings, involvement in teaching and examinations and also such activities as journal clubs. Of those surveyed, about 1200 replied and 90% indicated that they were involved in teaching at some level.

A journal club is a useful way of keeping up to date and also finding out what was going on around the city if the members came from different hospitals. I started one which continued for over thirty years. It proved useful as a source for speakers at meetings and courses as well as the discussion and information gleaned at them.

Continuing education was obviously going to become an important part of the process and our committee took over this role. Eventually we had a joint Faculty / ASA committee as well which was aimed to rationalise continuing education around the country. I also chaired that committee for some years. Although the Faculty and ASA functioned separately at national level they usually combined in the states to run an annual continuing education meeting.

My other major activity in the Faculty was as a Primary examiner in Pharmacology which I began in 1976. I enjoyed examining, especially the oral part. Everyone is aware of the stress the candidates go through but few realize that it can be difficult for the examiners to concentrate and ask good questions for several days so that they can fairly assess the candidates. At a course in New Zealand I was asked to conduct trial orals for students who were nearing the end of a five week intensive Physiology and Pharmacology course. Because I was a bit tired, having taught all day, I suggested that each of them would be my co-examiner for one of their colleagues and they would each have to ask one question. One third of them could not think of a question, one third asked the question so that the candidate did not know what answer was wanted and only one third managed to ask a straightforward question. It was an enlightening experience for us all. On another occasion I found out that not everyone, even doctors, has the capacity to assess and differentiate candidates at interview. Individuals lacking such ability should not be examiners as they lack the power to discriminate between candidates.

I had many interesting experiences and made some good

friends among my co-examiners. Sometimes we examined in New Zealand and other times in Perth, Singapore, Kuala Lumpur and Hong Kong as well as in Sydney and Melbourne. It was always a challenge to try to relax the candidates so that they could do their best. For some years we shook hands with the candidates when they entered. It began when one candidate mistook my standing and pointing to his chair as an invitation to shake hands. The idea caught on and became a routine. However, at my last exams in Sydney the lady supervising the candidates told us that they were suspicious of our motives. The candidates thought we were trying to assess how nervous they were! This was certainly not the motive, but it was a useful guide to apprehension, which enabled us to modify the opening question to make it easy, if necessary.

Occasionally we would have a candidate who was obviously not going to pass. I realized that people remember almost everything from these stressful occasions so I asked useful questions and gave some of the answers if they did not know them because I knew they would probably remember what I had told them for years. It gave them a small return for their efforts and expenditure in examination fees!

I had some challenging experiences. On one occasion a fellow burst out crying even though he was performing reasonably well. The stress was too much. Another candidate decided that he had failed the physiology in the morning and went to the pub and had what he described as a liquid lunch. He was persuaded by the lady overseeing their entrance to the examination that he should come in. He told me that he had had no intention of coming because he was "pissed". I asked him if he had done any interesting cases recently and was able to discuss the drugs he had used for one. I demonstrated to him that he had substantial knowledge and encouraged him not to give up so easily. I felt genuinely sorry for him. My co-examiners admitted that they would not have known how to handle these situations.

Some years later I was invited to help to set up the Master of Medicine examinations for the National University in Malaysia. As the qualifications were granted by universities I tried to persuade the two universities to use the same papers and external examiners so that the standard would be the same. The suggestion passed though several levels of bureaucracy but floundered at the top level when agreement was not forthcoming. Several years later I helped to set up the Diploma of Anaesthesia examinations for the South Pacific in Fiji. This was the first post-graduate medical qualification in the South Pacific.

Our early departmental scientific meetings at the hospital, to which the registrars conrtributed, were successful. Because of my involvement in the Faculty courses I decided that we should have a Registrars (trainees) meeting. The first one in 1971 attracted about 120 people and was sufficiently successful that they have continued. The first ones in Melbourne were run at the Royal Childrens Hospital. In alternate years we arranged for them to be run in Sydney, initially by Brian Clarke and then by Tom Torda. We received a little funding, from Parke Davis, who were promoting ketamine, and Abbott, who were promoting methoxyflurane (Penthrane) at the time. Now the latter is a historical drug. The funds assisted two interstate speakers to attend and present a paper. The idea was to have the meetings at the end of the course for the final examination candidates so that the interstate trainees could attend without the expense of another fare. Many of Australia's leading anaesthetists made their anaesthesia speaking debut at these meetings.

The *Travers Professorship* was instituted in the Faculty of Anaesthetists in honour of Lennard Travers, one of the founders, who came from Melbourne. He had begun his career as a surgeon but troublesome dermatitis from scrubbing before surgery led him to change to anaesthesia during the War. Following his death funds were raised by donation but they were insufficient to maintain a permanent chair, so the position is awarded about every three years to an applicant who has some status and a suitable project to undertake. I was appointed to this position in 1985. It enabled me to take some time off from the hospital to work in the museum and to undertake dissections for my work on nerve blocks, which became the basis for some of my teaching videos.

The appointee is also expected to visit some other states lecturing as well as delivering the Travers Oration at the Faculty, now College Annual Scientific Meeting. I travelled quite extensively in Queensland and in Western Australia. I drove up to Toowoomba, Townsville, Rockhampton and Brisbane where I lectured or ran workshops on paediatric anaesthesia. I also visited the anaesthetists and had dinner with them in Mackay and Nambour. It enjoyed visiting the country anaesthetists in their home cities. It is something that they appreciate and should be done more often. One side benefit of the trip was seeing three large flocks of 50 to 60 brolgas — tall crane type birds, mainly grey with some red on the head. They were magnificent sights.

In Western Australia I visited Perth, and did a trip with Ian Millar, who had formerly been a vet in the south west, and Nerida Dilworth who was Director of Anaesthesia at the Princess Margaret Childrens Hospital for 30 years. I lectured in Albany and Bunbury and we visited a number of other places of interest. Ian entertained us with commentaries of his vet life — he dealt with a bull here and another animal there!

I also visited Kalgoorlie for a day on my way back by train from an ASA meeting in Perth with my friend Carlos Riquelme from Chile. I helped the anaesthetist there with a couple of paediatric cases in the morning and gave a lecture in the evening. He lent us an old car which enabled us to see much more of the town. It was an interesting place to visit with its history going back to the gold rush. We visited old mines and it was amazing to see some of the former glory — for instance, the theatre with red velvet seats, and to be able to visit the 'two up' school. The next day I was not feeling too well and fell asleep on the train. I nearly missed the Nullarbor where the train runs dead straight for about 500km.

I had a busy year as I was also invited to New Zealand and Adelaide, where I gave the Travers Oration at the Faculty of Anaesthetists annual meeting.

In 1992 the Faculty of Anaesthetists separated from the College of Surgeons and became the independent Australian and New Zealand College of Anaesthetists. They moved to their new headquarters in St. Kilda Road — a magnificent old Victorian mansion called Ulimaroa. Since then they have built a six storey building behind it funded by having the fellows pay their subscriptions a year in advance.

I received the Orton Medal for outstanding service to anaesthesia at the College meeting in Canberra in 1992. (Figure C16) A few months later I received an honorary fellowship from the Royal College of Anaesthetists in London. (Figure C17) It was nice that my sister and her husband were able to attend in Canberra and my brother and his wife in London. Following the latter presentation we had tea at the Royal Geographical Society which was interesting because of its great collection of old maps and other memorabilia. On a later occasion I visited it because I wanted to see the paintings by Edward Wilson who went with Scott to the South Pole in 1912. Many of his wonderful watercolours of the Antarctic are kept at the RGS. You can only view them by special arrangement and have to wear cotton gloves to handle them. These were of particular interest to me as I had also painted extensively in the Antarctic during a trip to the Ross Sea where I had the wonderful experience of visiting the huts of Scott (1911), Shackleton (1907) and Borschgrevink (1899) as well as seeing the great beauty of that pristine continent. Other collections of Wilson's paintings can be found at the Scott Polar Research Institute in Cambridge, where his sketch books are also kept, and at his old school, Cheltenham Boys College.

In 2002, I was presented another honorary fellowship, from the South African College of Anaesthetists in Johannesburg, by their president, David Morrell.(72) This I very much appreciated because they recognised my contribution to, and association with Africa.

My teaching involvement with the Faculty/College continued until I retired from my full time position in 2000, a period of 32 years. Many changes in staff and accommodation had occurred over that time — from two secretaries to a large organisation, from an office in the College of Surgeons to a mansion and a six storey block with offices and lecture rooms. I believe that the training and examination system which it runs is not surpassed anywhere in the world.

Chapter 29

Australian Society of Anaesthetists

My first involvement with the Australian Society of Anaesthetists (ASA) was a presentation to the state section a few months after I arrived in Melbourne. I spoke on rheumatoid arthritis and anaesthesia. I highlighted the deformities in the neck and the arthritic involvement of the temporomandibular joints and the larynx which could lead to difficult intubation. Veins are often fragile and not easy to access for intravenous cannulation. Careful posturing on the operating table is essential to prevent pressure areas. The disease also causes general debility. Severe cases can be very difficult for the anaesthetist.

The Societies Annual Meetings rotate around the states. I have attended them regularly since 1968 when I have been in the country. They have always been interesting and the atmosphere is always congenial and friendly. In this chapter I will mention some of the highlights and organization of these meetings as it is interesting to follow developments in our specialty through them and become acquainted with some of the leading participants. I will also recall how I became involved in overseas aid and the committee which was established.

The annual meeting was in Hobart in 1967. It was a few days before my final examinations so I was not able to attend. My former mentor in Vancouver, Len Jenkins, attended and then visited us over the weekend between my written exams and the orals. I was a little tense about this but he reassured me that I had nothing to worry about. As it turned out I had Tess Brophy and someone else examining me and she asked about oesophageal atresia which I knew a lot about by then. It is amazing how one can remember the questions in exams 30–40 years later.

I attended the annual meeting for the first time when it was in Melbourne in 1968. I gave my first paper on the Winliz nebulizer which was developed by the respiratory technicians at the Hospital for Sick Children in Toronto. It was named after their wives. It was a simple but ingenious device with a water bath, in which floated a structure with a small hole for gas to emerge at a constant depth just below the water level. This raised the water which then hit a bar over the hole and shattered the drops into a fine mist which could moisten the inspired gases. I don't think it caught on before heated humidifiers, which saturated the gas with water vapour, came into use.

The following year we met in Brisbane. It was a notable meeting because Ben Barry was elected secretary. It was the last contested election in the ASA. He established a Society office in Sydney in a room in the basement of a house owned by the Elizabeth Bay Road anaesthetic group, itself the provider of many office bearers, including Presidents of the ASA. For the first time they employed a full time secretary, Sue Butterworth, who gave several years of good service and helped to establish the Society on a stable basis. They later purchased a Victorian terrace house in Gurner Street, Paddington before moving to their larger offices at Edgecliff. The consequence was that the Secretary always came from Sydney thereafter.

Ben also established the journal, *Anaesthesia and Intensive Care* and became its first Editor. He became President of the Society in 1985-6.

Tess Brophy, who made the resounding comment about prolonged intubation in Toronto in 1964, ran the meeting program in 1969. She introduced the idea of having a refresher course on Saturday, the AGM on Sunday and later Sunday afternoon was a social outing before the main meeting on Monday to Wednesday. She later became the first Professor of Anaesthesia in Queensland.

In 1970 the ASA meeting was replaced by the Asian Australasian Congress in Canberra organized by Doug Joseph, who was the Nuffield Professor of Anaesthetics in Sydney, and the red headed Judy Nicholas, who was an excellent Secretary. They became the first recipients of the Gilbert Brown award, for organizing this conference.

In 1971 Graham Fisk took over and invited me to help him. Little did I realize where this was leading. The meeting was in Perth. It was notable for the length of the Annual General Meeting which began at 9am on Sunday. I left with it still going on at 5.30pm. Since then the meetings have been curtailed never to exceed 3 hours.

Tom Shakespeare gave a talk on Compound 469 — isoflurane. I was able to back it up by showing the uptake curves for it because we had Bill Ward from New Zealand working with us. He had built an electrical analogue which used capacitors and resistors to generate the uptake and distribution curves for various agents in the body. I had the isoflurane figures and asked him to include them. It was a very advanced model at the time. Unfortunately isoflurane went under a cloud for several years because of some suspicion of toxicity in rats which was later proved not to be relevant. It was also the first meeting when medico legal issues were discussed in a panel chaired by Harry Cohen from Perth. I was also surprised at the dinner when my neighbour and a member of our journal club, Alec Kilgour, refused to stand for the toast to the Queen — the first signs of republicanism. Alec was a very nice fellow who, I found out later, came from a mining town on the New South Wales coast. He died in Broken Hill not long afterwards.

Graham Fisk proposed that a committee of three should organise the program and that each year one would rotate off. Millar Forbes from Perth and I were invited to join in 1972. The rotation idea did not work as the people who replaced Graham

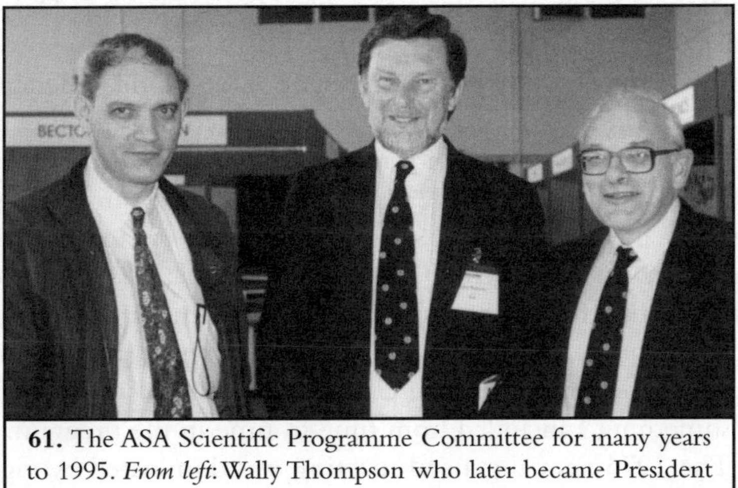

61. The ASA Scientific Programme Committee for many years to 1995. *From left*: Wally Thompson who later became President of ASA and member of College Council, John Roberts, Editor in Chief of *Anaesthesia and Intensive Care*, and Kester Brown. They jointly received the Gilbert Troup Prize in 1996.

and Millar departed before they took part in the organization. For the next twenty three years eight people were members of the committee for varying periods with a nominee from the state where the meeting was being held to help us. I was convenor for over twenty years except when we had a joint meeting with New Zealand in 1977 and 1989 and with the Canadians in 1985. In 1986 the Society awarded me the Gilbert Brown Award for my efforts. The other main contributors were John Roberts (61), Wally Thompson (61), Neville Davis, and Michael Cousins (Figure C28)

The refresher course evolved to have lectures in the morning and panels or discussion groups in the afternoon. It was amazing how most of the papers offered fell into groups which formed topic related sessions. These became commonplace from 1975. Some were built around the visiting speakers and sometimes a panel was included to change the pace.

The 1972 ASA meeting had several interesting features. The name of the journal, Anaesthesia and Intensive Care, was suggested by Ben Barry, the founding editor, was confirmed at a meeting attended by a small group including Maurice Sando, then the Director at Royal Adelaide Hospital and the head of a very organised training program. He strongly supported the inclusion of Intensive Care in the title. He later became Dean of the Faculty, but died relatively young.

It was the first time that a President of the World Federation-Ted Mayrhoffer (76) from Austria — attended our meeting. Jim Treloar, who had trained with me in Vancouver and subsequently went into practice with Peter Klassen doing day procedures in a private medical building, presented the first paper on Day Surgery in Australia before this became popular. I presented a paper on the use of sodium nitroprusside in cardiac surgery which might also have been a first. Bryn Thomas, a well known anaesthetic historian from the UK. spoke at a history session. This was something I included from time to time in the program.

The 1973 annual general meeting was dominated by vigorous discussion about how we should counteract the government's plan to introduce Medibank and its obvious desire to nationalize medicine. We had a labour government for the first time in many years led by Gough Whitlam. We still have Medibank but also maintain a significant private practice component.

I was overseas in 1974 when Michael Rosen came as overseas visitor. The 1975 meeting had a session on hypotensive anaesthesia. Interest in this topic had been stimulated by Ron Katz's talk in 1971 on sodium nitroprusside. The speakers spoke on a variety of hypotensive drugs and techniques which they had used. One, for instance, used the ganglion blocker, pentolinium. Another session was devoted to pollution in the operating theatre, a hot topic at the time.

The 1976 meeting was in Surfers Paradise. Because swimming is better in the morning it was suggested that we start later. The meeting ran from 11 am. to 6 pm. This proved successful, as people could recover from their social activities and have time for a swim or a leisurely breakfast with their friends if they wished. The attendance at the final session was the best of any meeting that I have ever attended — 60% at least of the registrants.

It was at this meeting that I gave the first paper on computers in recording theatre utilization. I well remember one friend almost denigrating me for talking on this. He later became a computer maniac. I gave what was supposed to be a light hearted and entertaining paper on anaesthesia in unusual locations. It was a disaster, because I was preceded by a country GP anaesthetist, Charles Wood, who gave a hilarious talk about his work in the country. I learnt never to have Charles speak before me again. He gave another couple of talks on unusual topics at later meetings. I once visited him in Kyogle in northern New South Wales, where he practiced, when I was on my way to Brisbane. I developed a great respect for him.

In 1978 the meeting was in Perth where Mary Durak, a member of one of the old outback Western Australian pioneering families, gave a wonderful exposition of the early days at one of the social functions. Our outing on Sunday was to the Spanish monastery at New Norcia, about 100 km from Perth. The most interesting feature to me was finding two paintings by the famous Spanish painter, Ribera, in their art collection. He is one of my favorite portrait painters. They are the only ones I am aware of in Australia.

The 1980 meeting was in Sydney. Ken Leighton from

Vancouver (Figure C3), who had started his training shortly after I did in Vancouver, and Bernard Brandstater (48), who gave the first paper on prolonged intubation in children in 1962, were the visitors. Ken Leighton spoke on the kidney in anaesthesia during which he postulated that the diminished urine output in shock may be associated with a decrease in catecholamines (adrenaline and nor adrenaline). Bill Runciman spoke next. He is a brilliant man trained in South Africa who has infused Australian anaesthesia with some great science, and founded the Australian Patient Safety Foundation. His topic was the kidney in septic shock, where he produced the scientific evidence for what Ken Leighton had postulated — that catecholamine blood levels were low. It was a fantastic sequence of papers.

In 1981 in Melbourne I heard a paper which had a great influence on me because I had never heard this important topic presented before. It was on *ergonomics* by a very stimulating surgeon from Whyalla called Michael Patkin. Years later I found out that Nahama, who is well known in music circles, and who had taught our girls in Yamaha classes when they were small, was his sister.

Another important component of most medical meetings is the trade display, where companies who sell equipment and drugs show their wares. At this meeting it was decided that the Society should have a Trade Liaison Committee. I thought Rod Westhorpe would be an ideal person for it so he and Tom Torda were appointed. Rod continued for many years as the liaison person. This proved particularly valuable when we were approaching the World Congress as some companies were being diffident about participating. Rod's personal relationship with many of the representatives helped to overcome the difficulties.

The memorable paper in 1982 was one by David Griffiths on the respiratory complications in the recovery room. He explained the set up of their Recovery room and then told us that 2% of patients on their backs but only 0.7% on their left side had problems. We knew it was better to have the patients on their sides. But then he said that 3.2% on their right side had problems. At first we were puzzled until he pointed out that they were facing away from the nurses desk. It was one of those wonderfully simple talks with a very practical message which are often the best remembered. The nurses must be able to see their patients. David was one of the people who had a delightful way of seeing through problems and putting a different slant on them. He worked in Zambia before coming to Tasmania. He did some of his training in our department. David headed the department in Hobart for some time before going into hyperbaric medicine in Townsville.

The next year in Brisbane we had our first Pioneer Lecture. There are several memorial lectures at the ASA and College meetings. The presidents do a two year term and give a presidential address in the second year. It was named the Geoffrey Kaye oration after our first secretary. It seemed to me that the best way to honour other pioneers rather than have a proliferation of named lectures was to have a pioneer lecture in the intervening year and when it was due, to honour a pioneer from the state where the meeting is being held. Roger Bennett, Greta McClelland and Gilbert Troup have been so honoured.

At this meeting Charles Wood talked on transactional analysis and the preoperative visit! We had a session on anaesthesia for animals which I chaired. Just before the session I found a large koala suit in the office. The chairman of the organising committee, John Hains (63) agreed it would be appropriate for me to wear it. (Cover) I agreed provided he announced at the start that the chairman had been delayed but he had found a suitable substitute! I then walked on to the stage. It was hot as it was lined with 5 cm of foam rubber. I lasted until I had introduced the second speaker. At the end there was a discussion period. I concluded by asking one of the speakers if koalas were susceptible to malignant hyperthermia (a rare condition where body temperature rises during anaesthesia). He didn't know but when he heard someone sniggering in the audience he said he thought the big ones might. The session ended with much laughter.

In January 1984 we held a special Jubilee Meeting in Sydney. It was just after the World Congress in the Philippines. I was given full responsibility for the program so I selected four topics to which I thought Australian anaesthetists had made significant contributions. These were history, education, pharmacology and intensive care. I selected the top local people on the topics, plus

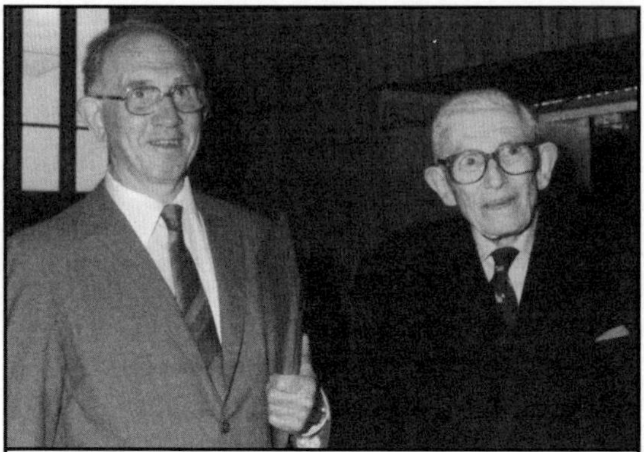

62. Geoffrey Kaye (R) and Denis Smith (Leeds,UK) during the ASA Jubillee meeting in Sydney, 1984.

an internationally renowned Australian working overseas and/or an international figure for each session. It was a wonderful program. The meeting was opened by Geoffrey Kaye (62), our original secretary, who was 84. He was very apprehensive about it and only planned to go to Sydney to give his talk. He spoke for 20 minutes without notes (he couldn't see them to read!) and then stayed for the whole meeting because he became so enthralled with it all. It was an excellent meeting.

By this time the meeting regularly attracted 200-250 registrants later going up to about 300 before MOPS (maintenance of professional standards) came in.

In 1986 the meeting was in Perth. The theme of the meeting was "accept the challenge" because they were holding the America's Cup there that year. We made a special fun award to Michael Waterfield for the best non scientific effort in relation to the meeting — he had cycled from Melbourne to Perth in 28 days, 26 of them into a headwind. The prize was a puncture repair outfit. He made a very gracious acceptance speech and said that if anyone had a problem with jet lag he thought he had the answer! Cycle!

For many years there was discussion about going to the Centre of Australia or offshore for our meeting, so eventually in 1987, we met in Alice Springs with a precongress meeting on anaesthesia for orthopaedics at Ayers Rock. Janet , Ken and I flew to Darwin and drove down to Alice Springs and Ayers Rock. It was a wonderful trip and provided plenty of scenery for photographs and painting. Kings Canyon with its brick red cliff on one side and lighter one on the other was enhanced during our visit by three German girls singing songs from *Sound of Music* by the waterfall.

Mike Waterfield rode up from Melbourne.

I took our overseas visitor, Alastair Spence and his wife, Maureen, out one morning for an early breakfast in the bush to see some rocks with aboriginal carvings. We became good friends and it was he who presented my FRCA in London some years later. (Figure C17) At lunch beforehand he said to me, "Now Kester, this is a serious affair so we don't want any of your nonsense." I must have developed some strange reputation with my friends. During the citation by David Hatch he mentioned my interest in photography and the hazard of having a photograph taken by me. This related to one I had taken of him sitting on a very grand commode in Rotterdam, a copy of which arrived on his desk when he became professor.(44)

In 1988 I managed one of my most complex arrangements for overseas visitors. The meeting was in Ballarat, an old gold mining town 110 km west of Melbourne. It has some interesting tourist sites which we made use of. The welcome reception was held in the Fine Art Gallery, one of the best country galleries in Australia. The social afternoon was at Sovereign Hill, a historical park on an old mine site, followed by a concert with singers from the Victorian Opera at the South Street Theatre, which had just been renovated. One of our anaesthetists, John Marum, sang in the Victorian Opera. He asked four of them to sing. Spare seats were sold to members of the community and the money was donated towards the renovations, which were nearing completion. This was followed by supper in the recently renovated Craig's Hotel which was built at the beginning of Ballarat in the 1850s. Tuesday was Melbourne Cup day when Melbourne has a holiday for a horse race. We had our own frivolities during the afternoon at the Ballarat racecourse. The "Ballarat Cup", human sprint race was won by Denis Clare, our research scientist. The team competition trophy, a mounted Goldman vaporiser, was won by Victoria. The overall meeting was very successful. It was attended and contributed to by members of the Association of Paediatric Anaesthetists whom I invited for one of our Paediatric Anaesthetic meetings the following weekend in Melbourne (41). They had a two-day trip via the Grampians and Great Ocean Road with its wonderful scenery to Melbourne. (Figure C8)

The ASA had a joint meeting with the Canadians in Toronto in 1985. I won the first prize for a video on nerve blocks and anatomy. The Canadians came to Brisbane in 1991. A provocative comment at the welcome reception that year from Di Khursandi from Queensland to me, gave me food for thought. She said " Although you have spoken to me every ASA meeting for the past ten years you have never had a conversation with me!" I realized that I hadn't and although I thought I knew her quite well I really knew very little about her. We often go to meetings and greet many people but with how many do we stop to have a real conversation? I have since always tried to stop to talk at greater length with some of those I meet. Of course, afterwards she was rather embarrassed about being so outspoken but I reassured her that her comment was a very valuable one.

I had driven up with Italo Zamudio from Chile (Figure C4), who was working with us, and my sister and her husband. On the return I took three days so that my companion Gunnar Bo from Oslo (28) could see a bit of the country. We had a great trip home coming over the Snowy mountains.

In 1992 I accepted a paper on morbid obesity from K. Swe from Alice Springs. We had never had a paper from there before. He described how a man weighing 278 kg was brought in on the back of a truck. He couldn't walk. They placed two operating tables together for the operation where they did an apronectomy. He had 70 kg of fat hanging from his belly which was removed. He walked out of the hospital!

In 1994 we decided to have a joint meeting with the Pacific and New Zealand Societies in Fiji. It was an interesting event concluding with a local choir singing most beautifully to us. That evening I went out to dinner with some of my friends from the Pacific and some who had taught and worked out there. A little after we arrived two other couples came in. One was President of the ASA. I told the waitress mischievously that he was the president and she should address him as such. When he was leaving at the end she opened the door and said "Good night, President Clinton!

Organizing these meetings was a challenge. I used to put aside time for about two weeks each year to put the program together.

It amazed me how we usually received about the right number of papers and how I could fill gaps and make an interesting program. We always invited some people for specific topics and often had one or two non anaesthetists contributing. Times were changing and continuing education began to be monitored with MOPS points so after the World Congress in 1996 it was time for new , younger and enthusiastic people to take over. Jim Bradley, who later became President of the ASA and Dennis Hayward took over from us converting the meeting into a much bigger National Scientific Congress which was able to cater for the expanding maintenance of professional standard (MOPS) requirements. My concluding contribution was to chair the scientific committee for the World Congress, a task which took 6 years.

I was fortunate to be allowed to perform this task which I enjoyed so much for so long. It is unlikely that anyone will have the privilege or opportunity of doing so again. My colleagues in the Society gave me a great honour when they revamped the program by naming the special opening lecture, "The Kester Brown Lecture."

I served on a number of committees. My other roles for the Society were to represent them on the Faculty's continuing education committee, the Joint continuing education committee which I chaired for several years, The Peer Review committee, which I also chaired, and the Overseas Aid Committee, which I convened for nine years. The latter coincided with my time as Chair of the WFSA Education Committee which was convenient as I could obtain funds from two sources. When we began we had no funds so I asked the Society to give us $1 per head of the membership, then $3 and then $5, after which they decided to look at our requests and fund as reasonably necessary.

In 1985 I made my first medical visit to Fiji on my way back from North America. It was the first of my overseas teaching visits. I was by then on the WFSA Education Committee. Tu Mua, who was the head of the department at the Colonial War Memorial Hospital in Suva had visited our department a few months before and invited me. Things were far more backward then.

When I arrived I was told that they had a patient with phaeochromocytoma for me to anaesthetise. This is a tumour which produces adrenaline and causes rises in blood pressure. They had obtained the drugs to lower blood pressure for me so I was optimistic. I saw the patient, a 34 year-old man. He was a bit anaemic so I thought I would give him some phenoxybenzamine which dilates the vessels and lowers the blood pressure. This was given intravenously the day before with two units of blood to fill the dilated circulation. I asked what monitoring equipment they had. "A blood pressure cuff" was the reply. Then they thought they may have an ECG. Eventually they found it — it had lead plates which were attached at the wrist and ankles. There were no special devices to administer the infusions of drugs — just an ordinary drip set. Then they told me that the man had been taking aspirin for his headaches for three weeks. This interferes with blood clotting. Could I get the necessary platelets from the blood bank? "Yes,"` but in the event they were not available and I had to get fresh blood. Fortunately I was used to using hypotension without too much sophisticated monitoring, and the operation went well. The use of phenoxybenzamine was to dilate the circulation and fill it with extra blood because the constant overstimulation with adrenaline reduces the blood volume. When the tumour is removed this stops. Unless blood has been given and an adequate blood volume established at the time problems related to low blood pressure will occur.

Anthea Hatfield had run a course in Fiji for the Pacific Islanders. Subsequently the ASA ran these with support from WFSA. To enable the island anaesthetists to attend a number of people went out for a week or two to provide locums for them. After a few years we managed to obtain government aid funding, because we had demonstrated that we were running something useful which was effective aid. Later, the government gave support for a lecturer to spend two years in Suva. Steve Kinnear, from Adelaide, went and managed to set up a Diploma of Anaesthesia course and examinations in the medical school.

I went out as the chair of the inaugural DA. examinations with Dick Willis, John Hains and Ted Ward from New

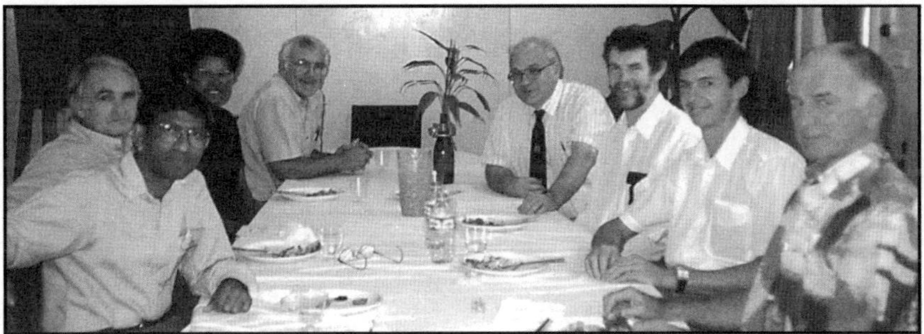

63. The examiners at the first South Pacific DA Examinations: John Hains (Former President ASA), Ganesh Rao (Physician, Fiji), Serima Bale (Senior anaesthetist, Fiji), Ted Ward (New Zealand), Kester Brown (Chairman), Dick Willis (Later President ANZCA), Steve Kinnear (Lecturrer and organiser of the exminations. Later Chair of ASA Overseas Aid Committee), Ron Hunton (physician).

Zealand.(63) We had all examined for the Faculty of Anaesthetists. Six out of seven candidates passed. One of the medical examiners commented to me that he was amazed how quickly they could make a medical assessment of the patient. I explained to him that we had to be able to do that because our available time or pre-operative visits was limited. I told anaesthetists that if they wanted to be good at their job they had to be *super physicians* so that they could make rapid assessments. Narco Tatula from the Soloman Islands (64) won the prize. He is very musical. He stayed with us once and told us he worked in a two-doctor hospital and that they often swapped jobs in theatre, so that when one was away the other would be competent to do both the anaesthesia and surgery with a nurses help — the reality of the third world. One evening, while he was staying with us, he complained of headache. Janet, who is a physiotherapist, though it was a postural problem and told him to put his hands behind his head and push it back into them. His headache disppeared. Narco and I were amazed!

The Diploma of Anaesthetics was the first post-graduate diploma awarded by the Fiji School of Medicine (64). Now there is a Masters program which was interrupted by the political conflicts in Fiji but recently the first students have graduated.

I taught on one of the courses with Hugh Spencer and Chris Sparks. It was a great experience to work with such wonderful and dedicated people. Chris had worked in Vanuatu and at

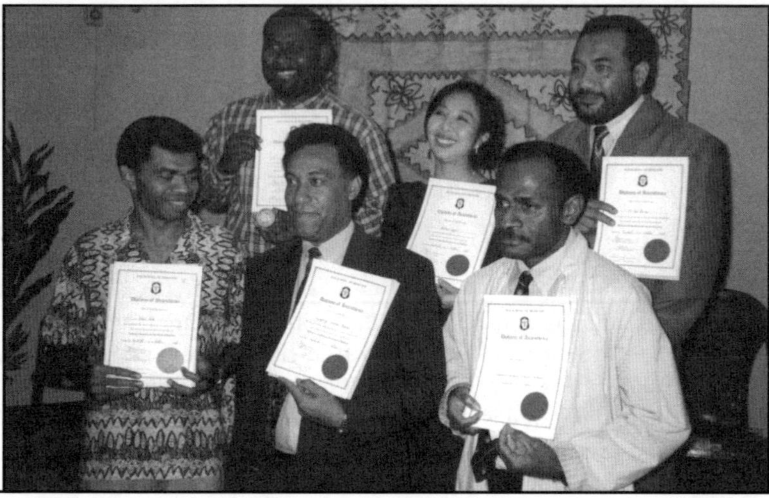

64. The first graduates of the Diploma of Anaesthetics at the Fiji School of Medicine with their diplomas. Standing — from left : Narko Tatuo (Soloman Islands — Prize winner), Heidi Cayari, Ali Biribo, Eloni Tora, Talia'uli (Geoffrey) Afeaki (Tonga), Inia Seseni.

that time was in the Soloman Islands for two years. Hugh is a very thoughtful, unassuming man who had studied history before medicine — he has been an "anaesthesia treasure", like some countries (e.g. Japan) have national treasures. He has since arranged short term appointments (6-12 months) at Waikato Hospital in New Zealand for several Pacific Island anesthetists.

One of the topics was nerve blocks, which turned out to be the best sessions I ever attended on the subject. Hugh Spencer worked in Hamilton , New Zealand. He was a great teacher and had learnt his block techniques by studying Grant's Atlas of Anatomy. He confirmed the desirability of injecting local anaesthetic in two layers during an ilio-inguinal block for hernia repair. The classic teaching had been to feel the loss of resistance when penetrating the external oblique aponeurosis, and then injecting the local anaesthetic which would block the nerves coming through to the surrounding skin. Two weeks before this someone had shown me the diagram in Grant's Atlas of Anatomy which showed that we should also penetrate the next muscle and inject into that space as well, so that local anaesthetic reached the neck of the hernial sac which the surgeon dissects. The same week a surgeon at the hospital found a pool of fluid around the sac — the local anaesthetic had inadvertently been injected into that space. This changed our teaching on how to do ilio-inguinal blocks.

Hugh taught us another useful trick. When injecting nerves around the wrist or ankle, which do not have clear landmarks, he instills the local anaesthetic at one point and then squeezes it around between two fingers of one hand with an finger from the other hand. This causes less tissue damage than injecting all round with a needle. It is a very simple but clever idea.

Although I taught on this course I felt my main contribution in the Pacific was as a catalyst to help others achieve these goals, because I did not have time to go more often. Later we started courses for the anaesthetists in Micronesia as well, as it was a long way for them to come to Fiji. Then things changed and government funding was directed through other channels so that the ASA was less directly involved. The courses and teaching we established continue, overseen by the senior anaesthetist, Sereima Bale. (15,63)

I worked with some wonderful people on this committee such as Haydn Perndt (65), Chris Sparks, Steve Kinnear, Peter Armstrong, who had all worked for at least two years in the Pacific, and several others including David Mawter, who took over the Chairmanship from me. Haydn had worked in Vanuatu as well as doing six month stints in Soloman Islands, Cook Islands and Tonga. He has worked with Red Cross and the Army in many other places such as East Timor and Somalia.

Later Haydn Perndt and George Meridew (cover) decided to run courses with practical tuition for people contemplating working in the third world. These have been very successful, alternating between Hobart and Launceston and now Darwin. I have been included in the teaching team to talk on paediatric anaesthesia and how to teach which I have greatly appreciated.

It has been a wonderful experience to have been so involved in various activities of the Society and an honour to have been entrusted with these activities for so long. They honoured me in many ways including making me a Life Member.

Chapter 29

World Federation of Societies of Anaesthesiologists

For many years I did not relish the idea of attending very large meetings such as a World Congress where I would be lost in the crowd and not be able to find the people I knew or wanted to meet. However, in 1984 I decided to go to the World Congress in Manila. Some events at this congress changed my life significantly.

Australia had bid for this congress, which was to be held in Sydney, but due to lack of adequate facilities nearer the time they pulled out and the Philippine Society took it on. They did very well considering that they had some major problems. First, most of the Americans did not come at the last minute because their government did not approve of the Marcos regime and they were frightened of the demonstrations. These turned out only to be people singing in the streets on Friday afternoons. Then some of the registration fees were siphoned off in banks in Hong Kong and Los Angeles.

The failure of the Americans to attend left many gaps in the program. I tried to help in the paediatric anaesthesia section by giving an extra paper and when one session was about to be closed about 30 minutes early I offered to run an impromtu panel, as there were several of the world's leading paediatric anaesthetists in the room. The audience would otherwise not have had the chance of hearing them speak. These included Jackson Rees, Gordon Bush (Liverpool), Ted Sumner (Great Ormond St, London), Claude St Maurice (Paris), Jeremy Sloan (Toronto) and Rob Eyres (Melbourne).

During the Congress Richard Walsh, then secretary of the Australian Society of Anaesthetists, asked if I would be prepared to be nominated for the Education Committee of WFSA. I thought about it and agreed as by then I had been involved with our Society' scientific program for twelve years. I was appointed and so began what turned out to be something I never contemplated — 20 years of involvement with the Federation.

Another simple but significant event took place. During the General Assembly I decided to greet the person sitting behind me, who I did not know. It turned out to be Jorge Urzua from Chile. Afterwards I engaged him in conversation, asking him where he worked. He was at the Catholic University in Santiago. Later I found out that this was one of the best departments in South America. When I told him that I worked at the Childrens Hospital in Melbourne he immediately asked me to come to a workshop that they were organizing. Chile was a poor country in 1984. I had to ask our Society to help me with the fare and I stayed in a very quaint but inexpensive hotel — Foresta. There were suits of armour and original oil paintings in the hall. This was the beginning of my association with South America. I have been seven times on teaching and lecturing trips covering much of the continent.

Jorge turned out to be an outstanding cardiac anaesthetist and physiologist whose approach to discussions on these topics was refreshingly different. He later came to Australia as our overseas visitor and became a member of the WFSA Education Committee.

The World Federation of Societies of Anaesthesiologists evolved from discussions by a group of anaesthetists who met at the International Anaesthesia Congress in Paris in 1951. They concluded that a world organization would help communication among anaesthetists in different parts of the world. An interim committee was set up with Harold Griffith as chairman. The other members of the committee were Alexandre Goldblatt (Belgium), John Gillies (U.K.), Jacques Boureau (France), Alexander Low (UK) and Torsten Gordh (Sweden) who, at the age of almost 90, came to the World Congress in Sydney (Figure C24). Jean Francisque Delafresnaye from the Council for International Medical Organisations was invited to join them as a consultant. There were observers from other countries including Dr Frank Leventhal from Australia. He was undertaking post graduate studies in Britain at the time. The interim committee met in Brussels in June1953 with some others, including Ellis Gillespie representing Australia, and again in 1954 in the Netherlands. It was decided to hold the First World Congress in the Netherlands in 1955. Ritsema van Eck chaired the organising committee and the Congress was held at Scheveningen in September 1955. There were twenty six founding member Societies when the Federation was established, including Australia which was represented by Norman James. He was Director of Anaesthesia at the Royal Melbourne Hospital for some years and was involved in the development of the Harrington — James ventilator which produced a negative pressure phase in expiration which was thought to be useful in Neurosurgery. Actually it increased the hazard of air embolus.

These founders of the Federation defined its aims. The object of the Federation is to make available the highest standard of anaesthesia to all the peoples throughout the world. To achieve this it is (1) to assist and encourage the formation of national societies of anaesthesiologists, (2) to promote the dissemination of scientific information, (3) to recommend desirable standards of training, (4) to provide information on post-graduate training and research, (5) to encourage research, (6) to establish safety measures and standardisation of equipment , and (7) to advise national and international organisations.

Subsequent World Congresses before I attended were held in Toronto (1960), Sao Paulo, Brazil (1964), London (1968), Kyoto, Japan (1972), Mexico City (1976) and Hamburg, Germany (1980).

The new chair of the Education Committee in 1984 was Howard Zauder. The other members were Professor Luder from East Germany from whom we never heard again, John Couper (Figure C19) from South Africa, whose wife became ill, Anis Baraka (74) in Lebanon, who only received mail every 2 to 3 months because of the war there and Riccardo Samayoa de Leon from Guatamala, who attended all but one of the first twelve World Congresses. It was difficult to communicate and we did little apart from approve three visiting lecturers in the first three years. The chairman then resigned because he became President of the American Society. I was invited to take over. I accepted on condition that I remained Chairman until 1992. In that position I attended the Executive Committee meetings.

In Manila the invited speakers at the World Congress were entertained at an afternoon tea / musicale at the Palace with Imelda Marcos. Many of her child prodigy musicians performed — an 8 year old played a Mozart concerto for instance. Despite the antagonism to their regime, she was a great supporter of the arts, music in particular. At the end, groups from each country were photographed with her. I missed the Australians so eventually had my photograph taken with her alone. It nearly proved useful when we arrived at the airport on Sunday night to find our flight had been overbooked by sixty. I had to be in Sydney for our Society's Jubilee meeting on the following Wednesday morning and the next flight was on Tuesday evening. I had to catch the flight. I was thinking of going up to the man on the desk and flashing the photograph in front of him as I thought that might have an immediate effect on him. Rob Eyres was with me. He had another idea and he managed to persuade someone that I was important enough to get on the flight. He had a extra two days, hotel and some expenses paid in Manila.

My next big congress was in 1986. I attended the Asian-Australasian Congress in Hong Kong. For the first time I was an Australian delegate to the Assembly. I had been to Korea in 1982 and one of their delegates, who knew me, approached me to ask for support for Korea to have the next Congress. I was able to help and they were selected.

It was at a social function that I met four Communist China delegates, which was a first for me. I was amazed to find one spoke fluent French and another German which they had learnt at school before the war and the Communist regime came into power.

It was the first time I spoke on how to teach and present a paper — I felt I had failed somewhat when a Chinese gentleman went to sleep in the front row!

It was at that meeting that I met Quintin Gomez, who had

trained many of the Pacific anaesthetists at the Philippine Training Centre. He had been treasurer and later President of WFSA and was an outstanding man in the region.

The next World Congress was in Washington, D.C. in 1988. It was organised by Jack Moyers and was quite a lavish affair. I have a tendency to say what I think. Following one expensive drug company reception I thanked my host for an enjoyable evening but then said that I thought they were wasting their money. "Why?" he asked. I told him that it was a World Congress but many countries were not represented because they could not afford to come and that if a little less had been spent on the party they could have helped some people to come from the unrepresented countries. Some years later a colleague came back from a meeting overseas and told me he had met this man. My message had had a profound effect on him. He had changed the company's philosophy to become more philanthropic and since then they have helped many people to attend such congresses and in other ways by providing educational materials. When I eventually met him again his enthusiasm for the idea was amazing.

A refresher course was run concurrently with the Congress, which I think was a distraction from the main meeting, resulting in fewer delegates attending sessions To present a paper at a World Congress involves a considerable amount of preparation and for some they think it will be the pinnacle of their career or, at least, it should be an important event in their lifetime. It is so disappointing when there are only a few in the audience.

John Zorab (67), who had been Secretary for eight years since 1976, became President of WFSA. He had been a very effective secretary, well supported by his wife, Shirley. He had many innovative ideas. He edited a Lecture series of books twice a year, proposed the idea of refresher courses and the idea of bringing an anaesthetist from each Eastern European Country to the west for a month while communism was still in control. Two of these — Maria Janecsko from Hungary (Figure C20, 74)(who became chair of the Executive Committee, and Ivan Smilov from Bulgaria — have both made significant contributions to anaesthesia.

On the way to the World Congress in 1988 I decided to go via South America to find out the needs of that part of the world. At first I was going to visit three countries, but it gradually increased for a variety of reasons until I spent a month visiting Argentina, Uruguay, Chile, Bolivia, Peru, Ecuador where I attended their Congress, Costa Rica and Guatamala. I lectured in all the countries and ran workshops in several. I did an all-day one in Quito. I also learnt the value of using South American lecturers there as they speak the language and understand the working conditions which is important. There were some very good speakers.

In Washington I had the Education Committee expanded. We had several good people added including Roger Eltringham from UK and Philippe Scherpereel from France who both made major contributions towards increasing the effectiveness of the committee (Figure C19). In the next four years we had $50,000 per year with which we managed to send teachers from 25 countries to visit 50 countries to lecture and in many cases teach in the operating theatre. Probably about sixty countries benefited as anaesthetists from some other countries attended regional courses. Some smaller regional societies, particularly in UK, supported courses by sending an additional lecturer. This increase in educational activity changed the course of WFSA, making education its major thrust besides the World Congresses. It has continued and is the major expense on WFSA funds. The Federation was gradually being seen as doing something positive for many societies, especially those in less affluent countries.

Mitsugi Fujimori (Figure C19) from Japan took over the committee which continued to run the way I had set it up, with each person having an area of responsibility and funds to organise courses.

He was followed by Hadyn Perndt (65) from Hobart, Australia. Haydn had worked in Vanuatu and several other Pacific Islands as well as places like Somalia with Red Cross. He therefore had a very good understanding of the situation in less affluent and less well developed countries. He worked very hard to ensure the programs continued. He also introduced some train-

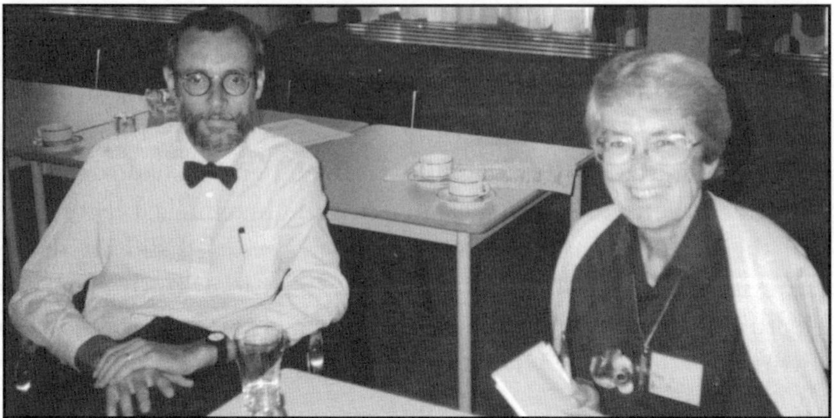

65. Two Australians, Haydn Perndt, chairman of WFSA Education Committee 1996-2000, and Patricia Coyle, who spent several difficult years in Uganda.

ing centres which provided basic or specialty training in regions where this was lacking or not easy to obtain. More recently he has been involved in East Timor. Few doctors have contributed so much in the less affluent world — another "anaesthesia treasure"!

Angela Enright (66) from Canada took over in 2000. She had been the Chair of the Montreal World Congress Organising Committee, had traveled promoting it and had made many contacts which were useful for someone who chairs the Education Committee. I had the pleasure of doing sessions on education in Singapore and Penang with her in 2002 on our way to the Asian Australasian Congress in Kuala Lumpur.

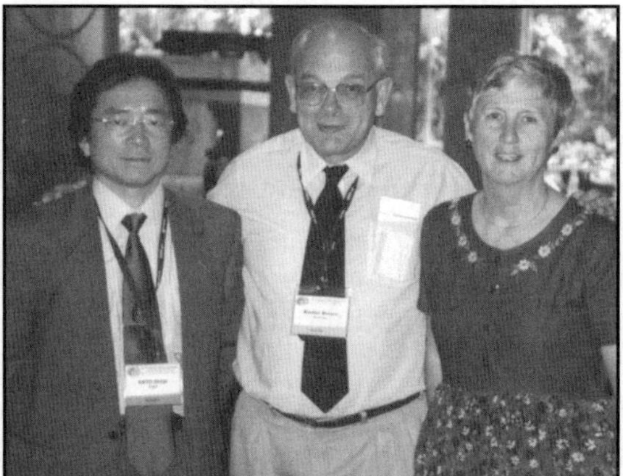

66. Shigeheto Sato (Japan — International Relations Committee), Kester Brown, Angela Enright (Canada — Chair, WFSA Education Committee 2000 and World Congress Committee 2000) In Kuala Lumpur 2002.

Between World Congresses Regional Congresses are held and the Executive Committee usually

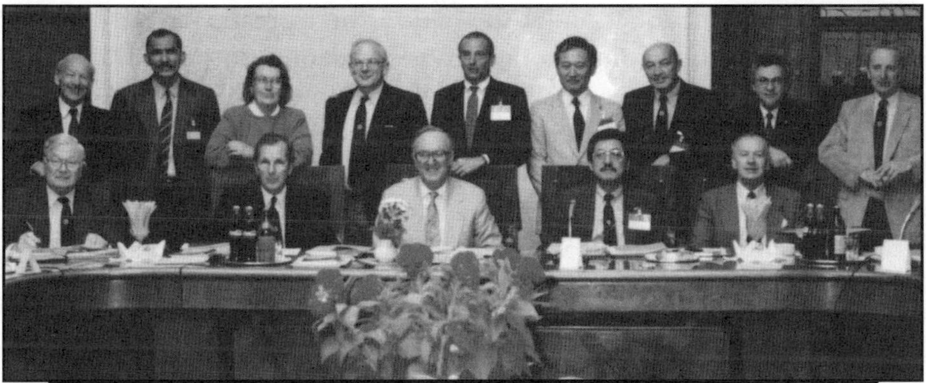

67. The WFSA Executive Committee meeting in Warsaw in 1990. *Standing from left*: Michael Rosen (Cardiff, UK), Manuel Silao (Philippines), Elena Damir (Moscow, Russia), Kester Brown (Australia), Bernie Wetchler (USA, Deputy Chairman, authority on day surgery), Kenjiro Mori (Kyoto, Japan), Jack Moyers (USA — organized the 1988 World Congress in Washington), Martin Marx (Uruguay, Secretary General, CLASA), Cedric Hoskins (New Zealand). *Sitting*: Richard Ament (Treasurer, USA), John Zorab (President, Bristol, UK), Michael Vickers (Chairman of Executive, Cardiff, UK), Lim Say Wan (Secretary, Malaysia), William Macrae (Chairman, Statutes and Bylaws, Scotland).

meet at one of these. In 1990 it was held in Warsaw (67). It was a bleak place at the time as communist domination had just ended. It was amazing to see how they had rebuilt the old town after it was completely demolished during World War II. On a city tour , one building was pointed out as one of six that survived the war. What devastation. One evening we went to Chopin's birthplace where they had a short piano recital. There was one seat short so I sat in the kitchen next door and sketched it while listening. Eventually I did a painting of the scene.

Following the European Congress I went on to the Asian — Australasian Congress in Seoul, South Korea. I had some involvement in helping the Koreans organise this congress. I gave a plenary lecture on "the role of the anaesthesiologist". At my suggestion they invited Horace Underwood to give a keynote address on "the Korean attitude". He was an outstanding man, the grandson of American missionaries who had come to Korea and founded Yonsei University. It now has one of the best medical schools in the country. He was still influential in the University. He had, as a young man, been one of the translators in the peace negotiations at the end of the Korean War.

During this Congress there was a meeting, to which I was invited, which led eventually to the formation of the South Asian Confederation of Anesthesiologists

The next world Congress was in Den Haag in the Netherlands in 1992. Harm Lip was the Chair of the Organising Committee and Anneke Meursing (34) was the secretary. Anneke and I were both elected to the Executive Committee of WFSA and with her support I became the Deputy Chairman. Lim Say Wan (68) from Malaysia became President. He was a very active man who held office in several organisations and encouraged the anaesthetists in his region to be more active. In his younger days he had been a leading badminton player. Michael Vickers (76) from Cardiff became Secretary.

We had the conference dinner at Schveningen, the site of the first World Congress. I renewed my acquaintance with one of the greatest lady anaesthetists, Dorothy Ffoulkes Crabbe

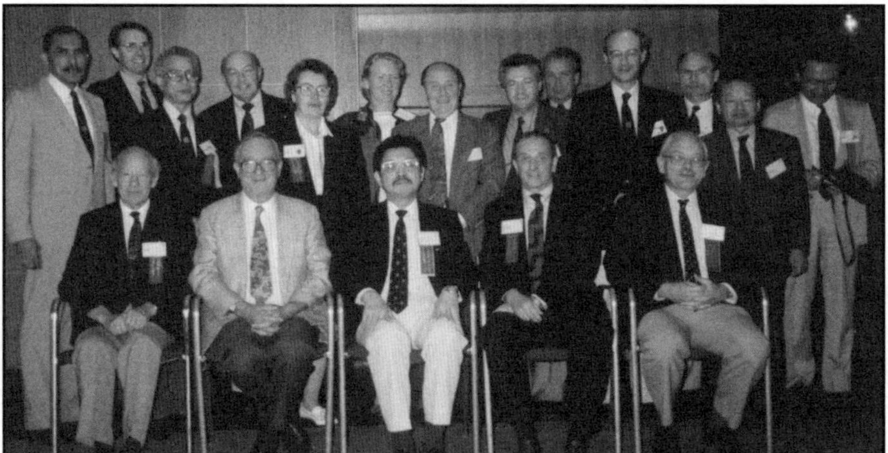

68. The new WFSA Executive Committee meeting in the Hague, Netherlands, 1992. *Standing*: M.Silao (Philippines), John Moyers (USA), Anis Baraka (Lebanon), Jack Moyers (USA), Elena Damir (Russia), Anneke Meursing (Netherlands), L. Blancato (Chair of Finance, USA), M. Marx (Uruguay), Gottfried Benad (Chair of Statutes, Germany), Patricio Kelly (Argentina), Harald Breivik (Norway), Mitsugo Fujimori (Chair of Education, Japan), Kenjiro Mori (Japan). *Sitting*: M.Rosen (Treasurer, UK), M.Vickers (Secretary, UK), Lim Say Wan (President, Malaysia) B.Wetchler (Chairman of Executive, USA), Kester Brown (Deputy Chairman).

(72,73) from Nigeria. I had known her since 1970 but she surprised me when I introduced her to anaesthetists from Finland and Beijing to find that she could greet them both in their own language. It turned out that she had been a medical student in London at the time when there were Turkish women refugees from Cyprus who couldn't communicate with the English nurses looking after them when they were having babies. Dorothy then decided that it would be useful to learn a few words and greetings in as many languages as possible so that she could communicate with patients wherever they came from. I have only caught her out once since. She is an amazing woman, a great orator and she became the first chair of the African Regional section of WFSA.

The biggest problem in the Hague was a lack of enough accommodation nearby. Otherwise it was an enjoyable congress. At the closing ceremony, the Australians had to invite everybody to the next Congress to be held in Sydney. I was asked to appear in a koala suit as I had worn one at previous meetings in Brisbane. I don't think that anyone suspected that one of the Executive Committee would be inside it! (70)

In 1994 the Executive met at the Asian Australasian Congress in Bangkok. It was here that Ruth Hutchison (69) made her first approach for financial assistance to organise a congress in Africa. Her request was more than the Federation could afford but she went ahead and organised it anyway — a wonderful effort. She has been one of the incredible women who have gone on working in Africa against the odds when there has been little equipment and few drugs. Another was Patricia Coyle (65) from Sydney, who worked alone as the anaesthetist at Makerere University in Kampala through an almost impossible period in Uganda. Despite everything she managed to train two Ugandans.

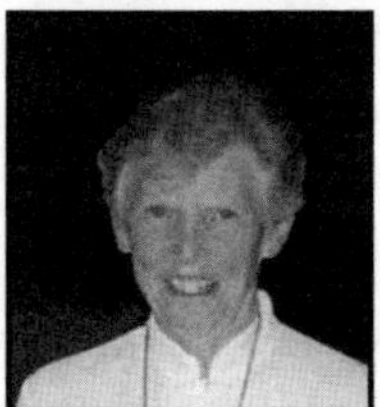

69. Ruth Hutchison (Zimbabwe)

Another memory from the AARS Board meeting in Bangkok was the chairman's brilliant speech in which he proposed dropping Australasian from the regions title. The Australians and New Zealanders were not in favour. I thought we had persuaded him not to make the proposal and when he did, it was difficult to know how best to counter it. I went back to the lesson I had learnt form my Nigerian friend, Bucknor, at university. I praised Manuel Silao's oratory and the content of his speech but said that it was not yet the appropriate time. He withdrew without argument. Later, at the big social event, we had a ride on an elephant together (cover) to show that there was no ill feeling.

The Thais manage to put on the most exotic shows at their final parties. At this one everybody had lit candles in holders which they placed on the lake. Then they had a fireworks display as a backdrop to the beautiful scene. At another meeting they had a parade of anaesthetic staff dressed in a very colourful collection of hill tribe costumes.

Preparations for the 1996 World Congress in Sydney began in 1990, six years before the event. I will discuss later the organisation of the scientific program for which I was responsible. The Congress was a great success with participants from over a hundred countries and speakers from about seventy. It was held at Darling Harbour looking out over the water of the famous Sydney Harbour. During the opening ceremony, attended by the Governor General, Sir William Deane, James Morrison, a well known Australian trumpeter appeared from the roof playing his trumpet while he was lowered to the stage. He then played a duet with someone playing the digeridoo. This was followed by a TV hook up with the Ether Dome in Boston, because we were celebrating the 150th anniversary of Morton's first successful public demonstration of ether anaesthesia there. The theme of the meeting was "Coming together — 150 years on". There was an evening at the Opera House with a choice of attractions. The final party was at the old Passenger terminal. The congress was successful in all ways and people around the world were still speaking about it years afterwards. Being involved with a congenial committee was a most enjoyable experience.

Michael Vickers from Cardiff became the President the Federation having previously been Chair of the Executive Committee and Secretary of the Federation following several years on other committees. He had a vast and valuable experience of the affairs of the WFSA. I became Chairman of the

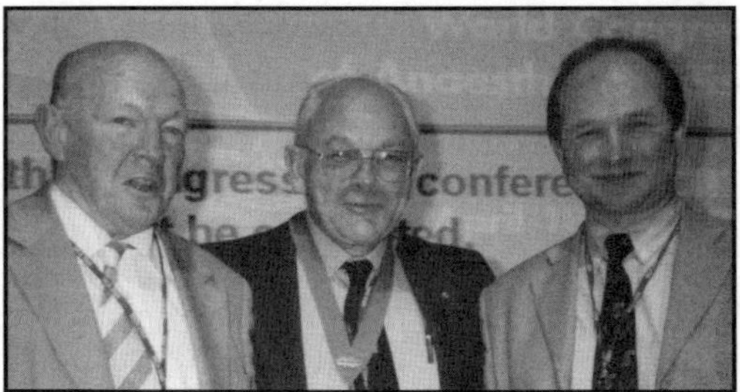

71. From left: Roger Eltringham, Kester Brown and Iain Wilson at the World Congress in Paris, 2004.

Executive and Anneke Meursing became secretary.

Roger Eltringham took over the Chair of what had been an ineffective Publications committee and made it into one of our most active ones. It became a significant extension of our educational activities. In collaboration with World Anaesthesia, a philanthropic group of anaesthetists based in UK, they produced a magazine called "Update in Anaesthesia", edited by Iain Wilson in Exeter (71). Iain had worked in Zambia for two years, so had practical experience of African conditions. It has been a very useful publication aimed to provide basic, practical information on anaesthesia for people who did not have ready access to books and journals. The Committee has also provided books for needy departments and has created a twinning arrangement for people to send their journals to needy recipients. It is all worthwhile work.

Michael Rosen (73) was treasurer. He proposed forming a WFSA Foundation to raise funds for some of our educational activities. He has an amazing aptitude for this and has successfully established the Foundation *to which people or organizations can contribute* towards these worldwide anaesthesia educational programmes. His first success was raising enough to support ten Eastern Europeans to visit pain centres in the West. He had already been President of the Association of Anaesthetists and the Royal College of Anaesthetists in London. He was awarded the CBE and an LLD from Dundee University, which was part of St Andrews University when we were students. By an amazing coincidence Michael Rosen, Roger Eltringham and I were all graduates of St Andrews University. It is also interesting that the first surgical anaesthetic in Britain involved another St. Andrews graduate — William Fraser, who brought the news form Boston to Dumfries in December 1846. Two more members of the WFSA Executive Committee, Mohamed Said Takrouri (77), now chairman, and Peter Kempthorne (62) did their anaesthetic training in Dundee and some years ago we also had the chairman of the Obstetrics committee, Trevor Thomas (1992-6).

Because I was originally from Kenya, I was also asked to convene a meeting of African delegates at the World Congress in Sydney to discuss setting up an African Regional Section of WFSA. This proved to be an interesting exercise. We met , discussed and eventually, having ascertained that this was to be for the common good of all countries, I arranged to meet one member from each country present two days later. When we met we elected a chairperson. After the first round there were two equal front runners — Dorothy Ffoulkes Crabbe (72) and Hannes Loots (72) from South Africa who were equal. When I called for the second round of voting Hannes Loots said he would stand aside so that Dorothy, who is Ghanian, could take the chair. I felt that this was a good omen for Africa.

The following year, at the African Congress, which had been organised by Ruth Hutchison (69) in Harare, Zimbabwe, Anneke Meursing and I helped the Africans who had drawn up their constitution to finalise it. It was accepted and the first Board was elected. Another gesture of good will occurred. There was a preponderence of South and East Africans. The French speaking West African candidate had not been successful in the election. There were three whites. One of them, Laurie Marks from Zimbabwe offered to stand aside and make way for French speaking Martin Chobli from Benin to take his place on the Board. Dorothy immediately said there was nothing in the constitution to deal with such a situation! I said " Just accept this generous offer and don't worry about the constitution." I am a great believer in practical resolutions. This provided a better balance. How rare it is for this to happen, especially for prestigeous positions in an international organisation. It is another example of the goodwill that exists among anaesthesiologists.

The Officers met in Harare in 1997 and took part in the establishment of the African Region.

In 1998, the Executive met near Frankfurt where the European Congress was held. I had thought that we would have a more effective meeting if the Committee met in a small place where we would all be together and have the opportunity to socialize as well as meet. I was in Europe the year before and visited Gunter Hempelman, who was organising the Congress and was a member of the Executive. We looked at a couple of venues and chose a small hotel in the beautiful village of *Braunfels*. A short walk up the street took us to the 16th century square and beyond that the castle perched on top of the hill surround-

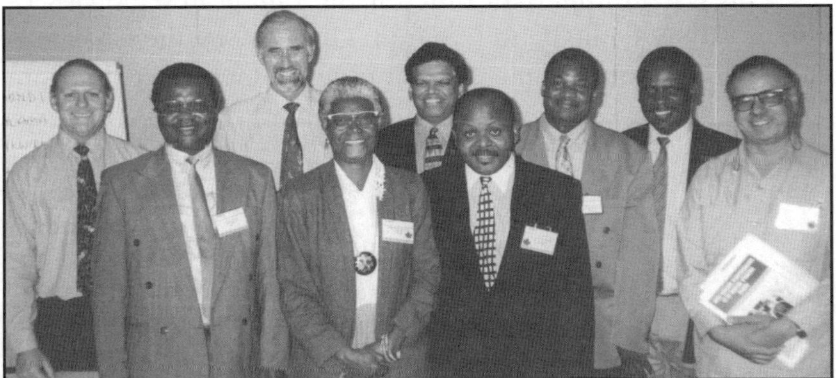

72. The first African Regional Board, Harare 1997: H.Loots (South Africa), C. Omondi (Kenya), David Morrell (South Africa), Dorothy Ffoulkes Crabbe (Nigeria, Chair),Vinod Nundloll (Mauritius),Victor Mwafongo (Tanzania), Martin Chobli (Benin), Henry Bukwirwa (Uganda), Ali Salama (Sudan).

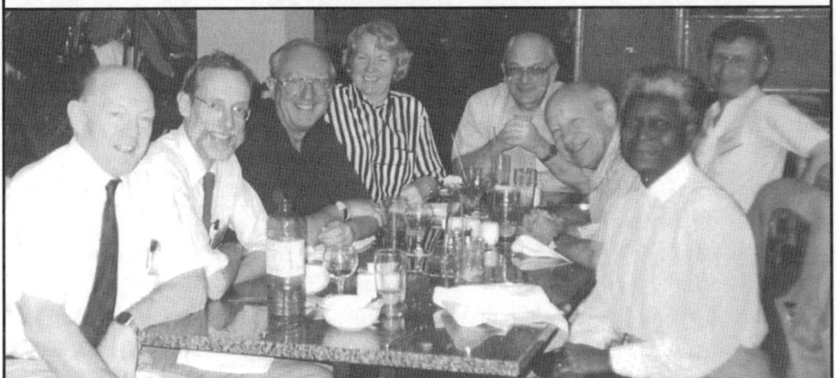

73. WFSA in Harare 1997. Roger Eltringham (UK, Chairman — Publications), Haydn Perndt (Australia, Chairman — Education), Michael Vickers (UK., President), Anneke Meursing (Netherlands, Secretary), Kester Brown (Chairman of Executive), Michael Rosen (Treasurer), Dorothy Ffoulkes-Crabbe (Nigeria, Chair ARS), Bill Casey (UK , Education Committee).

ed by beautiful gardens. It was an ideal setting for what was the best and most enjoyable executive meeting that I have attended (74). Everyone got to know each other and the discussion was much freer. It was also much less expensive than Frankfurt.

The European Congress was held in conjunction with the German Society Meeting in Frankfurt in 1998. Honorary Membership was conferred on me and several others, at the opening ceremony.

This was an important time for the European regional section of WFSA. Leslie Baird (75) from Glasgow was the Chairman had worked through some difficult times and resurrected it from

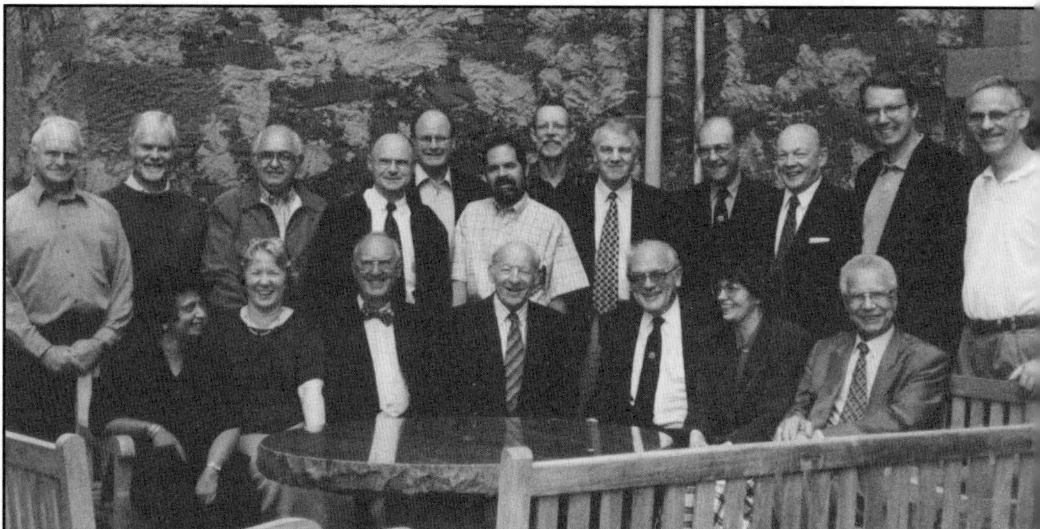

74. WFSA Executive committee at Braunfels, 1998. Committee Chairmen as well as Executive Committee attended.
Standing from L: Bill Runciman (Adelaide, Australia – Chairman of Safety and Quality of Practice Committee), Tony Rocke (South Africa – Chairman , Obstetrics and Chair of the 2nd. All Africa Congress in Durban, 2001), Jose Nocite (Brazil), Harald Breivik (Norway), David Bevan (Canada, Deputy Chairman Executive and Scientific Convenor, Montreal WCA 2000), Manuel Galindo (Colombia – Chair, Statutes and Bylaws), Haydn Perndt (Australia – Chair, Education), Jean Marie Desmonts (France), Patricio Kelly (Argentina), Roger Eltringham (UK – Chair, Publications), John Moyers (USA), Charlie Coté (USA – Chair, Paediatrics). *Sitting* : Anneke Meursing (Netherlands – Secretary), Michael Vickers (UK – President), Michael Rosen (UK – Treasurer), Kester Brown (Australia – Chairman, Executive), Maria Janecsko (Hungary – Became Deputy Chairman, 2000 and Chair in 2003) Anis Baraka (Lebanon).

an inactive period. It adopted a new name that I dreamt up with Maria Janecsko — Confederation of European National Societies of Anaesthesiologists (CENSA). It was also a time when discussions were beginning to take place about bringing the various European anaesthetic groups together. — European Society of Anaesthesiologists (ESA), CENSA and the European Academy (which runs the European Diploma). My speeches to the CENSA assembly were applauded so I assume I had made some helpful comments as applause is not common at such meetings.

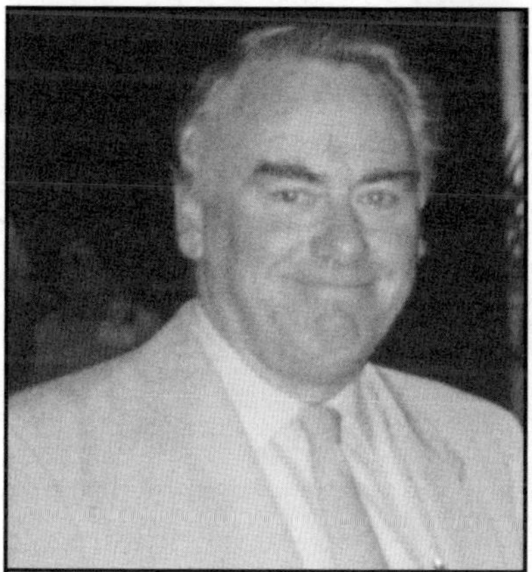

75. Leslie Baird — President of the Association of Anaesthetists of Great Britain and Ireland and Chair of CENSA.

ESA was relatively young and was managed from its Brussels headquarters. Its main aim seemed to be to run a professionally organized anaesthetic congress in Europe each year without any involvement of the local society in the country where it was held. It had gained the support of industry so that they could afford generous expenses for speakers more easily than meetings which did not have such industry support. While it would be good to have a unified organization in Europe it has not been easy to bring one together on an equitable basis. One has individuals as members, CENSA has national societies as members and the Academy organizes training and examinations across Europe. Their structures and financial situations are all different. Another problem is what happens to the countries which were part of the Soviet Union which are not strictly in Europe. At present the societies can be part of CENSA.

I have been involved in many discussions trying to smooth the way forward and I only hope that the end result is a harmonious organization which is controlled by the anaesthesiologists and works for the benefit of all Europe. The key to success is having trust between the groups.

Another important development at Frankfurt was the estab-

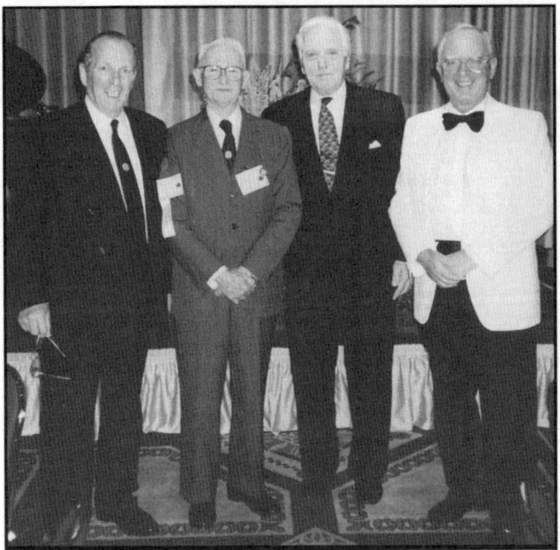

76. Four Presidents of WFSA in Frankfurt, 1998. *From left*: John Zorab (1988-92, UK), Carlos Parsloe (1984-8, Brazil), Ted Mayerhofer (1972-6, Austria), Michael Vickers (1996-2000, UK).

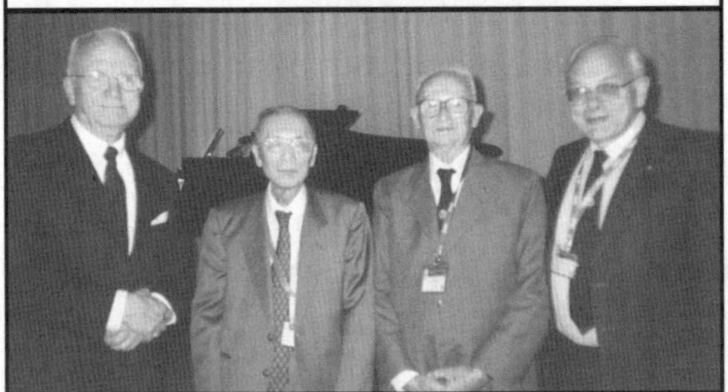

77. J. Gravenstein (USA), Hideo Yamamura (Japan), Carlos Parsloe (Brazil), Kester Brown (Australia) have a combined involvement in anaesthesia of 200 years. Taken at the Japanese Society Congress in 2003.

lishment of the International Patient Safety Foundation. I was involved with the discussions because I thought it would be sensible to have it affiliated with WFSA but in the end we did not pursue it because there were many people who were not anaesthesiologists who were involved and we did not have the funds to support it. J Gravenstein (77) from Florida, USA, a wonderful man, was on our Safety Committee. He was one of the prime movers in setting up the international organization with which the WFSA have good relationships.

The World Congress in 2000 took place in Montreal. It had a good programme, interesting events and the opportunity to meet colleagues from all over the world. Angela Enright was the chair of the Organizing Committee and she and others travelled extensively promoting the Congress. I was elected President of the WFSA.

The Canadians introduced a scholarship programme that

funded some young anaesthetists, who had leadership potential, from less affluent countries. It was a good innovation and provided great experience for those selected.

At the end of the Congress I had dinner with some of my friends from around he world. (Figure C22) The next day I joined the Paediatric anaesthetists tour. We went by bus to Quebec, train to Moncton, and then bus around Prince Edward Island and Nova Scotia to Halifax where we attended the fifth World Paediatric Anaesthetic meeting.

We planned to increase the number of Executive meetings

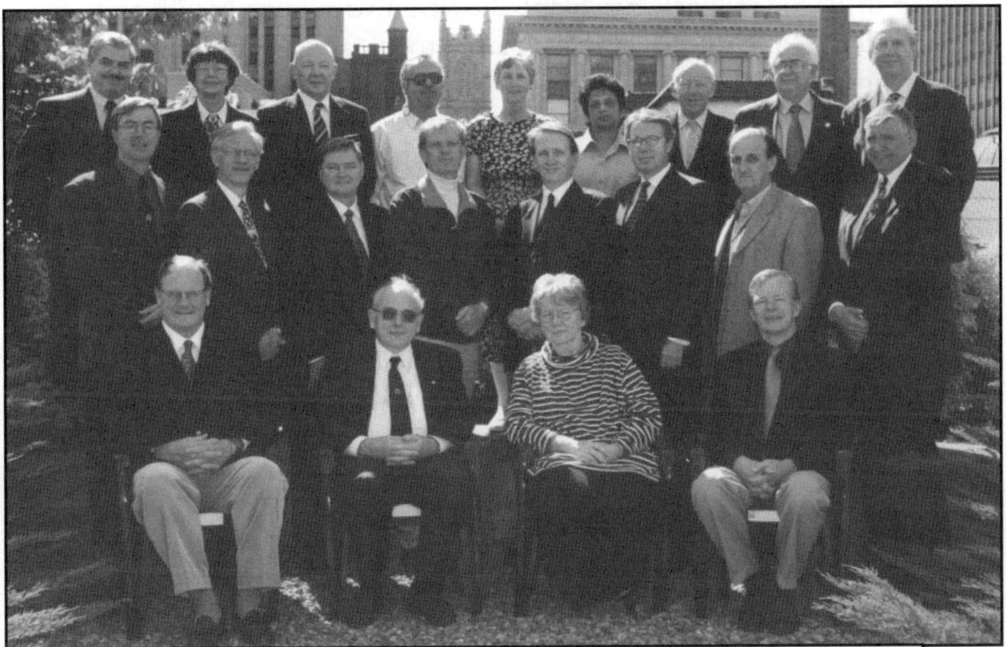

78. The WFSA Executive Committee 2000-4.
Back row: M.S.M.Takrouri (Saudi Arabia/Syria), Maria Janecsko (Hungary), Roger Eltringham (UK), Ali Salama (Sudan), Angela Enright (Canada), Deepthi Attygalle (Sri Lanka), Michael Rosen (UK), José Nocite (Brazil), Philippe Scherpereel (France).
Middle row: Peter Kempthorne (New Zealand), Charlie Coté (USA), Jerry Fontenot (USA), Gunter Hempelmann (Germany), Per Rosenberg (Finland), John Moyers (USA), Gonzalo Barreiro (Uruguay), David Wilkinson (UK). *Sitting*: Daivid Bevan (Canada — Chairman), Kester Brown (Australia — President), Anneke Meursing (Netherlands — Secretary), Richard Walsh (Australia — Treasurer).

between World Congresses and so met at the All African Congress in Durban the following year (2001). It was held two weeks after September 11th which made it difficult for two members to get there while another was to travel on a plane which was grounded for mechanical reasons. Again we went out of the city for the meeting to save on costs and to use the opportunity to get to know each other better.

At the opening ceremony I spoke on "Terrorism as a point of view" because the terrorist acts often emanate from a very deep seated grudge created by past treatment. It depends where you are- in the twin towers when the plane crashed into them or in Baghdad when it is being showered with huge bombs and rockets. Both were terrifying places to be and many innocent people died. The story told at my brother in law's funeral seemed relevant. He had been a District Officer during the Maumau uprising in Kenya. Some of the Maumau actions were definitely terrorist such as the family where the husband and then the son were killed in front of the mother who then had her abdomen slit open to expose her unborn child and left to die. The other point of view was that they were freedom fighters. So after independence in Kenya the gang leaders were immortalised by having streets in Nairobi named after them. Of course, there have always been people who have wanted to dominate the world using violent means such as war.

Years later my brother in law was at a parade where "General China", a gang leader he had hunted, took the salute. Afterwards he was introduced and was surprised when the old gang leader said "I know who you are. You were so close to me in the forest once I could have touched you. My men wanted to kill you but I would not allow them to." A compassionate terrorist or did he appreciate Bob's humanity?

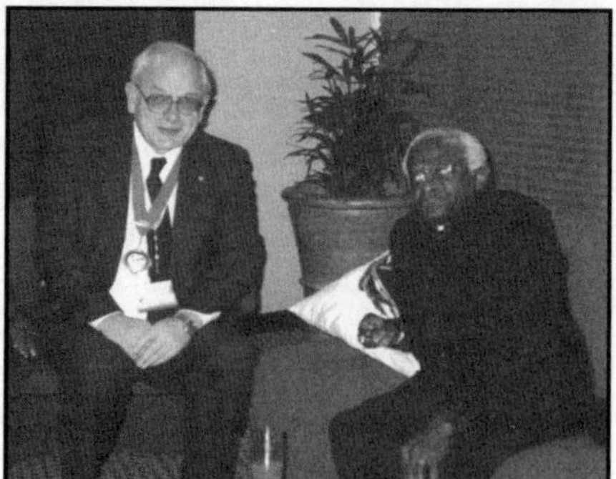

79. Conversing with Bishop Desmond Tutu before the Opening Ceremony in Durban, 2001.

Bishop Desmond Tutu (79) spoke at the Opening

Ceremony. I had the good fortune to meet this wonderful, cheerful man. It was understandable while he had such an influence in South Africa.

At the conference dinner I had a very representative group, as usual, at our table. I always believed at mixing different nationalities up at these functions so that they get to know other people. Kesete was evicted from Ethiopia where he ran the nurse anaesthetists training school, because he was born in Eritrea (at the time it was part of Ethiopia). He took one child but had to leave his other two with his wife. They were reunited about a year later. He now runs a nurse training school in Eritrea.

Farai has since had to leave Zimbabwe although at the time he was very actively involved in a distant learning project for those giving anaesthetics in Zimbabwe. This was an initiative of Michael Dobson in Oxford who has also been the WFSA liaison person with WHO. An Englishman who was helping with the technical computer side of the project was selected as an internationl observer for the much publicised elections. Two days before, he was jailed with many others. Fortunately he was released after payment of a small fine but it could have been much worse. I was Chairman of the Executive at the time and

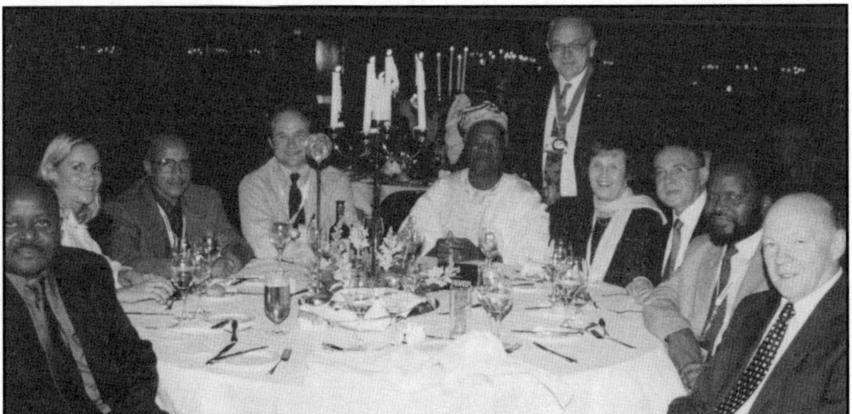

80. Conference dinner, All Africa Congress, Durban 2001.
From left: Victor Mwafongo (Tanzania), Iréna Dupire (Paris – Conference Organizing company), Kesete Teweldebrhan (Eritrea), Iain Wilson (UK – Editor, *Update in Anaesthesia*), Sam Upwonman (Nigeria), Kester Brown (standing), Yehia Khater (Egypt), Farai Madzimbamatu (Zimbabwe), Roger Eltringham (UK).

tried to keep in touch with the people there.

Sam Upwonman, who I had met in Nigeria when I went to teach there in 1989had been a great help getting me past a customs man who was trying to make me pay to have my passport stamped. Victor had worked with me but found it difficult returning to the poverty that existed in Tanzania at the time. Life is not easy in Africa. He has done well there.

In 2002 I attended the CENSA European Congress held in Florence. It was a great finale for Professor G.P.Novelli (81), who chaired the organizing committee, as he died less than two months later. He was a wonderful man and he knew he did not have long to live but made the most of the occasion. He even came to a special unplanned session that I ran for the trainees in Florence. I was a little concerned as I walked up the street to the conference as I developed a dysrhythmia (which I developed from time to time). I survived and apparently the trainees appreciated the session.

David Bevan, chairman of the Executive Committee, made it clear to us in Durban that the economic downturn in 2001 was going to threaten our financial stability unless we severely curtailed our proposed budget. We had set up an office jointly with the European Academy of Anaesthesia in 1994 but we had moved to a separate office in Kingsway in 1996 after the finan-

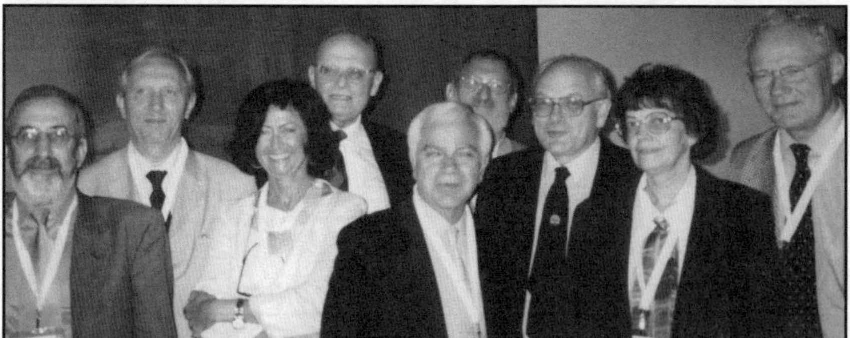

81. At European Congress in Florence, 2002. *From left*: A.Gullo (Trieste), Philippe Scherpereel (France – COC 13th World Congress, Paris 2004), [unknown] , Prof Novella (Florence – COC, European Congress 2002), R.Tufano (Italy – vice president, Italian Society), Gabriel Gurman (Israel –WFSA Education), Kester Brown, Maria Janecsko (Hungary – Deputy Chair WFSA Executive), Dietrich Kettler (Germany – President CENSA).

cially successful Congress in Sydney. At that time it seemed that the Federation had become big enough and had many newly developed activities to justify having a permanent office. With the declining economy we had to down size twice to reduce costs. We now have a good arrangement with the Association of Anaesthetists (AAGBI) at 21 Portland Place in central London (WC2B). Eventually, we decided that the executive committee should not meet in Glasgow in 2003 as proposed, in order to cut costs. The membership subscription had not been changed for twenty years. Maybe this was due to the fact that many thought the Federation did not do much for the Societies and they made enough from the World Congresses to support their programs. That all changed in the 1990s with the expansion of the educational activities.

The Officers met in Melbourne in 2001 (Figure C23). We met at the ANZ College of Anaesthetists, where we were guests of the College Executive Committee one day, and at my home on the other. In 2002 we met in at the AARS meeting in Kuala Lumpur where we also had the opportunity to meet several committee members (82). There was much of the discussion was around finances. David Bevan resigned in 2003 as he had too

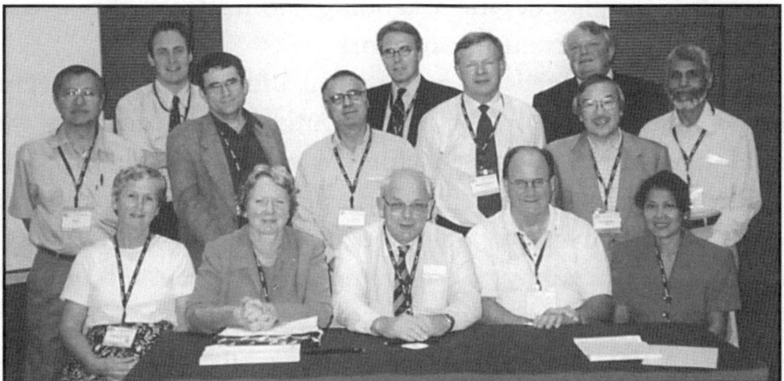

82. Officers meeting with WFSA committees members at Kuala Lumpur during the AARS Congress, 2002.
Standing: Thara Tritrakarn (Thailand, Education), Rob McDougall (Australia, Education), Alan Merry (New Zealand, Chair, Safety and Quality of Practice), Ali Salama (Sudan, Executive and Chair African Region), John Moyers (Assistant Secretary), Richard Walsh (Treasurer), John Richards (Australia, Statutes), Kazuo Hanaoka (Japan, Executive), Dilip Pawar (India – Chair, Pain).

many commitments when he became professor in Toronto. Maria Janecsko took over. Our meeting in 2003, (Figure C20) again in Melbourne, at the time of the Australian Society's National Congress where the officers were guests, was much more creative and hopefully some of the ideas generated will lead to a more effective organisation. In the end only some of our proposals were agreed to by the Executive Committee at the World Congress but at least the ideas were aired.

At the World Congress in Paris in April 2004 it was agreed to have a seven person Executive Management Group which would be authorised to run the day to day business rather than relying only on the officers. This would mean that fewer expensive Executive Committee meetings would be needed. The President would chair this group, giving the position a more active leadership role.

The Federation had two types of committee. Standing committees were Education, Publications, Finance and Statutes and Bylaws. The chairs attended the executive committees. Now the latter two will be chaired by members of the Executive Management Group. During the Congress I managed to persuade them that the now active Safety and Quality of Practice Committee should become a standing committee as this area has become very important in our work.

Special committees covered special and specialty areas. They seemed to take as long for the executive to construct as they would have time to meet before leaving the congress. They wouldn't meet until the next congress so, apart from a few individuals being active, they achieved dissappointingly little. These have been replaced by a co-ordinator who can set up small working parties of people who are willing and known to do the necessary work, to deal with specific tasks. They can also arrange for representatives from regional organisations in their special area to meet at the World Congresses.

Many good things have been done by the Federation. Haydn Perndt, a very hard working Chair of the Education Committee (1996-2000) promoted the development of training centres which have been established to give basic training in areas where the anaesthetic manpower is inadequate or negligible. One was

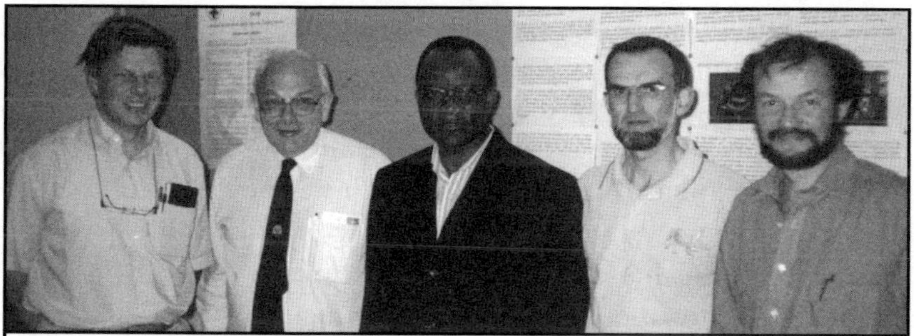

83. Philippe Baele, Kester Brown, a professor visiting from the Congo who had suffered significant hardship, Francis Veyckemans (WFSA Education Committee since 2002), Bernard le Polain from Louvaine University who support the Benin Training Centre.

established by Thara Tritrakarn (80) and his colleagues in Bangkok to train people from Laos, Cambodia, Vietnam, Myanmar and, recently, Mongolia. Nearly thirty people have been through this program. Thara has been a member of the WFSA Education Committee. I have stopped over there on several occasions to teach the students about teaching and organising training programs.

There are others in Ghana and Tanzania (with support from the American Society), Benin supported from Louvain University in Belgium (83), Senegal supported by the French and in the South Pacific supported by Australia and New Zealand. Gradually specialist training positions are being created as well. Charlie Cote (74) helped to establish one in Santiago, Chile for paediatrics which has taken people from Ecuador, Bolivia, Peru and Honduras. It is run by Sylvana Cavallieri.

Angela Enright, who chaired the organising Committee of the Montreal World Congress, took over from Haydn Perndt and has further developed the education programs so now many societies are reaping benefits from the Federation's activities.

In Uganda, Henry Bukwirwa (72) set up an Equipment Maintenance program when all those giving anaesthetics brought their equipment to a course where they were taught how to repair and maintain it. Ian Revell from the Penlon company has been an invaluable contributor to these courses. It is a good example of a company, which makes appropriate equipment for the less affluent world, following up with practical training in maintenance.

We produced an Appropriate Donations Document to help donors of equipment to match the needs of the recipients better because there are many places where inappropriate equipment has been given. There are store rooms around the less affluent world with expensive equipment which has never been used. It may need electricity where the supply is erratic, or gases where these are unavailable or parts which cannot be afforded in poor countries, or no one goes to show the recipient how to use it. Sometimes the instructions are not in the language of the recipients. It is such a waste. Our aim was to encourage donors to find out what is really needed. Our Document works through stages of development and sophistication of equipment used so that recipients can work through it level by level with the help of appropriate donations.

We also produced a document on space for anaesthetic departments. This followed a visit to a brand new hospital where the anaesthetic department had a space less that 2x2 metres in the recovery area to work out theatre allocations. How can anaesthetists develop teaching programmes or even an academic interest in the department if they have no space. They need office space, library, teaching and meeting areas and more if they are going to contribute more to the hospital than a few anaesthetics.

I have travelled extensively in the course of my work with the WFSA, giving lectures and teaching. I have been lucky because many of us in Australia are entitled to long service leave after 10 or 15 years service. This I have taken in segments and it has given me time to travel. I have found that when one goes to teach, the people want to look after you and show you round so that there is a mutual benefit. I have now lectured and taught in 66 countries. For example, in Bulgaria I participated in a FEAA course which revolves through all the topics every five years. It was a program started by Philippe Scherpereel in France and is now run in many countries. I was hosted by Ivan Smilov. I also met Gabriel Gurman from Israel there. He has made a huge contribution to Eastern Europe running a programme for ten years for anaesthetists to visit his department for periods of one to three months. This began as an expansion of the proposal of John

Zorab's to help the East Europeans in 1989 where each Eastern block country received one scholarship for someone to visit a Western department for a month. The Israelis offered to supplement this and take three from Romania each year. About a hundred anaesthetists from several Eastern block countries have benefited from it.

It has been a great privilege to be able to visit so many places. I have even taught and met the anaesthetists when passing by, in out of the way places like Punta Arenas (Chile), Ushuaia, Rio Grande and Rio Gallegos (Argentina) in the south of South America, and Arica in northern Chile where I visited with Carlos Riquelme on our way to Parque Lauca. The three anaesthetists there had never had anybody visit before. Sometimes such visits seem more fulfilling than ones to large centres where relatively few people turn up. All these visits have been a source of great pleasure. There are wonderful people all over the world and we as anaesthetists have an advantage of usually getting on with our colleagues wherever they come from.

In April 2004 the World Congress in Paris concluded my long and interesting association with the WFSA and its committees. It was an amazing occasion. On the social side we had an evening at the Louvre and another where we had a reception at the Hôtel de Ville (City Hall) followed by an organ recital at Notre Dame Cathedral. At the reception I was presented with a medal from the City of Paris by the Deputy Mayor. It was an unexpected honour as President of the Federation to receive this.

At the opening ceremony we were entertained by the Hospitals' Orchestra and a ballet group who put on a very imaginative performance. I gave a short summary of the WFSA activities and as dozens, maybe hundreds, of people came to thank me afterwards for the talk and express their appreciation I will include it here even though there will be some repetition of what I have already written.

Presidential address: Opening Ceremony — World Congress, Paris.

"Bienvenue á Paris en printemps. It is wonderful to have you all here where the seed was sown for the foundation of the

Federation in 1951. Four years later, in 1955, the WFSA came into existence at the First World Congress in the Netherlands. The details of the history are told in a book to be launched at this Congress.

The aims were to bring anaesthesiologists together every four years at the World Congresses and to improve the standards of anaesthesia all over the world. Certainly, anaesthesia has grown into a major medical specialty in that time and spawned off-spring in Intensive Care and Pain Management. There were 26 societies then, now 112.

That the standards have improved relates to better training. A major move forward was made by the production of obstetric and resuscitation manuals edited by John Bonica and Peter Safar respectively, and later paediatrics by Anneke Meursing, and the lecture series edited by John Zorab in the mid 80s. A memorial meeting to John Bonica, who did so much in the fields of regional analgesia and pain relief, will be held in Sicily this year.

The Federation really began to mean something to many Societies when it became proactive in running courses and sending teachers worldwide. Between 1988 and 1992 fifty countries were visited by teachers from 25 countries, a real international effort. Roger Eltringham and Philippe Scherpereel helped to make this happen. Successive chairs of Education, Mitsugu Fujimori, Haydn Perndt and Angela Enright have maintained this activity and added training centres in areas of need. They and many others have done wonderful work, sometimes in difficult circumstances.

In 1990, when I handed a copy of the proceedings of the European Congress in Warsaw to a Russian friend in Moscow, he said "This is like giving me diamonds". Literature and access to information is so important in learning and keeping up to date. The Publications Committee, under the chairmanship of Roger Eltringham, has achieved great things. We combined with a philanthropic group of anaesthetists, World Anaesthesia to produce and distribute *Update in Anesthesia* edited by Iain Wilson (71). It reaches hundreds of anaesthetists in less accessible areas, is now published in English, Spanish, French, Mandarin and Russian and is available on the internet where it has been accessed from over

140 countries. Dedicated people translate it so it can reach people in their regions. Roger Eltingham has also established a donor- recipient pairing arrangement for old journals.

What of the period of my presidency. It has not been easy because of the economic downturn from which we only now seem to be slowly emerging. Our investments have had poor returns. With the encouragement of our former chairman, David Bevan, we have cut back many expenditures but we have tried to maintain our education and publication activities as we regard these as so important.

There have been some exciting positive things happening. Henry Bukwirwa in Uganda initiated some equipment maintenance workshops with help from Penlon which have now been run in some neighbouring countries. You cannot give anesthesia if your equipment doesn't work. I remember when the Soloman Islands only had one functional operating facility because the Fluotecs had jammed in the other five. A competent technician from New Zealand, Laurie Dyball, fixed them quickly.

Primary trauma courses have been run in many countries. These were stimulated by Haydn Perndt and Michael Dobson who saw a need for simple courses in less affluent countries. Douglas Wilkinson in Oxford, Markus Skinner, Stephen Swallow and Rob McDougall (80) in Australia produced manuals and teaching kits and went out and taught them. The sale of paintings at a silent auction when I retired enabled us to pay for two Indonesians to come to Melbourne for a PTC trainers course. The following year a team went and ran some courses and trained some trainers there. In three years since then Eddy Rehardjo form Surubaya had revamped the manual to suit Indonesia, run 28 courses and trained about 850 people — a magnificent effort. This process aims to make the people able to run their own courses after initial instruction, which is so much better than continual spoon feeding.

Dilip Pawar (76), chair of the Pain committee, has set up a similar course on acute pain management it has been run in three South East Asian countries so far.

Alan Merry (76) and his Patient Safety and Quality of Practice committee, helped by Gonzalo Barreiro from Uruguay and

Florian Nuevo from the Philippines, are having a session at the World Congress to map out the future course for this committee.

These are exciting developments making a real contributions to improving standards.

Our documents, on appropriate donations which is aimed to make donations what the recipient needs rather than extravagant donations which cannot be used, and on appropriate space for anaesthesia departments, are two that I draw your attention to because they may be of significant help to you.

As your President I have visited 30 countries and all continents, spoken at meetings, done workshops and visited hospitals. I have stressed teaching and training, and understanding anatomy in relation to nerve blocks, both important and practical topics. I have learnt from those whom I have visited and I think helped to push anaesthesia forwards in some places.

Finally, I would like to say again what I said in Montreal when I became President. Make a friend at this Congress whose circumstances are different from yours. Those from affluent countries meet someone from a less affluent one and find out if you can help them. Maybe you have books, journals, computers or equipment which is still serviceable which would help them. You could visit them or invite and arrange for them to visit your department. You will be amazed at the possible consequences. It may give you something new in your life. Just go up and talk to someone, or talk to them on a bus or outing you may go on, but talk for long enough to find out about each other.

I would like to tell about an occasion in India when a young trainee approached me when I was there and asked if he could ask me a question. I said "Yes." " If you were to give me one piece of advice what would it be," I was speechless for a minute because I had never contemplated that question before. After some thought I said,

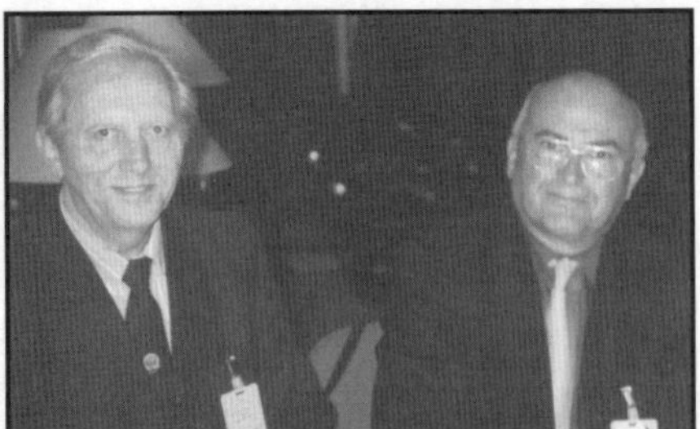

84. Philippe Scherpereel (chairman, Organizing committee 13th World Congress in Paris, April 2004) and Michel Pinaud (President, French society — SFAR) 2002.

"Don't forget to thank those who help you, no matter what their station is in life. It may make their day." Afterwards I thought that maybe it was a factor in making the work environment in our operating theatres more pleasant."

I then thanked the chairman of the Organizing Committee, Philippe Scherpereel (84), and presented him with a copy of the history of the "First Fifty Years of the WFSA" edited by A.Gullo and the WFSA archivist, Joseph Ruprecht (85). I then thanked the orchestra and dancers and finally Carolina, who showed us up to the stage, as a representative of all those who were helping in many ways around the congress.

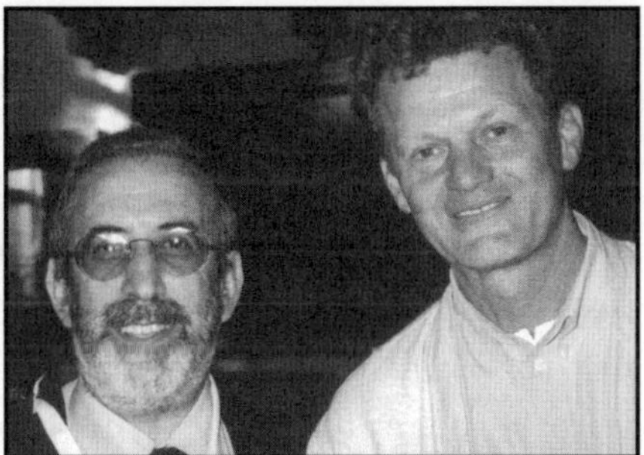

85. Antonino Gullo and Joseph Ruprecht, editors of World Federation of Societies of Anaesthesiologists — 50 years.

We had been through some difficult times financially during the previous four years because the American investments were not producing the necessary income. Our subscription had been $1.25 per society member for twenty years. At the General Assembly the treasurer, Richard Walsh (80, Figure C23) proposed an increase $2 and then after two years to $2.50. There was much negative debate. Could another formula be found which would be easier on less affluent countries, for example, basing it on GDP. After some time I suggested that the finance committee would look at other options but may not have time to come to a conclusion before we met again in two days. GDP did not help. At the next General Assembly I invited the treasurer to report and put his motion. While he was coming up to the podium I asked the delegates how many cups of coffee they could buy in their country for $2. One, two ,three and up to seven. Then I told them that that was the amount we were talking about. We expected a tight vote. In the event only two voted against the motion.

I have been involved in discussions which have required some diplomacy — among them the Peoples Republic of China and Taiwan, Cuba and a group in USA who were prohibited from having a planned joint meeting in Cuba by a presidential edict, and the process to unify the European organizations. These have been challenging and worthwhile especially if one can bring some sensitivity, hope and understanding to the discussions.

My Finale at the congress was to speak before handing over the presidential medallion of office to Anneke Meursing, who had been secretary for eight years. I talked about the Organ recital in Notre Dame, how there were people there from many religious backgrounds enjoying the immense performance there, how I had visited some of the most beautiful buildings belonging to many religions — the Mohamed Ali Mosque in Cairo with its beautiful domes; the Temple of the Emerald Buddha in Bangkok; the magnificent, marble Jain temples at Mt Abu and Ranakpur (86) in India. I hoped that coming together and meeting people of many nationalities and religions in a friendly atmosphere would help us contribute to a more peaceful world.

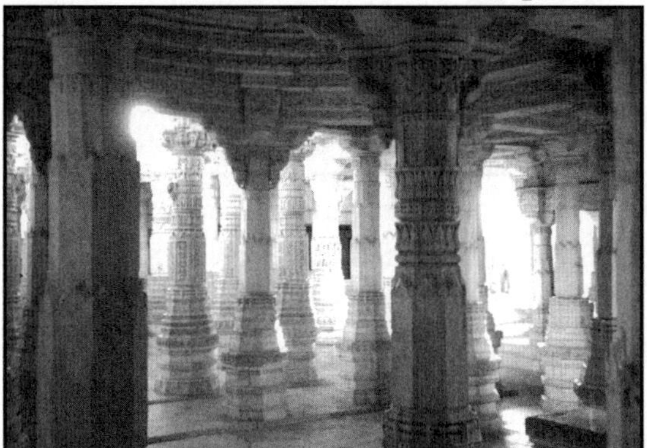

86. Interior of Jain Temple at Ranakpur. It was built in 1450-99 and has 1400 marble pillars in it.

I then thanked Janet, my wife, for all her help and support over the years that enabled me to do all that I had done. She received a generous applause which was well deserved. She received another when Anneke made a presentation to her, a very kind and thoughtful surprise.

There have been so many people with whom I have worked in the Federation and affiliated organizations who I have not been able to mention in the text but who have contributed in different ways, often giving freely of their time. I have recognised many, but by no means all of them by inclusion in the photographs selected, which were taken at various congresses.

Working for the WFSA was a wonderful experience, sometimes hard work and sometimes requiring very sensitive diplomacy. My aim has always been to help others, particularly those in less fortunate circumstances. I tried to enable others to achieve and do useful things, helping others. I think I managed to get good people into positions so that plenty of action occurred. I felt that I left the Federation with people who were keen to get on and help, so that the Federation's aims to improve the standard of anaesthesia around the world could be attained, and that the organization was more active and effective than when I joined it twenty years before. I think I have been a catalyst for many people to contribute and achieve.

Chapter 31

International Communication

When one is involved in an international organization, such as WFSA, understanding some of the differences in culture are interesting and important if one is going to communicate effectively and not cause offence.

Names can be a source of difficulty. In South America most countries are Spanish speaking. They put father's surname before the mother's but in Brazil and Portuguese speaking countries the mother's name precedes father's. Both are usually used. The problem arises when an English-speaking person who usually only uses the father's surname writes someone with a Spanish background. They often use the incorrect name. In Thailand the first name only is often used so an inquiry using the — usually long — second name may draw a blank. In Japan people are often called by their surname or an abbreviation or by a nickname or a shortened first name while in English-speaking countries the first name is often used. To an English speaker the use of the surname without a preceding title such as Mr. or Dr. is considered rather rude except in institutional situations such as schools or the armed forces!

In Iceland the father's first name followed by –son (male) or -dottir (female) is used as the surname. Genealogy is almost impossible in such a system. This system was also used more widely in Scandinavia in the past.

There are so many variations in the use of names it is sometimes better just to ask what people would like you to call them, having established what you are happy for them to call you.

The style of greeting is also variable. Japanese will usually offer you their card and bow as they present it. Others just offer a hand to shake. In some cultures, such as in the Middle East, a welcome hug is acceptable between men, especially between friends, while in others that would be regarded as strange behaviour. In some cultures, particularly in Asia, the Middle East and

Africa kissing a woman as a greeting is not usually acceptable while in South America and Latin countries it might be expected or at least accepted, usually on both cheeks. In some countries three kisses are given. Anglo Saxons are generally more inhibited.

Where do we stand for conversation? In some places people like to talk at close quarters (25-40 cm) whereas an Englishman likes to maintain his space (maybe 50-70cm). It is not surprising that someone who speaks at close quarters will offend the Englishman by invading his space. He will probably step back to regain his comfortable distance and in so doing offends the other person. What does one do to avoid offence?

Even the use of the head can cause confusion. Most people, particularly Europeans nod their head up and down when they indicate agreement. I understand that in Japan that means "we understand what you have said" but does not necessarily indicate agreement. This leads to much confusion in negotiations. In India a side to side roll of the head means agreement or yes but to most others cultures it means no.

And then the interpretation of words or expressions can make the difference between understanding and offence. 'Pulling your leg' is an expression used in Australia and some other countries to indicate that you are making some jovial fun of the other person. It is not meant to be taken as an offence. In Japan, on the contrary, it is translated literally and means that you are intentionally trying to de-stabilise the other person — a serious breach of etiquette!

Comments made in a lecture can be interpreted as criticism. For example, I said that because most people have a concentration span of about 20 minutes when listening to someone speaking it seemed that one hour lectures, especially several during a day, were not logical and we should have shorter ones. This was unfortunately looked on as criticism of the organization of the congress. Fortunately the organizers brought the matter up for discussion so that I could explain what I meant and that it applied all over the world. It would have been unfortunate if I had been considered critical without the opportunity of explanation.

Verbal communication needs the people to have a language that they both understand or else they need an interpreter. English is being used increasingly around the world so many people can at least understand some of it provided it is spoken *slowly*. Television is probably responsible for the increase in comprehension. People may not know a language well enough to be comfortable trying to speak it unless they know the other person has about the same aptitude in their language. There are things that a lecturer can do to help. Slow presentation is important for simultaneous translators to keep up, as well as the for the audience's direct comprehension. One can make slides in the audience's language — if you cannot read the script put both languages on the slide. Questions can be taken in the audience's language and someone can translate. This overcomes any shyness about speaking an unfamiliar tongue. It also lets the speaker better assess how much the audience understands of what is being said.

It is a gift to be able to speak a number of languages. People who live in areas where several languages are spoken are often multilingual, e.g.in Europe or India. There is no doubt that people appreciate your efforts if you speak even only a few words of their language. It helps to break the ice.

When serious negotiations are going on, it is better to keep the same negotiating team. It takes time for rapport, understanding and trust to develop. It is much easier to come to agreement with someone whom one trusts and knows than with a new negotiator each time. This is a good general principle but it is particularly important in eastern Asia.

Communication and trying to understand other people and their point of view is vital if we are going to reduce tensions in our troubled world. Many problems have arisen from failure to appreciate the other person's culture and use of words. We can make many friends if we succeed in communicating, even with a few words in their language.

Chapter 32

Congresses in Various Regions

I have attended National and Regional Congresses all over the world. The ones associated with WFSA have been mentioned in the previous chapter. There are several other regional groupings including the Pan Arab, ASEAN (Association of South East Asian Nations), SACA (South Asian Confederation of Anaesthesiologists, South American (includes only the South American countries), CLASA, which includes all Latin American countries in Central and South America, and Scandinavian. I will mention some of the events that occurred and people I met at some of the Congresses which I attended.

In 1990, at the Asian Australasian Congress in Seoul, I was asked to attend a meeting of a group from the South Asian countries (India, Pakistan, Bangladesh, Sri Lanka and Nepal) to help in their deliberations. They wanted to establish a regional organisation. After considerable discussion I was able to guide them — first, define their aims and objectives, set up a constitution and then, if they wanted to, allocate to one country to organize a Congress. This plan was agreed to and the next year they met again in India to make further plans. The South Asian Confederation of Anaesthetists (SACA) was formed and their first meeting was held in Dhaka in 1993. I have been treated as a sort of godfather to this organisation, and have been asked to help with constitutional and other problems at their Board meetings since. (87) It was a great privilege to be involved. It was wonderful to see the anaesthetists from countries with disparate politics getting together in this way. I attended the following meetings in Colombo and Karachi, but did not get to the Indian one in Chenai in 1999, and then back to Dhaka in 2003. Nepal could not hold their meeting so discussion arose whether the next one in 2005 should continue the rotation and go to Sri Lanka or let Nepal have a turn. I helped a reasonable and amicable solution to be reached, the compromise being that they would go to Sri Lanka next and then to Nepal.

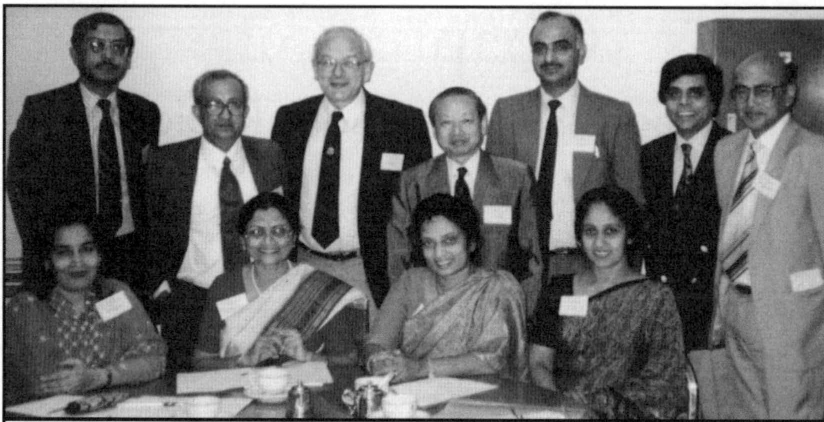

87. The first Board of the South Asian Confederation of Anaesthesiologists (SACA) in Dhaka, 1993.
Standing: Tipu Sultan (Pakistan), Sam Choudhury (Bangladesh), Kester Brown (as constitutional consultant!), M. Fujimori (WFSA), H Kaul (India), Battycharya (India), Tuladhar (Nepal).
Sitting: Roshana Kamal, (Pakistan), V Divekar (India), Deepthi Attygalle (Sri Lanka), Nalina Rodrigo (Sri Lanka).

I had some interesting experiences at the Pan Arab meeting in Tunis. My ear canal became blocked. This is a significant problem because one cannot assess how loudly one is speaking so I arranged to have it syringed out. The young Army anaesthetist, Souiden, kindly took me to a hospital. I asked him for advice about where to visit as we were staying an extra day after the congress. He said he would take me to his home town of Kiarouan which has a huge mosque and is the "Mecca" of north western Africa.. It was a fascinating trip. Imagine driving towards the desert and the land becoming more barren and bleak. Then suddenly a huge structure appears — what can it be? The colosseum at El Jem! It was the sixth biggest one built by the Romans, another sign of their empire spreading into north Africa. As we explored it Souiden told us that they sometimes had concerts there. When he took us home for a cup of tea after the trip he turned on the TV and there was a concert at El Jem. From there we went to Kiarouan. His home was a typical one built around a courtyard. The roof was flat and drained into the well from which they drew their water. His mother had prepared a specialty lunch — sheep's head chopped up in a stew. I carefully looked for mandible with some tongue and muscle attached. I did not feel up to eye or brain! His two boys were with us. Three years later I was looking at my photographs with my son Ken, who had been with me, and we talked about the boys. Two days later I had a letter from the older one telling me of his father's death. We subsequently corresponded from time to time. I was able to send them a nice photograph of their father taken framed by some Roman ruins at the old Roman town of Dougga where he had also taken us to visit. It was disappointing to see beautiful Roman mosaics there, unprotected.

The meeting was well run in French and English. I was impressed by Claude Ecoffey's presentations, because he spoke in French and had English slides. This was an interesting solution to a bilingual meeting. I have sometimes used slides in the audience's language, especially Spanish in South America, so that if there are translation problems the audience can at least get the essence of the lecture if I speak in English.

They held a practical session where several anaesthetists demonstrated practical anaesthesia in the operating theatres of one of the hospitals. The proceedings were televised back to the conference hall. It was a daunting experience. Public demonstrations in a strange environment often do not run smoothly as Horace Wells found out in 1844 when he tried to demonstrate nitrous oxide anaesthesia. I was asked to do a caudal anaesthetic. Occasionally the needle penetrates a blood vessel and blood comes back. One has to reposition the needle. It happened to me on that occasion! When asked to demonstrate in unfamiliar places I usually ask the local anaesthetist to give the anaesthetic and then guide them through some new technique which I may be showing them, having usually done a drawing of the procedure first.

I was invited to the next congress which was to have been in Bagdhad but the first Gulf war intervened.

I attended a South American Congress at Viña del Mar in Chile. We had a most impressive simultaneous translator, Sara Montecinos. She translated for hours from English to Spanish on her own. She is an anaesthetist in Santiago and a former international runner. I struck on the idea of taping her translation so that I would have a Spanish tape to go with my slides, also in Spanish, if I needed an extra talk or found I did not have a translator. I used one of these subsequently. It was only a matter of her turning on the tape recorder as she began, which she graciously agreed to do.

At that congress there were two Bolivians who were organising the next South American Congress two years later. They asked me to come to their meeting but I indicated that I already had a fairly full program that year. They invited me anyway. How could I refuse an invitation when I read the letter inviting me "as their *unique* non South American visitor because I was a special friend of Bolivian anesthesiologists". I had visited them before. So I went and found that I was the unique non South American — I was the only one! Then I found that they had neither simultaneous or sequential translation. What was I to do? I had 30 minute time slots and 30 minute talks. I only spoke *un piquito* (a very little) Spanish, but I did have translations of my papers in Spanish. I discussed my problem with some Argentinians who said that I should read the papers to them and they would help me. There was one small problem. Argentinians say j or ge instead of y when pronouncing ll in Spanish! I had to tell them that I had to speak Bolivian Spanish! Somehow I managed and they politely said that they could understand me. I think they appreciated my efforts. They were the most challenging presentations I ever had to make. Another time in Quito I took another approach — I had a friend read the Spanish text and I changed the slides. That was probably a little easier for the audience.

The first Scandinavian Congress which I attended was in Oslo in 1981. I had been to Topi Suutarinen's retirement meeting and tour in Finland, so took a tour around the north of the Baltic Sea and across Northern Sweden to Narvik by train. The fascinating part of the trip was crossing the mountains with snow and a frozen lake in northern Sweden and then descending down into Narvik Fjord between 10 and 12 at night, but it was still light. During the last hour we witnessed the development of spring with the first buds on the trees to full bloom at the bottom. It was an amazing experience. I then took the bus and train to Trondheim and the Hurtigruter (coastal steamer) on to Bergen. From there I took the train to Voss, a ski resort, where I spent the night before proceeding on to Oslo on the train — another great, scenic trip.

I presented my paper on small doses of suxamethonium in burns (see Chapter 23) to a small audience, but they were interested, as all the other papers seemed to come from Jorgen Viby Mogensen's department in Copenhagen. There was a film section in a separate room which was very poorly attended. This is a very unfortunate aspect of many meetings. Films should be shown in the general program, provided they are well made, because they often show very useful things. At that time the problem of theatre pollution was gaining some attention. There was a brilliant film showing leakage of gases from anaesthetic circuits using, I think, infra red photography. Hardly anyone saw it which was a pity as it was one of the most impressive presentations I have seen at a meeting.

I also met Bill Hain from Nottingham and Gunnar Bö (28), the leading paediatric anaesthetist in Norway who later came to visit us on several occasions. Bill could speak several languages and presented papers in French when in France, which was unusual at the time for an Englishman. He was also musical. Unfortunately he developed Parkinsonism which shortened his life.

Jorgen Viby Mogensen also visited us. I played tennis with him on en tout cas and grass in Melbourne, on wood in Copenhagen and on a rubberised matting in Manila during their coup in 1989. Playing on wood was very noisy and the ball tends to skid through. He was thrashing me until I decided to use a tactic which John Fitzgerald had employed against Nyström during the 1986 Davis Cup final. I went inside the baseline to take the first serve. If you can return it, it goes back very quickly and your opponent does not have time play his next shot. It worked and I managed to win a couple of games.

Years later I went to three more Scandinavian meetings. One was in Iceland in 1995 where I met a variety of people including many anaesthetists, lexicographers (they write dictionaries), the Norwegian ombudsman, the quality control manager of the LEGO factory and the Icelandic President, Vigdis Finnbogadottir

(Figure C21), who was a charming lady. She had three terms in office. She won 93% of the vote at her last election. I was fascinated with Icelandic thermal power and hot springs in a climate which could be very cold. One could sit in the hot water in Blue Lagoon while it snowed! Before the meeting I spent three days in the north of Iceland with its wild, stark and sometimes windy landscape, with cracks and upheavals across the land and sulphur coloured areas around hot springs.

The other Scandinavian Congresses which I attended were in Stockholm, where I was given strictly three minutes at the opening ceremony to tell them about WFSA, and in Tromso, beyond the Arctic Circle, where I finally saw the midnight sun. I spoke at the opening about Nansen and his trip with the specially built boat, the *Fram*, across the Arctic, telling some of the interesting stories from his trip, which I related to topics appearing on the program, including hypothermia. I met the young lady doctor who had survived the lowest recorded human body temperature of 13.7°C. It took several months for her to recover fully.

The Norwegians showed concern for some of the trouble spots and less affluent parts of the world. In Tromso I met the President of the Iraqi Society of Anaesthetists, Dr Haifa Ali. She had managed to get out through Jordan to make the trip. During the troubled years that followed the Norwegians paid the Iraqi subscription to WFSA so when eventually the Society regrouped after the war and asked to re-join they were given the news that their membership had not been allowed to lapse. There was also a group at the meeting concerned about the injuries people suffered from land mines.

I was invited to several ASEAN congresses but only managed to attend one in Chiang Mai in Thailand and two in the Philippines. The first was during the coup of 1989 and the second in Cebu. On that occasion I visited Tacloban where Angie Gapay, who spent six months in our department, had worked for many years. I had always told her that some day I would visit to do some teaching for her. It was an enjoyable visit begun with the amazing sight of welcome banners at the airport.. We then took the ferry across to Cebu for the Congress.

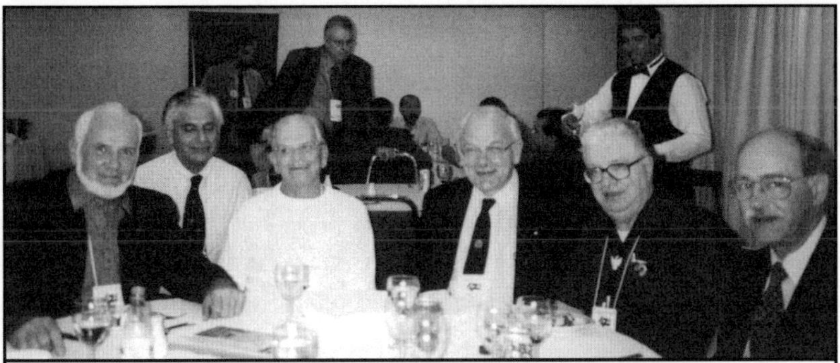

88. At the Brazilian Congress, Sao Paulo, 2002. Cedric Prys Roberts (Bristol UK — Musician, ornithologist, mountaineer, cardiovascular research etc, Former President, RCA in London), Narinder Rawal (Sweden — expert on regional anaesthesia), Zairo Vieira (Brazil/Chicago — practiced until 80, member of original WFSA executive), Carlos da Silva (Standing behind — Brazil — Paediatric anaesthetist in Florianopolis), KB., Armando Fortuna (Brazil. Wrote first paper on caudal anaesthesia from S. America in 1960s), Patricio Kelly (Argentina — WFSA Executive 1992-2000).

At some congresses I had to talk to groups about training programmes and teaching. At the Brazilian meeting in 2002 my comments lent support to increase their minimum training time from two to three years. One meets interesting people, both local and international speakers. (88) A group of us including Angela Enright, Jorge Urzua (Chile) and Gonzalo Barreiro (Uruguay) did a similar session at the Argentinian Congress in Mendoza in 2003.(89)

I went to several CLASA and South American Congresses. At

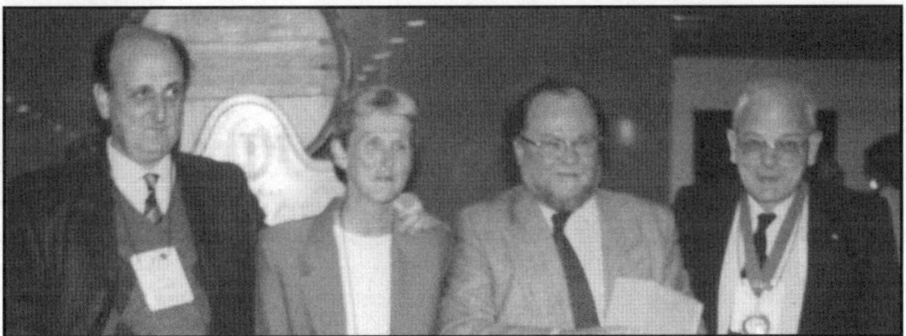

89. Gonzalo Barreiro (Uruguay, WFSA Executive), Angela Enright (Canada, Chair WFSA Education Committee), Jorge Urzua (Chile, WFSA Education Committee) and Kester Brown (WFSA President) after a discussion on Education In Mendoza, 2003.

these meetings we often met representatives of the regional organization, CLASA. One perennial problem that kept coming up for discussion was non physician anaesthetists. They were totally opposed even if their doctors had a shorter period of training than elsewhere. I eventually had to resort to my very limited Spanish to explain that in countries like Tanzania where there were only about ten local physician anaesthetists and a few foreigners for 30 million people one had to use some non physicians.

It was a pleasure and privilege to participate in these meetings and often I met former trainees or people who had done sabbatical leave with us. I attended many other meetings and did workshops and lectures in places when I was passing through a region. I tried to make my lectures practical so people could go home with something new to try. I used videos to demonstrate practical procedures because this is the next best to seeing demonstrations in the operating theatre and sometimes they were in the language of the country — e.g. Spanish or Japanese. People like to learn something that will be useful in their practice.

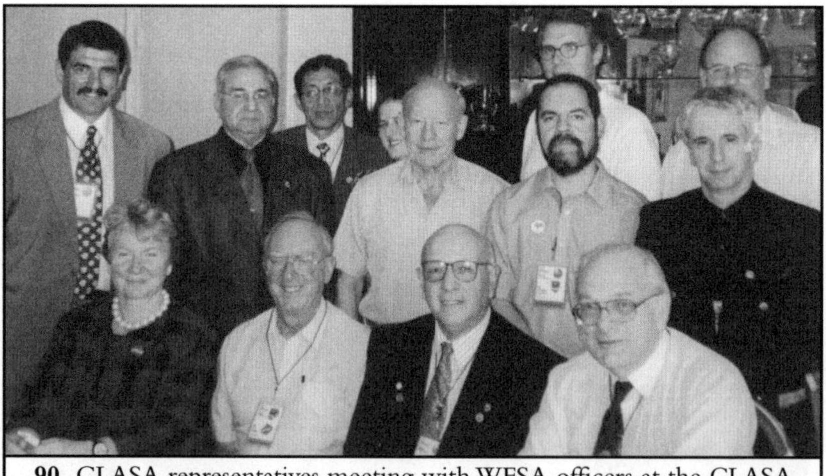

90. CLASA representatives meeting with WFSA officers at the CLASA Congress in Santo Domingo, 1999. *Standing*: A. Cataneo (Mendoza, Argentina), Alfredo Portella (Brazil), A.Cerroni (Peru —Vice President ,CLASA), Karen McMurchy (WFSA office, London and Cook Islands) Rosen (Treasurer, WFSA), M.Galindo (Colombia),J.Moyers (assistant Secretary), Alfredo Parietti (Argentina, President, CLASA), David Bevan (Deputy Chair, WFSA). *Sitting*: A Meursing, M.Vickers, Humberto Sainz Cabrera (Cuba), K. Brown (Chairman, WFSA).

Congresses are a great opportunity for people to meet with friends and people from other places. It is important that anaesthetists do not neglect the important part — the scientific and educational component. So much is available on the internet and through video conferencing that some may feel congresses are not necessary. This view fails to recognize the important information which is conveyed during discussion with knowledgeable people and the sharing of experiences with colleagues which is a very valuable component of these meetings. It would be a great loss not to be able to meet people personally.

It is also an opportunity to assess whether speakers with big reputations are as good as they are thought to be. It is amazing how often some well known person presents poorly, talks too fast, uses audiovisuals badly or is not actually doing much of the clinical work he is talking about.

Chapter 33
Organizing Conferences and a World Congress

Organizing the program for a conference can be a challenge. I was lucky to have a knack for doing this. It is important to group related topics together and maybe have more than one session devoted to a topic. Guest lecturers should be given times when the audience is attentive — during the first morning session or just after morning tea are best, and certainly not just after lunch. That is the time for a lively panel or an entertaining speaker so that the audience doesn't drift off to sleep. It is rather insulting to put a guest on at the end of the day although this is sometimes done to try to keep the audience there.

The guest speakers are invited because they are eminent, in which case they sometimes nominate their topics, or because they have a special area of expertise. If the meeting is topic driven then the choice is to present specific topics. Some speakers have a narrow range of research and expertise while others can speak on a wide variety of topics.

Starting time in the morning varies. I believe that if there is a social programme in the evenings too early a start is undesirable. Nine o'clock is my preferred time and 9.30am if there has been a dinner the night before. It is interesting that the best attended last session of all the four day meetings which I have attended was at Surfers Paradise when we began at 11am. The swimming was better in the morning!

No doubt ski meetings with early morning and late afternoon sessions are appealing for similar reasons but one hardly has to wonder what is the primary motivation to be there.

How long should the sessions run? Probably 1 to 2 hours is optimal, with most talks being kept to 20 to 30 minutes or less. It is often useful to have discussion time after a lecture but sometimes when a series of related topics are presented a longer discussion period at the end may be more productive, provided it has not been shortened by speakers going on too long. Three hour sessions are too long.

Should there be *concurrent sessions*? This depends on the size of the meeting. It will be necessary for big congresses. The key considerations are how much choice should there be and how many people will attend the smaller sessions if there are many from which to choose. For many years during the Australian Society of Anaesthetists meetings we had no choice except at the refresher course. Many people take a session or two off in four days so they tended to take them during sessions which did not interest them. Some choice, but not too much may be the solution unless one is trying to cater for all subspecialties such as at major regional or world congresses.

Should there be a *refresher course*? These can be useful but are sometimes used to generate extra revenue. They should NOT be during the main meeting. It is better to have a varied programme with a few short lectures (20-30 minutes), panels, workshops and discussion groups rather than a series of 50 minute lectures which are too long anyway in relation to average concentration span (15-20 minutes). It amazes me how many big meetings run courses which are six or seven 50 minute lectures in a day. The only good reason to do so is administrative ease for registration. It is certainly not for the efficient transfer of information.

Panel discussions where the panelists make brief introductory statements and the others comment and sometimes even members of the audience can comment creates a much more lively session than endless lectures. A good chairman who can keep the panel moving in a lively fashion is invaluable. Instead of a lecture on, say, obstetric anaesthesia one could have some anaesthetists and an obstetrician on the panel all contributing points. This has additional advantages in bringing different specialists together to hear the others' point of view on subjects. Panels or round tables where four or five speakers have 20 minutes each does not leave time for real discussion. It is better for them to have 5-10 minutes with 10 minutes at least for discussion on each topic by the panel or others. A series of speakers is not really a panel unless there is a lengthy discussion period at the end.

Group discussions, especially if the numbers are limited, provide a good learning forum especially if you have good leaders who can involve all the group and can catalyse discussion and give authoritative comment. Problem case discussions are always useful in medical meetings. Sessions where scenarios are set and a panel discusses them are usually entertaining and informative.

Several *free papers* on related topics may be offered and can be grouped to form a session. Sometimes there is room to invite someone with special expertise to fill out the session if another paper is needed.

I have been to many congresses where free papers are presented during sessions when some plenary lecture or panel is being held. The free paper session may only have half a dozen in the audience. This is a terrible disappointment, especially at large important congresses, because the speakers will have put considerable preparation into the paper thinking this presentation may be the pinnacle of their career. It is better to have sessions devoted to the free paper presentations without major competition or else have the free contributions presented as *posters* which people can study at leisure. Ideally there will be a time for them to be discussed. They should be presented in some readily accessible area and should be left up for a full day.

Practical workshops can also be held. These are becoming increasingly popular as the participants have hands on training.

In practical specialties like anaesthesia, demonstrating techniques with films, videos, CDs or even video conferencing from the operating theatre, can arouse great interest. At one conference which I attended, such a video conference attracted at least half the participants.

A meeting should be successful if it is well organised and has a varied program with good speakers. It is very important *to keep to time*. This requires good and effective chairmen and training of the participants. Speakers can be told beforehand that three double spaced typed pages are appropriate for a ten minute presentation. A warning and stop light can be used to make speakers keep to time. The chairman should then stop the speaker and if unsuccessful the microphone can be switched off! Strict discipline in this area makes conferences run more smoothly and eventually speakers will learn to keep to time. It is not fair on following speakers to go over time.

The *audiovisual facilities* must work smoothly. It can be a disaster if they don't. This means preparation beforehand, understanding the equipment and having efficient technical assistance on hand to ensure everything runs smoothly.

To assess the value of attending a meeting answer the question, "Did you learn anything that will modify your practice, help you to do your job better or understand some important concepts more clearly?" It is also important for the organizers to think about this so that programmes with some practical information are formulated.

When organizing teaching programmes or post graduate courses similar principles can be used. A series of lectures has limited value. It is better to create some interactive sessions, especially in post graduate programmes. Tutorials, case discussions, journal reviews, videos or CDs can all be used to create a variety which makes a programme more interesting.

The *World Congress of Anaesthesiologists* was held in Sydney in April 1996. I was asked to convene the scientific programme. It was a challenge which I relished because I felt previous congresses which I had attended had sessions on topics jumbled up so there was not a coherent programme. The theme was "Coming together — 150 years on." Coming together in my mind was the people from all over the world but also the different subspecialties and special interest groups. More and more these meet independently and there are regular specialty meetings. Anaesthesia is becoming fragmented. It seemed that if we could organise the Congress as a conglomerate of specialty and special interest meetings all the groups could get together and meet each other but still have their scientific preference and meeting to attend. So forty such meetings were organised, each with an Australian convenor and deputy and three others to help to develop the programme. The others had to come from different regions of the world. This was to ensure people from all over the world could contribute and no single country could become too dominant.

I planned the timing of each meeting and its venue so that *it was continuous in the same room for the time required* which was four days for cardiac physiology, pharmacology and anaesthesia. Meetings were arranged to follow logical sequences where possible. For instance Fluids was followed by Blood, then Trauma and finally Intensive Care covering three and a half days in all. Making this jig saw fit was one of the most challenging and exciting parts of the whole planning.

The convenors' brief was to provide update sessions which would make a refresher course unnecessary and cover other topics of interest. The speakers would be invited having been well recommended by one of the committee or anyone they chose to consult. They were told to try to make the program as international as possible. Only one convenor did not follow the guidelines. I checked all the proposed programmes and in only two or three did I have to suggest changes to make them more international. The end result was that there were 556 invited speakers from 56 countries. The paediatric anaesthesia component, which I convened, had speakers from 18 countries. The two day history meeting had speakers from 20 countries. When people said to me afterwards that they had enjoyed the Congress because they heard speakers from so many different countries I felt it had all been worthwhile.

Several other countries were represented by free paper selection or by a plan whereby each morning the first ten minutes was devoted in each room to a Society presentation about something to do with anaesthesia in their country. Days were allocated to Europe, Asia and the Pacific , South America and Africa and the Middle East to present. This enabled countries like Paraguay, Tanzania and Iceland, which most people would know little about, to participate.

Free papers were included if they fitted into the session programme. Otherwise most were shown as posters and some of these were selected for a brief presentation and discussion. The posters were in prominent positions in the industry exhibition where the coffee and lunch were provided. This gave them good exposure. There were 1400 posters which were each exhibited for one day.

The selection of posters to be presented was left to the section convenors and their deputies. They were asked to base the selection on merit but also to try include some from countries which might not have invited speakers. The selection was kept local because a complex selection system becomes complicated if too many judges are involved, especially if some do not work to schedule.

One area of weakness was film and video. These were shown away in a corner of the Industry Hall. I believe that good presentations on the screen need to be used more often in the main programmes because they can be just as informative and educational as someone speaking — sometimes even better.

We decided to give a commemorative medal to each speaker and chairman. This turned out to be a big job. The person originally allocated to do it withdrew as he gave up anaesthesia. My son had made a design for the logo which the committee did not select but it turned out to be an excellent one for the medal. He took the ASA logo of the caring hand holding a bowl from which the anaesthetic vapours rose. He put the opera House on the thumb and made the rising vapours into the supports on the Sydney Harbour bridge and the top of the bridge and hand carried the title of the Congress. On the obverse for the speakers medal was a picture of Morton's inhaler and "Coming together, 150 years on"- the theme of the congress — and the person's name. The medals were made by a Czech, Emil Haffner, who had emigrated to Australia many years ago. He had made medals for all sorts of occasions including Olympic Games. The next problem was having the names engraved on them. I found a retired man, Keith Grey, who had been a medal maker who inscribed medals for the hospital. He offered to do them without cost. I had to insist on a token payment. There were about 650 medals. The next problem was to sort them for distribution to 156 sessions. My dining room table looked like a model town with all the piles of them as the buildings. Then I had to pack them and transport them to Sydney in my VW Caravelle. They were quite heavy to move around! I think the speakers appreciated them.

The Congress was very successful, organised by a very congenial committee, chaired by Richard Walsh who has been a great contributor to the ASA, College as treasurer and President and now as treasurer of WFSA. It was a wonderful way to conclude my long association with the ASA scientific programmes.

Chapter 34
Not Always Plain Sailing

Teaching overseas is not always straightforward. Many unusual situations may develop.

On one occasion when I was doing a half-day workshop in Kuala Lumpur a neurosurgeon came to me at the morning tea interval and insisted on taking me to consult on a patient. It turned out to be Barlow, one of two Australians picked up with drugs which is a crime punishable by death in Malaysia. He had a chronic pain problem. All I could suggest was that they try to refer him back to his original doctor in Perth. Little did I realize the consequences of this little visit. Some months later, when Barlow and Chambers went on trial for carrying drugs I received a phone call from a reporter from a major Australian newspaper. She understood that I had met Chambers. I told her that I had never met him. She then accused me of being a liar. I had not met him. It was then that I began to learn what it is like to be verbally assaulted by the media. When I arrived home I received another phone call — from an anaesthetist friend in Sydney. "Did I know that my name was on the news up there — I was going to the trial in Kuala Lumpur."

Then I received another phone call from a Sydney radio station asking me to contact Karpal Singh, a well known Malaysian lawyer who was defending Barlow and Chambers. He wanted to subpoena me. I told the caller that I had no intention to call him. Then I was told that Karpal Singh had difficulty contacting me. I responded that the caller did not seem to have had any difficulty and so I thought Karpal Singh should be able to do so if it was really necessary. Next morning a newspaper reporter arrived at our front door with cameramen just after I had left for work. My wife answered the door and was harassed by the reporter's questions. That evening the front page informed everyone "that a distressed woman answered my door". Innuendo again. Who was she? They could easily have determined that it was my wife. I did not go to the trial because there was nothing that I could contribute that would have saved them. Janet then received a round of abuse from a relative because, she was told, I did not care about them. It was irrelevant in her eyes that I would have nothing to contribute. It was a small affair but it made me realize how unreasonably ruthless the press can be in seeking information. Trial by the media and verbal harassment by some of them is a serious infringement of privacy and is often contrary to the Australian adage of 'a fair go.'

Flexibility is needed if one is going to lecture around the world. Once, in Nepal, I was in Pokhara and had booked to fly back to Katmandu at 8am for an afternoon workshop. The flight was cancelled because of fog in Katmandu. Could I get the next flight at midday? "No, because they have extra passengers off a flight that ran off the runway at the next airport the day before!" I became a bit desperate. Knowing the locals are usually better at solving these problems I called one of the anaesthetists who finally got me on to the flight. I arrived at my hotel at the time I was to be picked up. When we reached the hospital we were informed that there was a power cut and as a result I could not show slides! I had to use the blackboard until the electricity came on two hours later.

On another occasion when I was doing a workshop in Ecuador we had to wait for someone who was supposed to open it. He never came but while waiting I found that the video projector did not work, so we had to find a replacement. Then I found that the bulb in the slide projector did not work. We obtained a new bulb but then I discovered that the carousel only went backwards! After finding another projector and putting a new bulb in it we were ready to start. The whole program was sequentially translated. One of the translators turned out to be an outstanding anaesthetist, Susana Cueva, who subsequently came to work with us.

Next stop was Guatamala. They assured me there would be no problems there. The video became stuck half way into the projector and we could not remove it. I had to change my whole programme and lecture all afternoon instead of having a video between my talks. Then the next day I had to show videos instead of breaking the programme up with talks!

The ultimate tactlessness was reached one evening when I was to address the Cape Society in South Africa. We arrived 10 minutes early to put my slides in the carousel. The only problem was that there wasn't one. It took 20 minutes to find one. Then they made a presentation to their former professor who was visiting and he replied. I was introduced at 8.45 pm. The chairman concluded his introduction by saying that we were running a bit late so could I cut my lecture short! I could have been mortally offended as an international guest speaker but the whole situation amused me. I began by saying that I would be delighted to cut my lecture from 90 to 45 minutes. Actually I was only going to speak for 45 minutes but he did not know that!

The ultimate catastrophe occurred in Jaipur in India. My host had been to check that all the audiovisual equipment was working. It was a special occasion — the 30th anniversary of their Trust hospital. It was the first of a series of meetings to celebrate the event. I felt so sorry for him during the events that followed. First the sound would not come through on the video. Then the slides would not feed out of the tray into the projector. They had four people trying to fix the problems. I decided that I could give the talk without slides. So I began. Then I realized that the audience were being so distracted by the people working on the projector that I stopped. At last the problems were fixed. Then someone decided to come round to the back of the stage to make some adjustment to the sound system. He tripped over the cable leading to the projectors and disconnected them all! Disaster! We finally succeeded and made our presentations. It is all part of the challenge of teaching.

Sometimes it was hazardous to go to places, but one was not always forewarned. In 1989 I was to be the plenary lecturer on Friday morning at the ASEAN meeting. In Manila I went down to the Conference Centre early to organize my slides. There was hardly anybody there when usually it would be bustling with people and there would be guards at the door. I went in to the slide room and was putting my slides into the carousel when a girl burst in saying, "there is a coup." The organizers arrived and were ready to cancel the meeting when I said that I was there. Some of the people would come and some wouldn't be able to but I could still give my talk. We continued and finished the Congress. At lunchtime we looked from the verandah across the bay to see the huge cloud of smoke rising from the fuel tanks. I painted the scene. (Figure C 26) The airport was closed so we all had to stay at the hotels. People could not come and go. Staff who were on duty remained there for three days. Some of the organizers had family members on both sides — a very worrying situation for them.

But out of bad situations comes some good. We had the chance to meet and dine with colleagues from the other countries so that we became better acquainted.

In 1997 I went to India and Pakistan. While in India the Government was defeated. Some countries (USA and Belgium) had told their citizens that Pakistan was not safe for travel. The South Asian Congress was due to be held in Karachi. There was a blow up between the Prime Minister and President, both threatening to sack the other. Tensions rose but we carried on. Driving in from the airport about midnight our driver went through red lights. He explained that it was too dangerous to stop.

I developed a severe case of gastroenteritis one night. The next lunchtime I was due to give a special memorial lecture. I did not have slides or a written speech — only notes about my subject. I was worried should I forget what I planned to say. Fortunately my friend, Tipu Sultan, saved the day and provided all that was required to cure me and replenish my fluids. I was able to give my lecture without any problems.

A small group of us, including Fritz Berry who is an American who ignores his government's advice, were going on to do workshops in Lahore and Islamabad. Crisis day arrived when we were in the capital, Islamabad. The President was ousted but there were none of the expected demonstrations. We could only conclude that the army supported the move. The next day we went on tour to the Swat Valley in Northern Pakistan where I took three great photographs. One was a rock in the river which I spotted as we drove by, beautifully sculpted by the greenish glacial water rushing by for centuries; one a wonderful portrait of an old man with his shawl around his head and another of a most intriguing building with six construction styles in one short stretch, overhanging a river. We could not photograph females because we were in country dominated by fundamentalists. In the most northern village which we visited there were stalls in the street. One shoemaker sat on the ground with his automatic weapon beside him. Next was a butcher in what was little more than a box with the meat out in the open. I decided to paint as I do when travelling so I took out my watercolours. One of my companions was with me. A crowd suddenly gathered around so I asked him to watch my left hand pocket which had my wallet in it. I felt slightly uneasy, especially as some of these men were armed, but then I figured I was probably doing something they maybe hadn't seen before and were just curious so I carried on. The crowd increased to about twenty. Fortunately I can produce watercolour paintings quickly. They seemed pleased with the result and I came to no harm.

On our return I had to catch a plane from Rawalpindi which is the nearest airport to Islamabad for international flights. We were running a bit late by the time we reached Rawalpindi. It was 5 o'clock rush hour and darkness was falling. Then we realized that the driver did not actually know the way to the airport. We struggled through the heavy traffic. Suddenly he decided to do a U turn in the traffic. A policeman stopped him and then a shouting match began. I was feeling less and less confident about catching my flight to Bangkok for another ASEAN Congress in Chiang Mai where I was to speak the next day. The argument became more heated. Then I thought I would produce my address card which indicated that I was Chairman of the WFSA Executive Committee. A man standing beside my window passed it to the policeman. He looked at it for a while, probably not able to read it, and eventually must have decided that it looked important and waved us on, much to our relief. We still did not seem to know where the airport was. Suddenly a plane flew overhead coming in to land. We knew we must be near and followed the general direction and there we were, beside the airport. I was in plenty of time.

On another occasion, when India and Pakistan were on the verge of going to war I was talking in Amritsar in the Punjab.

Despite the tensions between the countries I was taken to the border which is not far from Lahore. They told me that they still continued their daily 4.30 pm drill of both lowering their flags within a few yards of the other and then saluting each other before marching off. It struck me as a very friendly ritual when the countries were nearly at war. Maybe it is things like that that prevents the final step sometimes being taken.

Flying into Bogota airport was not totally encouraging as the runway is bordered by a row of retired planes. Bogota was not a tranquil place to visit. It is interesting to have been there and particularly to have visited their fantastic gold museum but the day we were there a car bomb exploded on the airport road. The next day we flew to Quito to find we had just missed by a day the local volcano having a little eruption.

I went to Turkey shortly after a big earthquake in 1991. I gave my hostess a stone carving from Kenya. Four days after I left they had another earthquake. Her house shook but only two things were broken — a cup and my carving.

In Kuala Lumpur in 1973 the customs man found my teaching movie on Paediatric Anaesthesia in a blue box. " Ah, Blue Movie!" he exclaimed. I then realized he wanted a bribe so I told him I was there under the Auspices of the Australian Government and if he wanted to make a fuss I would like to contact the Embassy. He soon backed down.

In Paraguay, there was no x ray machine to check the baggage. It was hot and I was sweating when I arrived to check through. The security man obviously thought I was suspicious. "What was I doing there?" I had to try to explain in Spanish that I had been giving lectures to doctors. He was still suspicious and searched me and had the sniffer dog check my baggage. It is a little more difficult if one is not very fluent in the language.

In 1990 I went to Moscow. I stayed with Elena Damir, President of the Russian Society. It was just after Perestroyka. When we left the apartment in the morning she gave me a key and explained that she left the broom across the hall to remind her to switch off the alarm when she came in. After visiting the hospital my guide, Sergei,who later came to work with me, took me around. Eventually we did not have lunch as we couldn't find a reasonable place because we were late. He took me back to the apartment. First I had trouble opening the door. I said goodbye and he left. I was in need of an urgent visit to the toilet so rushed in over the broom. When I came out I forgot about the alarm. A few minutes later there was a knock at the door. I couldn't understand the questions in Russian. According to the authorities I should not have been there. He asked for my passport, then the telephone. I was sweating profusely. Thank goodness the KGB were finished but I was not quite sure about this situation. After several phone calls he returned my passport and left. I was very embarrassed when Elena returned soon after. She had met him on the stairs. Apparently he had phoned her brother who wasn't sure but thought there may be a foreigner there. My imagination had run wild thinking about what it must have been like during the communist regime — frightening I imagine.

In Egypt we had to travel to Assuit and then to Luxor. Trouble with some fighting and shooting developed over the discovery of hashish among a mango plantation near our route. Our host was told at midnight that no foreigners were to travel. He managed to have that decision reversed but we had to travel by bus with a police escort rather than train from Assuit. Most of the passengers were unaware of the closeness of the problem.

The final trial was to have a metal object found in my bag during the screening at an airport not long after September 11th. Was I carrying a bomb? They asked me to identify what a strange metal object was showing up on the screen. I couldn't think what it could be. We hunted through the bag until I found the WFSA President's Medallion! It has caused me many hold ups — one of the disadvantages of high office but it is something one needs to carry, not put in the baggage that may be lost.

One needs to be flexible. My travels have not been dull!

Other Aspects

Chapter 35
Family and Other Interests

Anyone who has read this far will realize that I have had a very busy professional life. We also had five children over eleven years. All this would not have been possible without Janet, who supported me and was a very good mother to the children. She stayed at home to look after them when they were young. In Vancouver when the twins were small she sometimes worked at the Canadian Arthritis Society's evening clinic when I was home to look after them. Having twin girls who were born in Yellowknife was an advantage as they always had someone to play with. They were four when Fraser was born in Melbourne (1966) and thereafter were always old enough to be helpful to Janet with the younger boys. Kester was born in 1969 and Ken in 1973, by which time the girls were eleven.

When the children were all at school Janet went to work part time in the Physiotherapy Department at the Royal Childrens

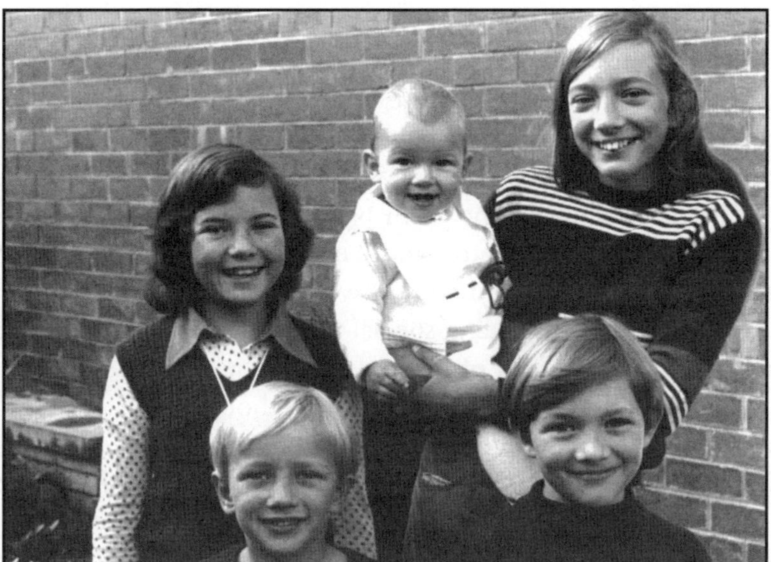

91. The author's children in 1974.
Behind from Left: Maryann, Ken, Catherine. *Front* : Kester, Fraser

Hospital where she stayed for five years. She was then asked to go to Queen Victoria Hospital as the paediatric physiotherapist where she spent several years, and when the hospital moved she went with it to Monash Medical Centre for a year. As her mother grew older Janet worked, for convenience, in a nearby old peoples home for five years before returning to a general practice with children. Eventually she closed her rooms and visited children with developmental delay in their homes. During her career she obtained a degree in special education from Monash University which proved useful in her work with children.

Administration took time on top of my clinical load. I continued doing about one night and weekend in five or six for many years, because we did not have a big staff and it was important to keep in touch with the emergency work. Only when the staff increased in my late fifties was I able to cut back and eventually stop being on call at night. I missed the work, but not the fatigue which it causes increasingly, as one grows older.

One has to be careful that work does not interfere too much with other aspects of ones life. It is important in a busy job to ensure that one always has time for family and other relaxing pursuits — outdoor activities such as sport, gardening, walking and cultural interests such as music or art. Although busy I managed to have time with my five children, especially taking them to various sporting activities and on various trips around the country, sometimes with a caravan or camping. In addition, I took each to Kenya alone or in pairs so that they could understand my background better and see where I was brought up. We usually visited other countries as well. These overseas trips were educational as well as being special times together with only one or two of them instead of in the mass of the whole family.

Our children went to a number of schools and each of them had some time at state primary schools. They all played hockey, Kester and Ken captaining their senior school teams. Kester had a state junior trial when under 13. They participated in and enjoyed a number of other sports, including tennis. Catherine and Kester, and to a lesser extent Ken, were the most competitive at sport and all played in junior tennis tournaments.

Maryann and Fraser played for pleasure. Catherine was school captain and the others held various other posts and were involved in a variety of activities such as music and plays. Fraser was the most practical. He had three days off school, when he was ten, to help the builder constructing our log house at the beach. We, and his teacher thought it would be more useful than three days at school! We had the frame and outside of this kit house constructed and then did the inside work ourselves. The bigger ones all helped in some way so it was a family project. The walls are all lined with veneer wood boards — each room is a different wood. Fraser also learnt electrical skills with his model trains and eventually learnt how to take engines out of cars and repair them. He also built train models. It is interesting how the talents in a family vary.

We had two cats which each lived about 18 years, several dogs, a rabbit, chickens, goldfish and mice. Kester and Ken also had an interesting selection of birds — we used to go to the Victoria market to buy them. All these added interest to our lives.

None of the children did medicine but they have all done interesting things. Catherine did Arts/Law and went on to do a Diploma of business administration. She eventually became a consultant to philanthropic groups, sometimes setting up some big projects for them including the Rural Foundation for Australia and a biosphere project returning land to its natural state near Mildura. Maryann became a teacher and then added special education. She later became a university lecturer training teachers. Fraser became a conservation architect who spent eight years in London before returning to Melbourne. Kester did science and commerce degrees and then became an accountant. Ken is a scientist with an interest in plant pathology. They are an interesting family. Apart from Ken, the youngest, they all have children. (Figure C25)

I continued to play hockey most years until I was 54, playing latterly in a team with Fraser and Ken. On one occasion all three boys played. One of the opposition asked how many sons I had as he was hearing "Dad" coming from all over the field. I had a break for three years when my front teeth were knocked out. I still play tennis.

I have done much travelling but mainly to attend meetings and to teach. On only five occasions did I travel without lecturing or going to a meeting. The first was to take Janet and the twins to see my family in Kenya in 1963. J.F.Kennedy was assasinated and Kenya became independent while we were there. The other trips were to see my father as he was dying in 1968, to take Fraser and Kester to see my mother and family in Kenya in 1979, when we stopped in Athens for two days on the way, and two trips, as I neared retirement and immediately afterwards, to the Antarctic. They were special treats and provided a great opportunity for photography and painting.

Photography has always been an interest since I was a teenager when my brother gave me a baby Brownie box camera. I am a believer that the eye of the photographer for a picture is the key to good photographs, not just or even the camera.

I began painting with oils in 1961 and since 1981 have carried watercolours everywhere I travel. I discovered, when at a school camp with one of my boys, that I could create a picture quickly in watercolour and that it dried in a short time so that one could easily do them when travelling. This has added to the pleasure of travel and has enabled me to absorb much more as one sees more detail when trying to record the subject.

Painting is a wonderful hobby for someone who is busy as it takes one's mind right away from the problems and stresses of life for a short time while painting. I learnt to paint very quickly because I had limited time. It has also provided me with a useful occupation in semi-retirement. I have passed on my enthusiasm for this to others looking for an outlet from their busy lives. I was amazed when several people came up to me at the World Congress in Paris to tell me how they were progressing.

While gardening has been something I have had to do, I enjoy it when I have no other more pressing things to do. A former Maths teacher of mine in Kenya, Jim Duff, who has lived in Adelaide for many years, was a very keen gardener and gave me some orchids which became another interest of mine. Jim Duff was an exceptional man. He taught me maths when I was 12 and 13. He was small, had red hair and was always immaculately dressed in a dark blue suit. He could control the class with just a glance at any mischief-maker, an exceptional skill. He knew just how to handle boys so that they respected him. In his geometry lessons he described how equilateral triangles were used to bomb dams during the war. He had been a pilot. He was a talented organist who could play with one hand and conduct a choir with the other. Our friendship has continued well into his eighties.

While I am not very musical I have enjoyed being in a city where we could attend concerts, ballet, opera and plays. Seeing and hearing Vladimir Ashkenazy conducting a Mozart concerto and then play the solo parts as well was one of the highlight performances I have witnessed. Carols by candlelight at the Myer Music Bowl in Melbourne where 25-30,000 people attend holding candles is another impressive show which is held each year on Christmas Eve.

I spent time on the mountains in Kenya as a child, particularly the Aberdares, and enjoyed hiking in the hills in Scotland when I was a student. I climbed Point Lenana (about 5000m) on Mt Kenya in 1958 but my greatest physical effort was to reach the top of Kilimanjaro, the highest point in Africa, the day after my 50th birthday. In retrospect, reaching the top was one of the great achievements of my life — to have survived such low oxygen tension gave me a new lease of life and I took up hockey again.

I enjoy taking people around Melbourne and other places in Victoria such as Ballarat, an old gold mining town. They have beautiful gardens which are a major attraction especially in March, when the begonias are in full bloom. There are masses of huge and colourful flowers. (Figure C28)

Interests outside one's work are important because without these retirement can be very boring and empty. One needs activities which one enjoys to make life meaningful.

I think one's family can be the greatest asset we have, provided we have nurtured them and the members get along well together. While children bring great pleasure, particularly when they are small, they can also bring worries and difficulties, especially as they grow up. It is very important to give them enough time and attention when they are young so that happy rapport is maintained.

Chapter 36
My Philosophies

My life has been a full of interest, accomplishment and satisfaction. I feel sad when I hear people say they wish they could have their life again, they would do things so differently. I don't. I have had a wonderful wife and family, good colleagues and friends and interesting, sometimes fascinating, work. I have travelled widely, seen some exotic places, people, animals, birds, plants, mountains, deserts, beaches, islands and many other things. I have been able to photograph and paint pictures which have given me and many others pleasure. I have indulged in sports which I have enjoyed and been to the top of Africa, Mt. Kilimanjaro and beyond 70 degrees north and south. Who could want more?

This book has been about my professional life. *The rest was too much for one book so the other stories will come in another one.* Few people would have had the opportunities that I have been fortunate to have had in my clinical work, teaching, research, administration and involvement in organizations. One of the greatest pleasures has been helping others from around the world — training them in our department or going and teaching them in their own countries. To have had anaesthetists and medical students from forty countries and to have lectured and taught in sixty six means that I have reached much of the anaesthetic community around the world. I have friends across the globe, with no boundaries related to colour, religion and nationality.

How did all this come about? Sometimes I wonder if it was luck, or my willingness to take opportunities or was I destined to do it all. I was lucky to get to university which I struggled through academically. I had an enquiring mind and when I finally began to mature intellectually in my late twenties my knowledge started to fall into place. People sometimes don't believe me when I tell them this but I went from getting 25% in my second year Physiology exam to being sent overseas to teach a whole course of Physiology and Pharmacology to post graduate students 17 years later. I had learnt to use what information I had gained and apply it to the task. I learnt much from discussion or from books rather than from formal training. Painting, teaching and tennis were largely learnt that way too.

I suppose I was fairly conventional but I was non-conformist in some ways, by which I mean that I did not accept that I had to do or accept things just because it was what the majority of people did or believed. I made up my own mind and said what I thought, even though my comments were sometimes considered controversial. My upbringing in Africa influenced my views on some matters. This probably helped when I became involved in world affairs in anaesthesia.

I learnt many of my attitudes from my parents. My father was hard working, kind, generous and caring towards his patients and didn't mind standing up for what he thought was right even if he was in a minority. My mother taught me other things, including having a belief in prayer and thus, to me, an indefinable higher being.

It is sad that so many people are taught to be antagonistic to those with other religious views. So much of the conflict in the world emanates from that and yet most religions have a significant amount in common including caring for your fellow man. There have been religious conflicts for centuries and suppression of people — the Spanish inquisition, for example. I remember being taken to visit the beautiful Mohamed Ali Mosque in Cairo and my friend, Samy Saleh, saying to me as we emerged " I am a Moslem because I was born as one here but I suppose if I had been born in different circumstances somewhere else I might be something else." How true this is for most of us. And yet so much conflict has resulted from religious intolerance even among Christians. I think the problem is that men have interpreted the original teachings of Christ, Mohamed, or any others so that very different interpretations from the original teachings have developed to suit their ends.

I have always tried to help to bring people together, looking for common ground, even if they worship differently. My views have become simpler. I find deep philosophical debate on the subject fruitless to me because none of us can conceive what we are debating — God and whether one exists. One either believes as a matter of faith or one doesn't. Jesus taught some useful principles — love your neighbour as yourself; treat others as you would like to be treated; use your talents; if someone offends you turn the other cheek. They are useful principles by which to live.

I have a few other ideas which I have found useful.

Always remember to thank those who help you, whatever their station in life may be.

When someone is being antagonistic, look for their good points and give them credit for them. It often helps one to feel less antagonistic. If their intent is to bully it may be that they lack something themselves, maybe a little humanity. They want to exert control at all costs. They are unlikely to gain respect by their actions.

I was often involved in conflict resolution. I always tried to look at both sides of the argument. If the individuals can be shown the reasons behind each other's actions and can accept them, even if it differs from their own view, a compromise and resolution can often be reached.

In the wider situation in our troubled world conflict resolution is difficult if one or both sides fail to realize or recognize that they seem to be the aggressors to the other side. Maybe their antagonism is too deep rooted to be able to see that peaceful negotiation is a possible, although idealistic, approach. If people are brainwashed enough they believe and it is hard to change deep-seated beliefs whatever side they are on. We should each try to appreciate the others point of view.

Out of most bad situations comes some good. In my own case I learnt this when I missed out on an appointment but, as a result, was able to participate in several other useful activities which opened the door to better opportunities later. Often I have consoled people who have missed out on appointments and in the end they have been better off or have got a better position. It is common for disappointment to be followed by consolation — something better turns up.

If you want something, ask. The worst that can happen is refusal and you have lost nothing but often you are granted your request which may not have happened if you had not made your wish known.

You can save time and energy by applying ergonomic principles — working out how to do things most efficiently.

'Use your head to save your legs!' I developed this in relation to sport. Work out where to be so that you had the least difficulty reaching the desired spot when needed. Jaroslav Drobny was regarded as a tennis phenomenon when he won Wimbledon in 1954 because he was 33. How did he do it? He didn't run for anything he couldn't reach and so conserved his energy for when he needed it most. In anaesthesia it suggests you sit down during a long case so you don't become tired standing.

Don't believe all you read or are told. There is much conflicting information provided and it is important to consider whether it is logical and reasonable before accepting it. Even anaesthesia textbooks contain comments which don't stand up to logical analysis — in fact, they may contain concepts which are rubbish! Learn to critically appraise information before accepting it..

I suppose I developed the ethic of hard work. I did work hard but I also used my time to live a full life. Sometimes that meant sleeping when I was tired. I was fortunate to be able to take short sleeps, sometimes only ten minutes , to revive myself.

In research one needs to be patient. In addition never give up. If a paper is rejected it is not the end of the world. I have mentioned several such situations earlier where rejection led to other positive outcomes.

Medicine has advanced in many ways during my time. Maybe it has developed too much, because we now often don't receive the care and attention which we used to receive when things were simpler. Even in affluent countries we do not have the manpower, the facilities or the funds to provide for all the amazing, modern developments.

Anaesthesia is safer. More anaesthetists are better trained and the monitoring equipment has improved considerably but they must not lose their clinical and technical skills, which are so important in their work. And they must always remember that their patients are people with feelings. They must be respected as individuals and treated with kindness.

I hope you, my reader, have had pleasure in reading this, have gained some useful information and, even better, have been inspired in some way because inspiration is a source of interest and enjoyment of life.

Chapter 37
The Views of Others

My memoirs are necessarily a record of the events in my life, the things I have done, the people I have met and developed relationships with, fortunately mostly friendly ones. I find it hard to express my feelings openly or to write a self assessment, such as an independent biographer might do, but I know I have enjoyed my life and many people have written appreciative and complimentary letters to me. Some of these along with a great array of photographs of anaesthetists all over the world were presented to me in a wonderful present, "Brown's Book", when I retired from full time work in 2000. It opened my eyes to the influences I had had on many people's lives of which I was unaware. Teachers often don't know what influence they actually have on their pupils. I am therefore including a few comments from others to conclude my story.

Janet was amazed when I finally said that I have done so much that it would not have been easy to live with me. She has been a remarkably tolerant and supportive wife and companion. She said that if she ever wrote a book about me it would be called "Chasing after Kester"! The reason has been that I am often in a hurry trying to fit everything in and I like to be punctual, something my mother instilled into me — my father was often late!

On my sixtieth birthday she organized a wonderful party for me. She told all the guests "No presents, just bring a poem about you and Kester. What a hilarious and enjoyable evening we had as they were read out. I responded by telling my life story with a selection of my (about one hundred) ties, many of which I have been given!

An example of one of these poems may give an unbiased view of a professional colleague and friend of over thirty years at the hospital, Justin Kelly.

The 'Childrens' is a funny place
Administration leads the race
To have less staff and yet more meetings
Then to wish all Season's Greetings.

T.C.K.Brown, my stalwart friend
Has tried for years to call an end
To senseless waste and overspending
And budget cuts at each years ending

But if sometimes he doesn't win
He tries and tries through thick and thin
To make important things his ends
And most of all he's loyal to his friends

I've worked with Kester now for years
He's never lost for good ideas
And though at home he's well respected
His worldwide fame was unsuspected
Until his type of good relations
Made anaesthesia the United Nations.

For he comes across fair and square
And people come from everywhere
To learn and marvel at
The way he works and also that
He can be such a clever man
And write books as so few can
And yet be husband, father and
A friend to those who need a friend.

Kester Brown , I owe you much
As a friend and fellow doctor such
As few are lucky to have met
In twenty lifetimes, but as yet
I'm not too sure they even know
Or realize the debt they owe,
The kids, the parents and their friends,
The world right to its furthest ends.

A Curriculum Vitae is a factual, lifeless, historical record of one's achievements and activities. Sometimes these are acquired from co-operative secretaries and someone puts some life and comment into what they record. They dress them up. This then appears as a citation when some honour is being bestowed. The following are some excerpts from the one read when I was awarded the Orton Medal by the Australian and New Zealand College of Anaesthetists in 1992. It was presented by Michael Hodgson who later became President of both the College and the Australian Society of Anaesthetists.

"Mr President, Kester Brown , M.B.Ch.B. (St Andrews), MD (Melbourne), Fellow of the Australian and New Zealand College of Anesthetists, has spent a significant and formative part of his life in four countries- Kenya, Scotland, Canada and Australia. Fortunately for Australian Anaesthesia he settled in, and spent most of his life here ---- (As an author's aside; it is interesting that several leading contributors to Australasian anaesthesia spent their early years in Africa — Bill Runciman, Wally Thompson, Alan Merry, Johan Van der Walt, Dave Fenwick and others.)

Kester is a quiet family man who has friends all over the world.

He can be gentle and tolerant, independent, persuasive and stubborn, all ingredients for success.

He can do the unusual and unexpected. As a student he worked as a grouse beater for Her Majesty, the Queen Mother during university holidays, and once appeared in a koala suit whilst chairing a session at a national anaesthetic meeting.

The Orton Medal is awarded for distinguished service to anaesthesia and I wish to indicate to you why Council believes this to be deserved.

Two words could best describe Kester's achievements, as an educator and teacher. His activities have been directed and acknowledged at the local, national and international levels.

His publications have never ceased since his early days in anaesthesia and now total almost one hundred in some twenty journals. They have been on topics of a general nature directed at all medical practitioners, on topics directed to a purely anaesthetic readership and to specialty groups.

He has been a forerunner in the anaesthetics world, in this country at least, in the development and use of teaching aids such as films, videos and anatomical dissections."

And so on —

He finished: "Some years ago, when introducing Kester to an anaesthetic audience in Tasmania, I described him as a friend of Tasmanian anaesthesia for the help and assistance he had given us.(I arranged a rotation for Tasmanian registrars to Melbourne for paediatric and obstetric experience) I truly believe today I can describe him as THE FRIEND OF ANAESTHESIA for the distinguished service he has given."

Following the World Congress in Paris in April 2004 where I handed over the Presidency to Anneke Meursing, she wrote the following comments in a very kind letter to Janet and me.

"Now that the World Congress dust has hopefully settled and you look back on one of the best World Congresses ever, I have come to express my heartfelt thanks on behalf of all the members in the global anaesthesia community for your contributions to improve anaesthesia worldwide.

Sometimes people have failed to comprehend your altruistic and dedicated approach to life. Hand in hand with your altruism is your down to earth, no nonsense attitude. The words arrogance or condescending are strange to you and your family.

All these traits have shaped you into the unique and truly World President you have been. In my WFSA lifetime, General Assemblies have never been so smooth and entertaining whilst at the same time difficult decisions were guided through.

What a wonderful teacher and trainer you have been to me and many others."

I was very touched by these and many other kind comments that I have received.

I hope these memoirs have conveyed some of the interest I have had in my life. With the photographs they should form part of the history of anaesthesia during the past forty years.

Appendix

A SELECTION OF MY IMPORTANT PERSONAL PAPERS

1. Respiratory insufficiency and its treatment following pediatric cardiovascular surgery. Canadian Anaesth.Soc.J (1966) 13: 342. With A.E.Johnson, A.W.Conn

2. The Pharmacological Basis of Drug Interactions.The Australian and New Zealand Journal of Surgery (1971), 41:79, with NM Cass.

3. Biochemical Changes During Surface Cooling for Deep Hypothermic Open Heart Surgery. Journal of Thoracic and Cardiovascular Surgery (1973), 65: 402, with ME Dunlop, BJ Stevens, EA Shanahan & CP Clarke.

4. The Use of Sodium Bicarbonate in the Treatment of Tricyclic Antidepressant Induced Arrhythmias. Anaesthesia and Intensive Care (1973), 1, 203 with GA Barker, ME Dunlop, and PM Loughnan.

5. Overdosage – Rise and Fall of Tricyclic Antidepressants. Australian Paediatric Journal (1975), 11: 190.

6. Tracheostomy and prolonged intubation in children in Gray C. and Rees G.J. (eds) Paediatric Anaesthesia – Current Trends Chapter 11 (Butterworths) 1981.

7. Anaesthesia and the Mucopolysaccharidoses: A Survey of Techniques and Problems. Anaesthesia and Intensive Care (1983), 11: 203, with PM Kempthorne.

9. Neural Blockade for Paediatric Surgery. Chapter 21 in Neural Blockade. (1988) 2nd ed. MJ Cousins, P Bridenbaugh. Lippincott & Co. With O Schulte Steinberg

10. Dorsal Nerve of Penis Block – Anatomical and Radiological Studies. Anaesthesia and Intensive Care (1989), 17: 34-8, with NJ Weidner and J Bouwmeester.

11. .Liver tumours and muscle relaxants: Electromyographic studies in children: Anaesthesia (1987), Volume 42, pp 1284-6, with M Gregory, B Bell and PC Campbell.

12. Anaesthetic considerations in liver tumour resection in children. Pediatric Surgical Int (1988), 4: 11-15, with PD Davidson and AW Auldist.

13. Suxamethonium – electromyographic studies in children. Anaesthesia and

Intensive Care (1990), 18: 473-6, with OA Meretoja, B Bell and D Clare.

14. Electromyographic responses to small doses of suxamethonium in children after burns. British Journal of Anaesthesia (1987), 59: 1017-21, with B Bell.

15. Basic science applied to paediatric anaesthesia. Update in Anaesthesia (2000) 11. 73-77

16. Local and regional anaesthesia in children. British J Anaesthesia (1999) 88 65-77 with RL Eyres and RJ McDougall.

17. The use of summary answers as the basis for tutorials. Anaesthesia and Intensive Care (1976) 4:322

OTHER REFERENCES

1. J.G.Stocks. Management of respiratory failure in infancy. Anaesthesia and Intensive Care (1973) 1: 486-506.

2. J.H.Humphrey, M.McClelland. Cranial nerve palsies with herpes following general anaesthesia with Trilene. Report of the Central Middlesex County Hospital. Brit. J. Anaesth. (1944) 1: 315.

3. R.Dery, J.Pelletier, A Jacques, M Clavet, J Houde. Alveolar collapse induced by denitrogenation. Canadian Anaesth. Soc. J, (1965) 12: 531

4. T.W.Baillie. From Boston to Dumfries (1969)

5. Gwen Wilson. Fifty Years – the Australian Society of Anaesthetists 1934-1984.

6. A.Gullo, J Ruprecht. World Federation of Societies of Anaesthesiologists – 50 Years. (2004) Springer.

OTHER BOOKS BY THE AUTHOR

Anaesthesia for Children, with G.C. Fisk. Blackwells. 1st Edition 1979, 2nd Edition 1992

Anaesthesia and Patient Care, Blackwells, 1983

Second volume of Kester Brown's memoirs forthcoming

The second volume recounts his life growing up in Kenya in the 1940s and 50s, his years in Scotland and Canada where he worked and travelled in some less commonly visited places, and finally the period in Australia working as a paediatric anaesthetist and travelling extensively lecturing and teaching. He tells of people who he met or who influenced his life. The book is extensively illustrated.

Email Kester Brown: tckbrown@netspace.net.au